Springer Series on
REHABILITATION

Editor: Thomas E. Backer, Ph.D.
Human Interaction Research Institute, Los Angeles

Advisory Board: Carolyn L. Vash, Ph.D., Elizabeth L. Pan, Ph.D.,
Donald E. Galvin, Ph.D., Ray L. Jones, Ph.D., James F. Garrett, Ph.D.,
Patricia G. Forsythe, and Henry Viscardi, Jr.

Paul W. Power, Sc.D., C.R.C., N.C.C., is a Professor and Director, Rehabilitation Counseling Program, University of Maryland. He received his M.S. in rehabilitation counseling from San Diego State University and his Doctor of Science degree from Boston University in 1975. Dr. Power is the author of numerous articles and book chapters on the topic of family and disability. Significant publications since 1980 include *A Guide to Vocational Assessment* (1984), *Mental Health Counseling* with David Hershenson (1987), and *The Role of the Family in the Rehabilitation of the Physically Disabled* with Arthur Dell Orto (1980). His speeches and workshops on both national and international levels have also focused on the role of the family in the treatment and rehabilitation process. Dr. Power serves as a member of the editorial advisory board of the journal *Rehabilitation Education*, and has served as the contributing editor for the *Journal of Pediatric Social Work* and for the *Journal of Allied Health and Behavioral Sciences.*

Arthur E. Dell Orto, Ph.D., C.R.C., is Professor and Chairperson of the Department of Rehabilitation Counseling at Sargent College of Allied Health Professions, Boston University. He received his M.A. in rehabilitation counseling from Seton Hall University, and his Ph.D. from Michigan State University in 1970. Professionally, Dr. Dell Orto has worked in a variety of settings, both as a rehabilitation consultant and as a licensed psychologist. He is the coauthor of three books: *The Psychological and Social Impact of Physical Disability* with Robert P. Marinelli (Springer Publishing Co., 1977), *Group Counseling and Physical Disability* with Robert Lasky (1979), and *The Role of the Family in the Rehabilitation of the Physically Disabled* with Paul Power (1980). He has published numerous articles and given national workshops on the topic of the family and disability.

Martha Blechar Gibbons, R.N., M.S., C.P.N.P., received her B.S. in Nursing from San Jose State University, and her M.S. in Maternal-Child Nursing from the Medical College of Virginia, Virginia Commonwealth University. She is currently the editor of *Children's Hospice International Newsletter,* and a doctoral candidate in Human Development at the University of Maryland. Ms. Gibbons has worked as a clinical nurse specialist, and a pediatric nurse practitioner in a number of areas, including pediatric urology, community health, and pediatric oncology. She is a Fellow of the National Association of Pediatric Nurse Associates and Practitioners (NAPNAP), and a member of the Association for the Care of Children's Health (ACCH), Children's Hospice International (CHO), and Sigma Theta Tau.

Family Interventions Throughout Chronic Illness and Disability

Paul W. Power
Sc.D., C.R.C., N.C.C.

Arthur E. Dell Orto
Ph.D., C.R.C.

Martha Blechar Gibbons
R.N., M.S., C.P.N.P.

Editors

SPRINGER PUBLISHING COMPANY
New York

This book is dedicated to Marilyn Price Spivak, founder of the National Head Injury Foundation, who traveled where there was no path and left a trail for others challenged by the enormity of illness and disability.

Copyright © 1988 by Springer Publishing Company, Inc.

All rights reserved

Springer Publishing Company, Inc.
536 Broadway
New York, NY 10012

88 89 90 91 92 / 5 4 3 2 1

Library of Congress Cataloging-in-Publication Data
Family interventions throughout chronic illness and disability.
   (Springer series on rehabilitation; v. 7)
   Includes bibliography and index.
   1. Chronically ill—Family relationships.
2. Chronically ill—Rehabilitation. I. Power, Paul W. II. Dell Orto,
Arthur E., 1943-   . III. Gibbons, Martha Blechar. IV. Series. [DNLM:
1. Adaptation, psychological. 2. Chronic Disease—psychology. 3. Family.
4. Handicapped—psychology.
W1 SP685SF v. 7 / WB 320 F198]
RC108.F36 1988   155.9′16   88-8634
ISBN 0-8261-5580-4

Printed in the United States of America

Contents

PART III: Emerging Family Issues
During Adolescence and Adulthood

PART IV: Selected Challenges of the Later Years

Preface

Disability is a family affair. Any family is affected by the onset of a disabling condition in one of its members, and the entire family usually begins a struggle to retain its equilibrium and to adapt to the given situation. Family factors also directly influence the mental and emotional functioning of the disabled individual. The disabled person's reaction to treatment and performance in rehabilitation efforts is a function of both the person and the family environment (Power & Dell Orto, 1980). The family bears the day-by-day burden of coping with the disability or illness. Thus the family can become a major help to an individual's rehabilitation or adjustment, or a significant stumbling block to the attainment of treatment goals.

In recent years the family has received increased attention in intervention approaches and in the literature, and the family's role for the parent's adaptation is becoming pivotal for human service interventions (Bray, 1987; Cohen, 1982; English, 1982; Jacus, 1981; Kerosky, 1984; Sutton, 1985). The family plays an important role at every stage of an illness, though too often the total rehabilitation and treatment efforts have only focused on helping the patient. In spite of the increased attention, there is a paucity of literature depicting how the family can assist in the patient's adjustment to disability, trauma, or illness. (Caroff & Mailick, 1985).

This book shows how appropriate interventions can put an illness or disability into perspective, and how an intervention can create an option for the family to live its life as fully as possible. It also provides different helping approaches for varied family situations. It offers the reader knowledge about selected disabilities and disease entities, and how they affect family dynamics and adjustmental concerns. Further, the book identifies the needs of family members in selected, disability, and disease-related situations and explains assessment approaches that focus both on family adjustment goals and the utilization of the family for support and/or rehabilitation purposes. Importantly, this book provides insights for helping a family as it comes to terms with the reality of a chronic illness and explains what helping skills could be most effective for coping with the disability or illness trauma.

The intended audience for this book includes health, allied health, and other helping professionals whose work responsibilities will bring them into contact with families as they pursue their interventions with the identified patient. It is also written for those still in training in a health or allied-health-professional field—social workers, psychologists, clergy, nurses, rehabilitation counselors, occupational therapists, and physical therapists. All of these people have, in the estimation of the authors, an excellent opportunity to assess the family dynamics as they affect the person with disability or illness, to provide support for the family, and to share information about effective coping strategies and community resources.

The chapters cover a wide range of disabilities and chronic illnesses. Many were selected becouse of the emerging interest in health-care and rehabilitation-delivery systems of specific topic areas, such as infant apnea, young children with AIDS (a second generation of AIDS victims), the disabled child's impact on siblings, the impact of substance abuse on the family, respite care, Alzheimer's disease, and the adolescent in transition from school to work. Other chapters were included because of the continued necessity to explore fresh insights into how families can cope with specific issues that are related to certain diseases or disabilities, such as women with physical disabilities, the sexual needs of the disabled adolescent, coping with childhood cancer, and the child and deafness. The chapters are grouped into four parts: Family Assessment and Intervention Issues; Child and Family Issues; Emerging Family Issues During Adolescence and Adulthood; and Selected Challenges of the Later Years. Complementing each part of the book are personal statements which illustrate in a realistic manner much of the content contained in the related chapters. Written by individuals who are directly or indirectly experiencing the impact of illness or disability, each statement identifies family and personal issues that must be confronted by family members. These statements add a unique focus to the book, for they translate the theory embodied in each chapter into the practice of everyday concerns. At the end of each chapter, moreover, is a list of available resources that may be utilized by helping professionals to assist families. Finally, each part includes a group of study questions and suggested activities that could be used for classroom purposes. All of the material contained in the four parts expresses the viewpoint that the family should be included in the domain of the allied health professional. They emphasize that progress toward treatment and adjustment goals cannot be made without considering and evaluating the total family system.

The chapters in this book are original contributions by the authors, and they articulate the philosophy that all family members must usually learn to deal with the same dimensions of coping as does the disabled person. These dimensions include emotional reactions, dealing with other people, the presence of guilt and anger, and family readaptation. The chapters further embrace the conviction that helping professionals need to expand their clinical practice boundaries to appropriately include the family as integral to treatment and rehabilitation efforts. One of the primary goals of treatment and rehabilitation is to help the ill or disabled individual to come to terms with the reality of the situation, and then to achieve as much as possible an optimal style of life. This transition takes place more readily when both family members and helping professionals can discover within the family environment the resources that increase the family's and, in turn, the patient's ability to cope with the crisis of illness or disability.

REFERENCES

Bray, G. P. (1987). Family adaptation to chronic illness. In B. Caplan (Ed.), *Rehabilitation psychology desk reference*. Rockville, MD: Aspen Publishers.

Caroff, P., & Mailick, M. D. (1985). The patient has a family: Re-affirming social work's domain. *Social work in health care, 10*, 17–34.

Cohen, S. (1982). Supporting families through respite care. *Rehabilitation Literature, 43*, 7–11.

English, W. (1982). The role of the family in rehabilitation. *Rehabilitation Research Reviews*. Washington, DC: National Rehabilitation Information Center.

Jacus, C. (1981). Working with families in a rehabilitation setting. *Rehabilitation Nursing, 6*, 10–14.

Kerosky, M. (1984). Family counseling in the rehabilitation setting. *Journal of Appied Rehabilitation Counseling, 15*, 50–51.

Power, P. W., & Dell Orto, A. (Eds.) (1980). *Role of the family in the rehabilitation of the physically disabled*, Austin, TX: Pro-Ed.

Sutton, J. (1985). The need for family involvement in client rehabilitation. *Journal of Applied Rehabilitation Counseling, 16*, 42–45.

Acknowledgments

This book is the result of the combined efforts of many persons. We would like to thank Paul, Janet, Robert, Tosca, and Linda who gave us their personal statements to be included in this volume. We would also like to acknowledge the support of our wives, Barbara Ann and Barbara Ann, and husband David, all of whom provided valuable suggestions. Special mention must be given to Mrs. Pat Baker, University of Maryland, whose typing helped bring the book nearer to its completion; and Ken Paruti, Denise Henson, Doreen Correia, and Keith Pijanowski of the Department of Rehabilitation Counseling, Sargent College, Boston University, for their assistance in the preparation of the manuscript and in the library research.

Contributors

Tosca Appel, M.S., received her degree in rehabilitation counseling from Boston University. Professionally, she has been active in many self-help groups for the physically disabled, and has particularly focused her efforts on assisting persons with multiple sclerosis.

Sue Bregman, Ph.D., is a licensed psychologist in private practice in Lanham, Maryland. She has specialized in marriage and family therapy and adjustment to disability since 1971 and is currently president-elect of the Middle Atlantic Division of the American Association of Marriage and Family Therapists (AAMFT). Dr. Bregman has written a book and several articles on the subject of sexual adjustment to disability.

Elaine E. Castles, Ph.D., received her degree in clinical psychology from the Catholic University of America and has had more than ten years of experience in working with mentally handicapped individuals. In addition to her private practice and consulting work, Dr. Castles is supervision psychologist at the Rock Creek Foundation, an agency which provides comprehensive services to dually diagnosed mentally retarded/mentally ill individuals. Dr. Castles is a member of the American Psychological Association and the American Association on Mental Retardation.

Beverly Celotta, Ph.D., is a licensed psychologist and president of Celotta, Jacobs & Keys Associates, Inc., a consulting group specializing in mental-health program development services. She received her B.A. in psychology from Queens College, her M.A. and Advanced Certificate in school psychology from Brooklyn College, and her Ph.D. in Educational Psychology from the University of Colorado. Dr. Celotta has served as a school psychologist, educational research and evaluation specialist, and faculty member at the University of Maryland. She has authored or coauthored over thirty articles, chapters, and manuals in the area of the application of the systems approach to mental health program development, and is currently on the editorial board of *Measurement and Evaluation in Counseling and Development*.

Marita McKenna Danek, Ph.D., C.R.C., has been director of the rehabilitation counseling program (deafness emphasis) at Gallaudet University since 1981. She is a 1985 Switzer scholar and recipient of the 1986 National Council on Rehabilitation Education (NCRE) Rehabilitation Eduacator of the Year award. She has published book chapters and articles in the field of rehabilitation counseling and is active in numerous professional organizations.

Paul F. Egan, M.S., earned his B.S.W. at Suffolk University and the master's degree at Boston University Sargent College of Allied Health Professions. Upon graduation, Mr. Egan became employed with Blinded Veterans' Association as a Field Representative based in Boston, and now travels extensively, visiting with blinded veterans in their homes and assisting with related benefit allocations with V.A. and State officials.

Rennie Rogers Golec, M.A., is the Assistant Director for Internships and Volunteer Service at the University of Maryland. She has a master's degree in community counseling and is a doctoral candidate in counseling and consultation. A coauthor of *A Workbook for the Practice-to-Theory-to-Practice Model* and *The Mattering Scale*, she has worked with colleagues at the University of Maryland to develop a support-group sequence for family caregivers of Alzheimer's disease patients. Her father was a victim of Alzheimer's disease.

David B. Hershenson, Ph.D., C.R.C., is a national certified counselor and is listed in the National Register of Health Service Providers in Psychology. He holds a Ph.D. in counseling psychology from Boston University and has been involved in counselor education for the past 20 years. Dr. Hershenson has authored over 40 book chapters and journal articles in the field of counseling, as well as being the co-editor of the *Psychology of Vocational Development: Reading in Theory and Practice* and the coauthor of *Mental Health Counseling.* He is currently chairperson of the Department of Counseling and Personnel Services at the University of Maryland. His professional interests are counselor education, career development, and mental health rehabilitation.

Allen F. Johnson, Ph.D., B.C.C.S.W., is Director of the Auburn Family Institute, MA, and Clinical Supervisor of Morningstar Home, Oxford, MA. He is author of *Developmental Achievement in the Child with Spina Bifida* (1980) and other professional publications. He founded and is currently treasurer of the International Association for Pediatric Social Services, Inc., serves on the Editorial Review Board of the journal, *Pediatric Social Work*, teaches courses on disability issues at Clark University, Worcester, MA, and is in the private practice of family, marriage, and child psychotherapy of both the challenged and the able-bodied.

Carol Keydel, L.C.S.W., is a psychiatric social worker and Associate Professor of Psychology and Human Services at Anne Arundel Community College in Arnold, Maryland. She is also a psychotherapist and works with troubled families in her private practice.

Kay Harris Kriegsman, Ph.D., provides counseling and psychological services for the Psychological Sciences Institute, Baltimore, MD. She is also the training manager for the Attendant Care Program of Easter Seal Society of Washington, D.C. and is a consultant to the HOW (Handicap is Only a Word) Conference, an annual meeting for teenagers with physical disabilities and their families. She received her B.A. from the University of Denver, and her M.A. and Ph.D. in counseling from the University of Maryland. Dr. Kriegsman organized and facilitated coping groups for women with physical disabilities. She serves as a member of state advisory boards on special education and attendant care services. Dr. Kriegsman has authored or coauthored four articles on women with physical disabilities and on college students with disabilities.

Ann D. Lassalle, M.A., is a doctoral student in Counseling and Consultation at the University of Maryland. She received her master's degree in Community Counseling. Ms. Lassale is currently interning as a training-evaluation specialist at the United States General Accounting Office. She is a coauthor of *The Mattering Scale* and *The Mattering Scale for Adult Students in Higher Education.*

Susan Leibold, RN, B.S., M.S., is a clinical specialist in charge of the Spina Bifida Program, Children's Hospital, Washington, D.C. She received her B.S. degree from DePauw University and her M.S. degree is from the Medical College of Virginia. She has served as nurse coordinator in charge of the Apnea Program, Children's Hospital, Washington, D.C., and her professional focus is pediatric nursing.

Janet Miller, M.S., brings a unique perspective to the illness and disability experience. In her multiple roles as mother, consumer, and rehabilitation professional, she is able to understand the complexity of issues that impact families challenged by the rehabilitation process. Ms. Miller was awarded her Master of Science degree in Rehabilitation Counseling from Boston University Sargent College of Allied Health Professions in 1983, and has since worked as a Rehabilitation Consultant.

Robert Neumann, Ph.D., is currently Coordinator of Counseling Services at Access Living of Metropolitan Chicago, where he administers a peer-counseling program for spinal-cord-injured patients at the Rehabilitation Institute of Chicago, provides counseling for Access Living clients, teaches classes on independent living and personal growth, and conducts support groups. Additionally, Dr. Neumann is a leader for self-help courses sponsored by the Arthritis Foundation. Before coming to Access Living, Dr. Neumann served as psychologist in the Departments of Physical Medicine and Rehabilitation at Memorial Hospital, Gary, Indiana. He received his Ph.D. in counseling psychology from Northwestern University in 1980.

Linda Pelletier, M.A., received her B.A. in English in 1974 and her M.A. degree in teaching from Salem State College in 1976, her M.A. degree in Rehabilitation Counseling from Assumption College in Worcester, MA in 1980, and is presently a doctoral candidate in Rehabilitation Counseling at Boston University. She has worked as a counselor and advocate at various independent living programs. In addition, she gives frequent lectures on the psychosocial and sexual aspects of physical disability. She is currently employed as a research and teaching assistant at Sargent College Boston University.

Edna Mora Szymanski, M.S., is a senior vocational rehabilitation counselor with the New York State Office of Vocational Rehabilitation. She received her degree in Rehabilitation Counseling at the University of Scranton in 1974 and is currently a doctoral student in the field at University of Texas at Austin. Ms. Szymanski was president of the American Rehabilitation Counseling Association from July 1985 to June 1986. She currently serves as a commissioner on the Commission on Rehabilitation Counselor Certification, as an editorial board member for the *Journal of Applied Rehabilitation Counseling*, and as a member of the President's Committee for Employment of the Handicapped.

Judith Teplow, B.S., received her degree in Education from Wheelock College and is currently completing her master's degree in Social Work at Boston College. She resides in Boston with her husband and 16-year-old daughter and is committed to meeting the needs of families challenged by amyotrophic lateral sclerosis (ALS) through education, support, and political action.

Dorothy Ward-Wimmer, R.N., is the Immunology Clinical Specialist for Children's Hospital National Medical Center, Washington, D.C. As one of the Hospital's primary resources for information regarding Human Immunodeficiency Virus (HIV) infection in children, Ms. Ward-Wimmer assesses issues surrounding HIV-infected children and develops appropriate responses/programs to them. Currently a master's candidate in Thanatologic Counseling, Ms. Ward-Wimmer's background includes 6 years as the Coordinator of the Hospice and Special Services for the Jersey Shore Medical Center, 4 years as a Nurse and Family Worker for New Jersey's Ocean County Head Start Program, and 13 years as a nurse in pediatrics, Intensive Care and Coronary Care.

I
Family Assessment and Intervention Issues

Introduction

"The family is the most central and potent external force, not only in shaping the individual personality but also in the expression of physical illness" (Jaffe, 1978, p. 170). These words represent a challenge for treatment and rehabilitation-care providers, for they imply that family members can shape the way a person adjusts to an illness or disability, and, as well, can offer a support system to the disabled individual. Contact with the family, consequently, can serve a most useful purpose. But if this contact is to be effective, assessment and intervention approaches must be developed that are in harmony with family and patient needs, and with time-limited opportunities that are available to allied-health professionals in their varied work settings.

Chapters 1 and 2 explain an intervention approach that responds to these demands. Though the assessment and intervention topics are separate chapters, assessment is actually an indispensable, interchangeable ingredient of effective intervention. One builds upon the other. In Chapter 1, moreover, a definite viewpoint for exploring family dynamics and illness and disability factors is emphasized. This perspective highlights the author's premise that a family assessment should usually be undertaken at certain critical points in the patient's treatment and rehabilitation. Within this suggested time framework, the helping professional can begin to identify family needs, family strengths, information, and management concerns. An understanding of these issues can provide a stimulus to the helping professional to utilize appropriately the patient's family in his or her own rehabilitation efforts.

Chaper 2 presents an intervention approach that continues to use this time framework of critical points in the patient's treatment. During these particular intervention opportunities, allied health professionals can assume certain roles. The enactment of each role becomes a pathway for family assistance.

Though other chapters in this book will suggest particular intervention approaches respective to a specific disability or illness, Chapters 1 and 2 give to the reader many general selected guidelines for what to look for and what to do when disability or illness strike a family. These chapters provide certain core considerations when assisting a family with an ill or disabled member.

The utilization of designated roles when meeting with family members, the implementation of such basic helping skills as listening, attending, and responding to family needs, and the selection of opportune times to meet with family members are all threads that are present throughout the tapestry of family intervention. The other chapters in this book build on these core considerations.

Part I concludes with a personal statement from a man with a long-standing disability. It emphasizes to the helping professional the value of an insightful family assessment that includes the identification of family strengths. His account raises the questions: What might have been without family support? What could have happened? Would this man have found his niche in the employment world with earlier family intervention? The discussion questions following the personal statement gives the reader the opportunity to answer these questions.

REFERENCE

Jaffe, D. T. (1978). The role of family therapy in treating physical illnesses. *Hospital and Community Psychiatry*, 29, 170–174.

1 An Assessment Approach to Family Intervention

Paul W. Power

The family can be a valuable resource in the patient's treatment and rehabilitation; more than ever before, health and allied health professionals are focusing their attention on the family environment. This trend has led to new perspectives in illness, disability, and rehabilitation intervention. The disabled or ill person, the family and the health professional form a therapeutic triad. All three are necessary for effective intervention, which in turn, depends on an appropriate assessment plan.

An appraisal of what it is in family life that influences the disabled family member can become the basis for the development of appropriate family helping strategies. Without an understanding of the family situation, intervention approaches often go awry. Yet family assessment is different, both in focus and emphasis, from individual patient appraisal. Most health professionals have been trained only to diagnose and understand the disabled or ill person. Until recently, academic curricula did not usually prepare the student to understand the family dynamics surrounding the health care of the patient. Today, many more training programs are assisting the future helping professionals to become aware of the difference between "patients and their family" and "the patient in the family."

This chapter explains a family-assessment approach that can be applicable to the different job functions of health and allied health professionals. Because family appraisal is often a complex process, such topics as the setting for an assessment and the role of the professional in performing assessment will also be discussed. An awareness of these areas can minimize the difficulties that are often present when one is performing family assessment.

Moreover, in the formulation of any family-assessment strategy, the "problem-to-be-worked" may be different for each professional. A nurse in a medical setting will focus on the interplay of the family members in relation to the care and treatment of the ill child or adult. A rehabilitation counselor may be more concerned with how family members influence the client's motivation toward the achievement of vocational-rehabilitation goals. Social workers and family counselors may often direct their attention to how the family can utilize community support systems for its own survival. Physical or occupational therapists may explore how the family can become a necessary partner of the patient for continuing a treatment regimen at home. Consequently, the reasons for attending to the family during the disabled person's treatment and/or rehabilitation my be different. The assessment approach explained in this chapter will attend to these differences, but at the same time will offer guidelines that are applicable for most family-appraisal opportunities by health and allied health professionals.

Within the context of the role of a health professional, there is usually some flexibility to perform other functions that, although they are not part of one's essential responsibilities, may enhance one's work with patients or clients. Such is the case with utilizing the family in the patient's treatment and/or rehabilitation process. Doherty and Baird (1983), in their discussion of primary care family counseling for family physicians and other health personnel, suggest three distinct functions: education, prevention, and support. In other words, during the performance of a particular role as a health professional, one may have the opportunity: (1) to educate families or couples, (2) to provide anticipatory guidance in order to prevent future problems, and (3) to give informal support to family members.

When contact with the family is possible, an understanding is needed of how the family influences the patient, and of what those family factors are that may facilitate or be disruptive to the disabled person's treatment or rehabilitation. Many diverse viewpoints have been developed in order to understand family dynamics, but we will use a rehabilitation-skill-based-theory approach described below. This theory can serve as the basis for an assessment approach that will be suggested later in this chapter.

REHABILITATION-SKILL-BASED THEORY

Based on the work of Anthony, Pierce, & Cohen (1979), with modifications and application to the family by the present author, this theory focuses on the need of family members to learn certain skills in order to adapt to the disability situation. The theory does not emphasize what has happened within the family in the past; rather, it stresses what family members can do in the present to help both the patient and themselves to maintain treatment needs and family life. Such factors as family role relations and expectations, interactional patterns, and family systems are all considered in this assessment model. They are: family strengths, needed family skills, and evaluation at psychosocial "trigger" points.

Family Strengths

Most of the assessment approaches to family dynamics have emphasized pathological or dysfunctional characteristics of the family unit (Wilcoxon, 1985). Yet, attention to positive family factors developed in the 1960s and 1970s as an outgrowth of the focus on preventive services. The identification of family strengths can pinpoint family resources, serve as reinforcements for family members, and indicate guidelines for intervention. From the author's clinical and research work with families and disability, he has identified the following family strengths, each of which suggests to the professional a needed area for appraisal and a possible pathway for intervention.

The Ability of the Family to Listen

Listening is a precious commodity in our society, and in this context of family and disability it means primarily the family members' ability to listen to each other and to helping professionals. Many families with a disabled family member are caught up with their own sense of loss and anxiety, especially during the early stages of health care intervention. But if family members have the ability, despite these emotions, to listen to each other and to the information provided by medical and related staff, then intervention planning may be implemented effectively.

Shared, Common Perceptions of Reality Within the Family

This family strength refers to a knowledge among family members of their own limitations, the physical and emotional resources to deal with any family change, and what the treatment and adjustment needs of the patient are. It includes an acceptance of each family member as what "he or she is," with personal assets and deficits. When all of these perceptions are present, then family members are able to understand what family accommodations are necessary, and what could be their own possible contributions to family adjustment. This understanding does not remove the reality of denial, for family members will usually deny selected aspects of a disease or disability, especially during the weeks immediately after a diagnosis or trauma. Such denying frequently buys them time to develop their own personal resources to confront the inescapable implications of the disability event.

The Ability of Family Members to Take Responsibility for Disability-Related Problems

What this strength implies is the attitude that "I can prevent problems if I can take responsibility." This strength is illustrated by such questions as: "If my mother has an accident and becomes disabled, what are the family needs that must be met for adequate family functioning?" Or, "Who will take over some of the family chores, such as caring for young children, paying bills, or attending to the treatment concerns of the disabled person?" The early assumption of selected family tasks may prevent later problems, such as neglect of the disabled person, resentment among younger family members, and isolation of family members from each other because of a perceived lack of attention. In other words, this strength implies that family members confront the demands of the disability situation and begin to tackle the many issues that arise when living with a disabled person.

The Ability of Family Members to Use Negotiation in Family Problem Solving

This family strength could be one that may have taken many years to develop and has been utilized many times before the occurrence of a disability or illness. It means that family members are willing to talk with each other about various options over a course of action, are able to compromise some of their own wishes, and are open to family-life suggestions from other family members. When a decision is reached about what should be done, it represents an action that has collective input.

Family Members' Willingness to Take Good Care of Themselves

This strength includes the family's ability to use well their leisure time, to relax and to seek a balance between family responsibilities, a paid job, and recreation. It implies that family members have the conviction that they must, to survive in living with a disability, take appropriate, good care of themselves. Frequently, however, family members become guilty if they attempt to seek legitimate respites from caring efforts. The author has heard often from a family member, "My work is 24 hours . . . this is my mission in life." But when the family has periodic, legitimate outlets, a renewed source of vitality is available. In turn, this energy often becomes the stimulus for family members to be supports for each other.

The Family's Ability to Focus on the Present, Rather Than on Past Events or Disappointments

Family members usually bring to a disability event much of their unfinished, emotional business. It might be a past regret, an unrequited anger, or a lingering resentment. Such business can get in the way of family togetherness. Anger often facilitates the isolation of family members from each other. Yet family members need to be encouraged to emphasize what is happening now;

to use constructively the present opportunities in the home, in the job, and with friends; and not to dwell constantly on the past or on an uncertain future. It is difficult for family members to forget or to suppress negative emotions, but when they can it is another pathway to their helping each other in this disability situation.

The Ability of Family Members to Provide Reinforcements to Each Other

Most families have a pattern of positive reinforcements that appear to make family life more satisfying. It may be spending some time playing with the children, or an hour of allowed private time, an outing together to a favorite restaurant, a delicious meal cooked by a wife or husband, or sexual love shared by the spouses. Whatever it may be, the onset of illness or disability does not have to eliminate completely such reinforcement. Frequently, family members have to be encouraged to restore these satisfactions to each other. Reinforcements, in turn, are expressions of support.

The Ability of the Family Members to Discuss Their Concerns

This strength is also called by the author *Family Expressiveness*. It involves the family members' capabilities to talk to other family members, extended family, selected friends, and helping professionals about the impact of the disability experience on themselves, to share their disappointments, and perhaps even to tell health care workers that they are torn between compassion, guilt, and anger when taking care of the disabled person.

The Ability of Family Members to Provide an Atmosphere of Belonging

This strength means the family's willingness to convey to the patient that "Really, you are still, basically, the same person: You are still an important member of our family." Work with families has often suggested that, after the onset of a serious illness or a traumatic disability, family members tend frequently to become isolated from the disabled person. They have difficulty adjusting to many illness manifestations, especially those associated with head and spinal-cord injury or a neurological disease. During intervention efforts, helping professionals might even encourage this family isolation by emphasizing patients' deficits, rather that their residual assets. Such an emphasis highlights the "differentness" of the disabled family member. But if both the patients and their families are going to adjust to the disability, then patients must feel that they "matter."

Family Members' Capacities to Use Everyday Experiences as Resources

Many disabled persons have mentioned to the author that, after being discharged to their home for outpatient care, they become discouraged upon realizing the time and effort required to return to some portion of their previous productivity, such as at a job, at home, or in social activities. Cogswell (1968) has called this transition the *resocialization process*, and explains that after hospital discharge the patient's home can become a refuge. Living in the home can become a moratorium between the hospital stay and a future way of life. But if time in the home is spent productively, then the utilization of this opportunity may provide the stimulus for renewed functioning.

The Family's Willingness to Have Hope and to Appreciate that a Change is Possible

This strength implies that there is a residue of hope among family members that life can be somewhat more peaceful, or that living can be more satisfying for the disabled family member, and even for the other members of the family. It also implies that family members at least understand that "If I can change just to a small degree, it might make a difference for my disabled family member." Accompanying this understanding is the family's willingness to stay together as a unit and to take the risk to see if their problems can be alleviated.

In summary, therefore, an emphasis on family strengths in this rehabilitation-skill model serves as a background for understanding many of those capabilities a family may possess to cope with a disability situation. Also, because a family assessment will usually be conducted by a helping professional in a variety of settings, this perspective of family strengths can contribute to an assessment approach that is both direct and easily applicable to these different helping situations.

Needed Family Skills

The family's adjustment to a disability implies the acquisition or possession of needed skills. The basic goal of family intervention, consequently, is to extend or enlarge the family's repertoire of these skills, or to modify the family community so that family members can perform at their optimum levels of skill functioning (Anthony et al., 1979). This skill identification encourages the observation of each individual family member's reaction to the disability and allows the helping professional to identify the adaptive function(s) the disability may play in the family system. Examples of skills that need to be identified in many families that are experiencing a disability are the following:

1. Ability to recognize family crises resulting from recurring adaptations to a disability
2. Ability to problem solve as a response to disability-adjustment demands
3. Ability to communicate with helping professionals
4. Ability to use community resources
5. Ability to respond to the treatment needs of the disabled person

Evaluation at Psychosocial "Trigger" Points

The family's adjustment to the disabled family member usually takes place over an extended period of time. A review of the literature reveals that the psychosocial consequences of the impact of the illness on both the patient and family are often conceptualized in stages or critical "trigger" points (Caroff & Mailick, 1985). Each stage brings with it a series of tasks for both patient and family, with the potential for adaptive and maladaptive patterns of coping. But because of the complexity of individual and family responses to a disability, as well as the range and diversity of diseases and disabilities, it is difficult to generalize how patients and families will experience the challenge of each stage of the illness (Caroff & Mailick, 1985).

Particular times during the treatment and/or rehabilitation period of an illness when the family can be especially vulnerable to excessive stress have been identified by Christ and Adams (1984). These eight points in the course of an illness and its treatment and/or rehabilitation are (1) the diagnostic process; (2) the onset of treatment; (3) negative physical reaction to treatment and treatment side effects; (4) termination of a treatment protocol; (5) reentry into school, social, and family life; (6) recurrence or metastasis of the disease; (7) initiation of researach treatment; and (8) termination of active treatment and terminal illness. Christ and Adams (1984) developed these stages after working with families that were attempting to cope with childhood cancer. This present chapter author, however, from his own clinical experience and research, has found that with many other illness and/or disabling conditions there are actually four points during which family members confront special stresses. Each point can trigger specific emotional reactions from the family or can highlight the existence of particular family needs. Any one of these points can also represent a unique crisis for family members, and they may require special help to enhance optimal coping with the disability. Specific assessment areas should be explored at each time. These trigger points are:

1. Diagnosis and beginning of treatment
2. The course of in-hospital treatment/rehabilitation

3. Termination of in-hospital treatment/rehabilitation and return to an available family
4. Outpatient status for treatment/rehabilitation

A FAMILY-ASSESSMENT APPROACH

The approach now to be explained suggests the evaluation of needed family information, dynamics, skills, and existing family strengths at the four trigger points in the patient's treatment and/or rehabilitation. To be noted, however, is that a professional's understanding of the patient's family can be gained in a variety of settings. For the nurse or physical therapist, knowledge of the family may be obtained in a hospital or clinic waiting room, or in the patient's room. Social workers, psychiatric nurses, or rehabilitation counselors may utilize an office to make a family appraisal, but this author believes that, when possible, an effective assessment should include a home and family visit. Family mealtime, for example, has a broad appeal as a source of information, but little research has been reported in this area. Minuchin (Minuchin, Roseman, & Baker, 1978) have done some original work on family luncheons with anorexics and their families. He has attempted to deal with underlying family dysfunctions and utilizes mealtimes to capture some of these family dynamics. Grossman, Pozanski, and Banegas (1983) have used the family luncheon, whether in the home, in a hospital cafeteria, or a picnic area, to study family interactions. They believe that observation of the family luncheon is a supplement to clinical observations, and is a valuable tool to learn about family dynamics. In these informal settings families appear to relax more easily and thus a more valid portrait of the family is often obtained. Yet if the helping professional is attuned to the importance of learning about one's family in order to achieve effective treatment, then almost any opportunity or place where the family is present can be advantageous for appraisal.

Also, any family assessment will usually be conducted within a brief time framework. Today, in many working environments—for example, the hospital and most rehabilitation counseling offices—the rapid flow of patients through these systems usually necessitates short-term, episodic care. Because families can often be seen only briefly, assistance to family members must be carefully designed to make effective use of this limited helping opportunity. Also, many health professionals (i.e., nurses, occupational and physical therapists, rehabilitation counselors, and certain social workers) focus primarily on the patients themselves, and so most family contact occurs in this context. When a family contact is made, attention to family members should really be an extension of one's work with the individual patient.

Because of the briefness of the helper's opportunity to meet with families, assessment information may not be obtained at only one meeting. To facilitate the family's verbal expression of important information, the helpers need to utilize such basic communication skills as (1) attentiveness; (2) a nonjudgmental attitude; (3) using understandable words when talking with family members; (4) using verbal reinforcers, such as "I see" or "yes"; (5) reflecting back and clarifying the family's statements; and (6) phrasing interpretations tentatively so as to elicit genuine feedback from family members (Okun, 1987). The helper should not assume anything, and ask only what she or he believes that the family member can answer so that the person feels competent and productive. Also, the helper should ask questions that family members can handle emotionally at the time (Satir, 1967). In other words, the helper must create a setting during a family meeting in which people can, perhaps for the first time, take the risk of sharing their emotions and seek information about their concerns. Table 1.1 outlines the family-assessment model explained in this chapter.

I. Diagnosis and Beginning of Treatment

Assessment can begin at the time when a diagnosis is made after a trauma or the beginning of an illness. For family members it can be a period of intense anxiety, uncertainty about the future, and accompanying feelings of helplessness, guilt, and perhaps anger. When the helping professional has the opportunity to contact the family at this time, four areas should be explored. They are:

(1) What is the Current Family Functioning?

The professional can begin to identify those family dynamics that may promote or hinder the patient's treatment and rehabilitation during initial contact with the family. For example, are there warm and trusting attitudes shown in familial interactions? Is there an open and mutual respect demonstrated toward each other by family members? Is there much confusion and disagreement about events affecting family life? Are there conflicts over the performance of family responsibilities? Is family communication characterized by frequent distorted or unrealistic views of each other? Included in this exploration is identification of who the family spokesperson is, who may be the principal caregivers for the patient, and what the strengths and pitfalls are in the family that could influence the patient's treatment and rehabilitation.

An awareness of these dynamics will begin to promote an understanding of what kind of family is part of the patient's life. Is it, for example, a *high-functioning*, normal family, characterized by an open communication among family members and the availability of many social and economic resources?

TABLE 1.1 Family-Assessment Model

I. Diagnosis and beginning of treatment
   1. What is the unique composition of the family?
   2. Have there been any previous crises in the family and how have they been handled?
   3. What is the emotional reaction of the patient?
   4. What does the family need at this time?

II. During the course of in-hospital treatment/rehabilitation
   1. What information does the family have about the disability or illness?
   2. What are the needs of the family while the family member is in the hospital?
   3. What has the family done so far to respond to the disability or illness?
   4. What are the resources available to the family?
   5. What is the perceived threat to family functioning because of the disability?

III. Termination of in-hospital treatment/rehabilitation and return to an available family
   1. What information and expectations does the family have for their affected family member?
   2. Who will be the family member mainly responsible for the "care" of the disabled person?
   3. What emotions does the family have about re-entry?
   4. How much energy does the family have at their disposal?
   5. What services does the family need?

IV. Outpatient status for treatment/rehabilitation
   1. Have new disruptions occurred within the family?
   2. Has the relationship to health care providers changed?

Though a high-functioning family is not immune to severe stress, living, as it may be, at the edge of crisis for an extended period of time, this family is able to seek out professional staff at times of crisis and is further able to utilize additional supports.

The *low-functioning* or vulnerable family, however, may provide problems for the patient, medical staff, and for each other once treatment occurs. Though this family may only provide members with a minimal-to-adequate level of support, care, and nurturance, customary family duties can usually be carried out. However, at the onset of an illness or disability, family members can be vulnerable to maladaptive living patterns and even show a hostile relationship to the disabled person. They may also have previously experienced severe illness with a family member, and there still may be much unfinished business in the form of residual anger or resentment because of such an illness's past impact on the family. Vulnerable families are also characterized by such factors as (1) having intellectually limited patients and family members; namely, they have achieved academically and socially only with the greatest effort; (2) having a disabled person who had other physical or mental handicaps prior to the diagnosis; and (3) having the presence of other serious illnesses in the family, especially another person with the same disease or one who has suffered the same type of accident trauma (Christ & Adams, 1984). For the low-functioning and vulnerable family it may be difficult to adapt to a disability situation, including the adjustment of many family roles, the development of a working relationship to health-care staff, and the utilization of necessary resources. Some family members may even prefer to avoid any personal contact with the disabled person and leave all treatment responsibilities to one family member. The low-functioning and vulnerable family may need more active monitoring to avoid coping failures and the development of chronic, maladaptive patterns (Futterman & Hoffman, 1978).

The helping professional may also identify a "disturbed" family, one that has, for example, the presence of an alcoholic family member who is continually bringing added stress, or a family member with a borderline character organization that is manifested in a variety of destructive behaviors, for example, a history of depressive neglect or increased interpersonal conflicts with staff (Christ & Adams, 1984). Because of these problems and because of continued treatment demands, the family members may be less able to deal effectively with the stress of a diagnosis or the disruption in family life caused by disability. When the disturbed family is identified by the helping professional, a referral for family therapy treatment may have to be made. The elements of a successful referral are discussed in Chapter 2.

(2) Have There Been Any Previous Crises in the Family, and How Have They Been Handled?

Because family members can behave with differential competence in different contexts, yet often transfer learning from one problem-solving situation to another when the latter is similar, it is useful to explore any history of crisis management (Dillon, 1985). The crisis history should include details of previous crises, descriptions of who is mobilized to carry out which adaptational tasks, and how situations and roles ultimately resolved themselves. It is also important to compare the family's experience of the current illness or disability with aspects of similar crises in the past. Players may change according to the demands and rewards inherent in each situation (Dillon, 1985).

When confronted by a number of unknown factors inherent in an illness episode, past experience can be a strong determinant in the family decision-making process. If past learning experiences have been positive, the family may be more innovative in exploring alternatives when faced with a new crisis situation. Effective intervention, consequently, requires an understanding of how a family has coped with a previous crisis. For example, what were the general characteristics of the family decision-making process? Was this a collaborative effort, or did one member exercise greater authority over the family group (MacVicor & Archbold, 1976)? These are just two of the questions that may be asked during this family exploration.

(3) What Is the Emotional Reaction of the Patient?

How the ill or disabled family member reacts emotionally to the condition will have an impact on family functioning. Though at the time of diagnosis, it may be too early to evaluate this reaction, the professional can still identify beginning signs that may suggest a continued emotional reaction that could become a deterrent to adjustment. The patient, for example, may be aware of a permanent occupational role change, and thus become quite angry. The nature of the disability, and its occurrence at a particular developmental stage, may signify for the patient that "my job usefulness is finished." From this realization, lingering grief and a continued depression may follow.

(4) What Does the Family Need at This Time?

Even though attention has been directed to the emotional reactions of family members to a trauma, the needs that flow from these reactions have been largely ignored (Power & Dell Orto, 1980). For example, at the time of diagnosis, family members may be experiencing feelings of uncertainty, shock, anxiety, and even anger at their beginning awareness of future, personal, and family losses. Each of these felt emotions suggests such needs as the desire to process information, to explore alternatives, to clarify frustrations, to be listened to empathically, and to receive support. A recognition of these needs may suggest guidelines or objectives for the helper's interventions.

II. During the Course of In-Hospital Treatment/Rehabilitation

At this crucial time in the patient's illness, there are many areas for the helping professional to explore. An understanding of each area can give an indication of what kind of intervention approach could be utilized. The five areas are:

(1) What Information Does the Family Have About the Disability or Illness?

The professional can explore whether family members are aware of the basic facts of the particular illness or disability, what the course of treatment may be, what the illness/disability implications for family life are, and what the residual strengths or assets of the patient are. Information about the disability may already have been given by health professionals. But family members, because of their anxieties, tend not to process information very well during their conferences with the physician (Polinko, 1985).

(2) What are the Needs of the Family While the Family Member is in the Hospital?

An awareness of these needs provides relevant suggestions on how health professionals can intervene with family members. Many of these needs include the following: (1) to be treated with respect and individuality, (2) to receive concrete services (e.g., available community resources, financial information), (3) to maintain a sense of competence in family life, (4) to be listened to and understood as concerned persons who are attempting to cope with a disability, (5) to process information provided by health professionals, (6) to know how to interact effectively with health professionals, (7) to recognize their own strengths, (8) to care for themselves, and (9) to recognize potential problems. There are perhaps other needs that emerge early in the treatment process, but the preceding are those that have been identified most often by this author.

(3) What has the Family Done So Far to Respond to the Disability or Illness?

Though treatment or rehabilitation may begin immediately or soon after the diagnosis, there is usually a period of time, even if it is one day, in which family members can begin to organize themselves to live with the new trauma. This organization may involve contacting someone for financial information, or a discussion among family members of what needs to be done by each family member to respond to the family demands of the illness or disability, or an identification of support systems available to the family.

(4) What are the Resources Available to the Family?

These resources include both those available from within the family, and those external to the family members. They include financial resources, the availability and willingness of extended family members, and the presence of community support systems, such as respite care, child day care, or programs for the elderly. The availability of these resources can make a difference in the family's adjustment to a trauma. Family members frequently state that the main reason they have adapted to a disability, and then have become a source of help to the ill family member, is that support external to the family itself is available.

(5) What is the Perceived Threat to Family Functioning Because of the Disability?

This is an important area to explore in any family assessment, because all families are especially vulnerable to unwelcomed stress and prolonged anxiety after the occurrence of a disability or illness. For example, if a newly disabled person's spouse must make repeated and long visits to the hospital, how will this absence from home affect the maintenance of family duties? Or, if a disability causes unemployment of the principal family wage earner, how will the family make up for this deficit? These are just two of the many issues that emerge with a disability in a family. In other words, how will family life change because of the disability? An awareness of what happens to a family in a disability situation can make a difference in whether family members can be utilized for the eventual rehabilitation of the disabled person.

The preceding areas of exploration are suggested directions to examine when a disabled or ill family member is undergoing in-hospital treatment or rehabilitation. To solicit information from family members in these areas, the following questions may be asked by the helping professional.

"How do you think your family will adjust to this disability?"
"How much have you been told about this disability or illness?"
"Can you describe your family life before the disability?"
"What do you think will be the most difficult problem area for your family now that this trauma has occurred?"
"Have you ever had the opportunity to use resources located with your church or other community centers? If so, what help was provided?"

III. Termination of In-Hospital Treatment/Rehabilitation and Return to an Available Family

When the in-hospital treatment phase is a long one, the family might find it all the more difficult to welcome the return of the patient. While expressing initial enthusiasm at the patient's discharge, family members may wonder if they have the energy, information, and competence to manage their ill or disabled family member.

When the family meets with the helping professional at the time of hospital discharge, the following areas could be explored:

(1) What Information and Expectations do the Family Members Have for the Patient?

Though family members received many important facts about the condition during the inpatient period, this information may have changed because of the patient's unexpected progress, or lack thereof, or because the family members' initial denial of certain implications of a disability has broken down and now the family is ready to confront the actual facts of the specific disability. The expectations that family members have for the patient's return to home should be identified, such as performance of family duties, resumption of any social life, and involvement in other aspects of family life.

(2) Who Will be the Family Member Responsible for the Care of the Disabled Person?

The principle caregiver is not always the disabled person's spouse or parent; they may have already relinquished such responsibilities because of emotional or physical reasons. Yet there is usually one person who assumes most of the care or responsibility for the disabled person. Whoever it is, this individual needs to be identified.

(3) What Emotions Does the Family Have About Reentry?

As stated earlier in this chapter, long hospitalization or only occasional visits to see the patient may make the disabled person seem a stranger to some family members. With a severe disabling condition, such as paraplegia, brain trauma, or related neurological deficits, the family may be ambivalent to have the patient at home because of caregiving responsibilities. Or, after institutionalization because of a chronic mental illness condition, family members may be very anxious because of their uncertainty over possible behavior problems at home. When meeting with the family, the helper can make a mental note of the number of openly hostile comments about the disabled person, especially those made in a way critical to any aspect of the patient's behavior. Such an identification provides a beginning understanding of the family's degree of emotional involvement with the patient.

Importantly, an exploration of what feelings the family has regarding the expected discharge of the patient might prevent the later occurrence of family adjustment problems. If family members are, for example, continually uncertain about their caregiving capabilities with their severely disabled member, or feel more comfortable in urging this person to be in the sick role, then the patient's efforts toward maximum independence will be often thwarted.

(4) How Much Energy Does the Family Have at Their Disposal?

This assessment question refers to the personal strengths that family members have for the home care of the patient. Caregiving for the severely disabled, for example, is a relentless responsibility. It does not necessarily end within a short time period after hospital discharge. Such areas as the physical capabilities of the principal caregiver and the financial and family network resources available to the immediate family need to be ascertained by the helping professional.

(5) What Services Does the Family Need?

At the time of discharge from the hospital, family members may need concrete services to aid them in their own caregiving efforts. The identification of financial resources, respite care opportunities, home nursing possibilities of day care centers: Each may be needed by a respective family. Often families are reluctant at patient-discharge time to voice their needs in these areas, and these needs may have to be anticipated. Moreover, a support group can often become a valuable resource for the family, but families may not be emotionally ready to enter such a group until they are caring for the patient at home. Earlier, they may find it difficult to confront the physical and emotional implications of a disability or disease, such as, for example, cognitive impairments, sexual limitations, reduced mobility, behavior disturbances, and there being no possibility of eventual return to full employment. Living daily with the disabled person, however, helps family members to gain more of a needed reality perspective and the realization that perhaps they could learn from others how to deal with these problems. All in all, the recognition of what concrete services are necessary can help considerably in a family's adjustment efforts and in their assistance to promote rehabilitation goals for the patient.

Hospital discharge is a critical time in a disabled person's rehabilitation. The helping professional can facilitate effective intervention by asking the family certain questions. For example:

1. How do you feel about having your family member at home? Do you foresee any problems?
2. What is family life going to be like, now that your family member has been discharged from the hospital?

3. Who do you believe is going to be mainly responsible for taking care of your family member while he or she is at home?
4. What are your expectations now for your family member?
5. Can you tell me your understanding of your family member's disability/illness?
6. What services do you feel you need now to help your family adjust to the family member's being at home?

IV. Outpatient Status for Treatment/Rehabilitation

Family contact by a helping professional does not necessarily have to end with the patient's discharge from the hospital. Many families may still be involved on an outpatient basis with particular health workers because of treatment necessities. When family contact is made, the helper may want to explore whether there has been a family response to previous identified areas of need, such as needed services and information, changes in the family members' expectations for the disabled person, and the family members' abilities to care for themselves. Is the family, when appropriate, actively involved in the patient's treatment or rehabilitation? Further areas of exploration might include:

1. Have new disruptions occurred within the family, such as the onset of excessive drinking, prolonged separations, or new resentments at having the disabled person at home?
2. Has the relationship to health care providers changed in a negative direction? Attitudes may change with a perceived delay in the patient's recovery or rehabilitation, or because of severe treatment side effects. The helping professional can ascertain whether the family's attitude is a temporary one, caused by unmet expectations or surprise events, or if it is a continuing mood.

In order to solicit information in these areas, the following questions are suggested:

1. Regarding the disability/chronic illness, what do you feel is the most difficult problem for your family at the present time?
2. How has your family changed since your family member has been at home?
3. Are there any other services that you feel you need at the present time?

CONCLUSION

When disability strikes a family, an adjustment is demanded not only from the client but also from the entire family. Disablement and chronic illness usually require new means of coping and interaction. If the family is going to be assisted in adjusting to those situations, as well as helped to become a resource for the disabled or ill person, then a family assessment should be undertaken by the helping professional. Depending on disability circumstances and the opportunities for family contact, this evaluation will vary both as to extensiveness and subject matter. Family needs will also change as adjustment attempts are made. This chapter has described a family-assessment approach that focuses attention on the family at critical times during treatment or rehabilitation. The approach provides a family-diagnostic structure that, in turn, provides a basis for effective intervention. Interventions with families and disability is discussed in Chapter 2.

REFERENCES

Anthony, W. A., Pierce, R. M., & Cohen, M. R. (1979). *The skills of diagnostic planning*. Amherst, MA: Carkhuff Institute of Human Technology.

Caroff, P., & Mailick, M. (1985). The patient has a family: Reaffirming social work's domain. *Social Work in Health Care, 10*(4), 17–34.

Christ, G., & Adams, M. A. (1984). Therapeutic stages at psycho-social crisis points in the treatment of childhood cancer. In A. E. Christ & K. Flomenhaft (Eds.), *Childhood cancer: Impact on the family*, pp. 109–130. New York: Plenum.

Cogswell, B. E. (1968). Self-socialization: Re-adjustment of paraplegics in the community. *Journal of Rehabilitation, 34*, 11–13.

Dillon, C. (1985). Families, transitions, and health: Another look. *Social Work in Health Care, 10*(4), 35–43.

Doherty, W., & Baird, M. (1983). *Family therapy and family medicine*. New York: Guilford.

Futterman, E., & Hoffman, J. (1978). Crisis and adaptation in the families of fatally ill children. In E. G. Anthony & C. Koupernik (Eds.), *The child in his family: The impact of disease and death*, pp. 127–144. New York: Wiley

Grossman, J. A., Pozanski, E. O., & Banegas, M. E. (1983). Lunch: Time to study family interactions. *Journal of Psychosocial Nursing and Mental Health Services, 21*, 19–23.

MacVicor, M. G., & Archbold, P. (1976). A framework for family assessment in chronic illness. *Nursing Forum, 15*, 180–194.

Minuchin, S., Roseman, B. L., & Baker, L. (1978). *Psychosomatic families: Anorexia nervosa in context*. Cambridge, MA: Harvard University Press.

Okun, B. F. (1987). *Effective helping: Interviewing and counseling techniques*. Monterey, CA: Brooks/Cole.

Polinko, R. (1985). Working with the family: The acute phase. In M. Ylvisaker (Ed.), *Head Injury Rehabilitation*. San Diego: College-Hill.

Power, P. W., & Dell Orto, A. E. (1980). *Role of the family in the rehabilitation of the physically disabled*. Austin, TX: Pro-Ed.

Satir, V. (1967). *Conjoint family therapy*. Palo Alto, CA: Science & Behavior Books.

Wilcoxon, S. A. (1985). Healthy family functioning: The other side of family pathology. *Journal of Counseling and Development, 63*, 495–499.

2 An Intervention Model for Families of the Disabled

Paul W. Power

Families who are confronted for the first time with a disability or chronic illness often need some kind of intervention by a helping professional. Disability and severe illness have a disequilibrating effect on patients and families. This chapter explains an approach to short-term intervention developed for those families challenged by new stressors, emerging patient needs, and difficult adjustments to the presence of severe illness or disability. It is difficult to establish an intervention approach based on a classification of diseases. For example, neurological illnesses are at different times considered either chronic or progressive. Some forms of cancer are now regarded as chronic by virtue of improved medical technology (Caroff & Mailick, 1985). The helping approach proposed in this chapter, consequently, will have a more broad-based application, and will identify basic strategies that can be applied to families in almost any disability situation. This approach will not be directly applicable to families who can be classified as seriously disturbed. With these families, prolonged family contact that focuses on changing or modifying family structure is usually necessary. Family therapists, utilizing varied methods, are achieving an enviable reputation for helping these disturbed families.

Often crucial to the effectiveness of any helping relationship, however, are the professional's attitudes toward a particular client or family. These attitudes can frequently inhibit the establishment of a working relationship with a family. For example, if the professional believes the notions expressed by "Don't worry, I'll save you," or "I know what is best for you," then the professional will usually allow for little input from family members regarding their roles in the patient's care. Family members can become resentful that more opportunity is not provided for expression of their opinions or plans. Consequently, before offering any assistance to the patient's family, helpers should examine their own possible prejudices associated with offering support, challenging the family, and providing information and anticipatory guidance.

For instance, a helper may identify with a family who needs to be taken care of temporarily and may overprotect the family or continue to protect the family when it is no longer necessary (Nelsen, 1980). Also, helpers who are fearful of not being able to do enough may withdraw from family members or blame them for being "weak." Helpers may also have difficulty accepting family members' behavior that conflicts with their own values.

Research indicates that certain traits and characteristics of helpers appear to positively affect helping relationships (Okun, 1987). The more in touch people are with their own behaviors, feelings, and beliefs, and the more able they are to communicate genuinely, clearly, and empathically their understanding of themselves to helpees and others, the more likely they are to be effective helpers.

AN INTERVENTION APPROACH

Effective, timely intervention is based on the facts learned from a family assessment. The helping approach presented in this chapter flows from the assessment model described in Chapter 1. This approach particularly highlights the professional's understanding of family needs at various times in the treatment and rehabilitations process. The identification of these needs, as well as an understanding of the type of disability, family functions, and the times available to provide the family with assistance, facilitate the development of intervention goals and suggest different types of intervention.

When the professional is assisting family members, the goals for intervention should be identified soon after an initial assessment. The targets of intervention focus on those family interactions that are affected by the illness and disability, and when appropriate, on how the family can assist the patient to achieve treatment and/or rehabilitation goals. Too often intervention efforts have been concentrated only on assisting family members to adjust to a traumatic condition. Yet there are also instances when the family can become a rehabilitation resource for the patient. There are three general ways in which a family can function as such a resource, namely: (1) by becoming a support system for the patient; (2) by diminishing stress for the patient; and (3) by facilitating, when possible, the disabled/ill family member's rehabilitation.

Within each of the three ways there are specific methods that can be used by a helping professional to involve the family for the patient's achievement of important goals. These methods represent different intervention forms, which are:

1. *Education*. Educating families or couples can include communicating a knowledge of community resources, such as peer support groups, respite care, and financial-aid opportunities, discussing with the family the patient's emotional concerns caused by a trauma (e.g., illness, accident, or unemployment), informing the family about illness, disability, or other trauma-related information, and assisting family members to learn behavior-management skills.

2. *Support*. When the family is undergoing changes because of a disability, the family members are usually under emotional strain. There may be many adjustment concerns and necessary changes in family roles, leisure activities, and other aspects of home life that can facilitate continued stress. Support can include listening to family members, sitting quietly with the family, conveying acceptance, and offering reassurance and expressed concern to family members on disability issues.

3. *Prevention*. This is often the weakest link in the delivery of services to family members. Prevention involves offering advice to family members on the importance of being aware of escalating, stress situations. The professional can assist the family to adjust the demands of caring for the ill or disabled family member to the strengths and limitations of their own resources, such as social support, confidence in caregiving responsibilities, and time-management skills. Any efforts to assist the family in their own mental health is a form of preventive maintenance that should render the family less vulnerable to stress-induced illness or prolonged fatigue. Effective intervention also involves early detection of possible problems. The professional can help family members to see the opportunities within the home environment for adjusting to a serious illness or disability and for assisting the patient to reach rehabilitation goals.

These three forms of intervention are incorporated into the helping model that follows. The model will also utilize the same trigger or critical points that were identified in Chapter 1 as necessary times for the collection of assessment information. Each point below represents a critical time for family members because certain needs emerge or important concerns are reexperienced. If these needs and concerns are responded to, it can make a difference both in the family's adjustment and the patient's achievement of rehabilitation goals. At each time, the helping professional can intervene with education, support, or prevention.

INTERVENING AT CRITICAL POINTS

First Critical Point: Diagnosis/Beginning of Treatment or Rehabilitation

The occurrence of a trauma or the diagnosis of a chronic disease is a critical time for families. Many emotions occur among family members, such as feelings of shock, anger, helplessness, intense anxiety over an uncertain future, guilt, and grief. Families at this time may find it difficult to face the day-to-day consequences of the disability or illness and they may not fully understand how life has really changed for them. All attention is usually on the ill family member. For many families, the onset of a disability can begin a period of intense crisis, when family members may find it difficult to meet their home and employment responsibilities, customary routines are disrupted, and the future appears uncertain.

An understanding of family needs at this time is crucial. In the author's experience, the dominant needs of family members at this time of diagnosis and/or beginning of treatment are: to receive support, to explore alternatives, and to process information. The emphasis for intervention is on support, because the family is usually attempting to bring itself together so that coping efforts can begin. Immediately after a trauma or diagnosis, family members may need comfort more than they need information or advice. Information can come later, when it is more easily absorbed. Then the communication of selected facts can make a difference for the family's adjustment.

When discussing support, Nelsen (1980) believes that sitting quietly with someone who is faced with a very disturbing situation shows a willingness to accept the person. Family members may simply want, for example, the kind of support shown by the soothing presence of the professional, the helper's listening skills, and the reassurance that the emotions induced by the trauma are understood and accepted. True listening is an expression of caring by the helping professional. Support can further be provided by using many "I-value-you"-type statements during the family interaction. Such statements assist the family to feel they are likable (Satir, 1967).

Information that could be communicated at this time can usually focus, when needed, on the basic facts of the illness or disability, the treatment alternatives, and the resources available to assist the family. The attending physician or nurse customarily explains the nature of the illness or disability and treatment plans and options, but family members may not have understood what was communicated. Repetition may be necessary. Family members, because of their anxieties, are often not prepared to listen to information about the disease or disability. Regardless of the circumstances, moreover, they frequently believe that their family member will get better. Denial operates very strongly around the time of accident occurrence and diagnosis. Though the professional may wish to provide as much information as possible about the disability or trauma, family members will usually hear what they want to hear. Their initial denial of selected information may give the family time to gather emotional resources with which to deal with the implications of what has happened.

During assessment, the professional may learn that the family appears very disturbed or quite vulnerable to a worsening of family functioning. If family members are to adjust to the demands on family life of the disability or illness, then they may need help in the forms of extended, personal counseling or family therapy. The helper realizes, consequently, that his or her intervention efforts should include motivating the family to seek further professional assistance. But it is usually difficult for family members to go through with any referral. When the family is convinced that their own seeking of assistance will make a difference in their family member's treatment and rehabilitation, and they are motivated to help the patient to get better, they are often willing to obtain some needed family assistance. The helper may also share perceptions with family members, such as "I believe you are going to find that coping with this situation is very difficult, and you might need someone who can give you help for a longer period of time than I can provide."

Advising families to seek assistance for their problems is a delicate matter. It can facilitate a referral when the helper identifies and carefully explains what professional counseling or family therapy usually involves, initiates the beginning contact (such as offering to make an initial appointment with the therapist), and then later contacts the family to ascertain whether a meeting with the therapist ever took place. But the family's response to any further help may be a reflection of several factors: the relationship they are establishing with the professional, the seriousness of the patient's condition, the availability of resources, and their own motivation to seek help for the patient's own adjustment and rehabilitation.

All in all, this time of diagnosis is an opportunity for the professional to promote a beginning relationship with family members. A helper's awareness of the importance of good listening and of showing respect for family viewpoints, combined with both encouraging family members to express their concerns and imparting relevant information, can promote the conviction among family members that the professional is a partner in their efforts to assist the patient to reach treatment and/or rehabilitation goals.

Second Critical Point: Course of Hospital Treatment and Rehabilitation

While the disabled or ill person is undergoing in-hospital treatment, adjustments are being made in family life to accommodate new or changing responsibilities. Family members are often trying to balance the needs of the disabled person with their own everyday demands of living. New considerations may also enter the family scene, such as financial issues, the necessary modification of family roles and duties, and the ever-present thought: "What is it going to be like living with our disabled family member?" Many emotions may have subsided that arose at the occurrence of the trauma, such as feelings of helplessness and hopelessness, particularly as more information is gained about treatment and possible rehabilitation. But other feelings usually linger, namely, anger, guilt, and anxiety over an uncertain future.

Certain needs may surface as the family balances the demands of the patient with the usual demands of a family life. These needs can be identified as: the necessity to reframe the situation in order to render it possibly less stressful; the need to marshal resources; the desire for more information on treatment and prognosis; the need to feel competent; and the growing necessity to establish a working relationship with health professionals. Communication with health professionals in a hospital setting is usually a new and frustrating experience for most family members. Their own worry over the patient's future, as well as their perception of the all-powerful role of the physician or nurse, so often inhibit a more initiating and assertive relationship with those responsible for the family member's care. All of these concerns and needs, consequently, help to shape an intervention approach that is aimed at assisting family members to reduce their stress, to receive support, to learn new ideas about coping with a disability or illness, and to gain information about their role in the patient's adjustment to the disability or illness. As support is the primary suggested intervention for the helping professional at the time of diagnosis or trauma, so the educating of family members and the imparting of information are the main foci of helping efforts in the second critical period for the family.

Helping by Educating

Attention to family needs at this time can begin with assisting family members to learn the useful skill of reframing or mentally restructuring the disability situation. Matheny, Aycock, Pugh, Curlette, and Cannella (1986) report from their extensive literature review of useful coping strategies that cognitive restructuring is the second most frequently cited coping strategy, next to relaxation exercises. A great deal of stress generated from a disability comes from stressful mental sets: from self-critical evaluations, from the fearful ballooning of potentially painful experiences, and from looking only at the worst eventualities caused by the onset of disability or illness (Matheny et al., 1986). Cognitive restructuring involves engaging family members in a gentle, rational confrontation of their irrational beliefs about the disability or illness, so as to replace those beliefs with ideas that are more adaptive (Mitchell & Krumboltz, 1987). It aims, for example, to reframe the disability or illness stressor as a challenge to overcome, and attempts to place these concerns into a perspective with other life responsibilities and advantages. The helping professional can provide insights into how to identify positive outcomes inherent in living with a disabled family member. The disability, though usually causing a severe emotional impact on family members, does not have to be viewed exclusively as trouble or as a hopeless reality. After encouraging family members to share their beliefs about what the onset of disability means to them, the professional can suggest that the family reflect on such ideas as: "Is it possible to identify the value to the family of what has happened?" "Is your own lot as onerous as that of others?" "Is it possible that if all of you are willing the family may grow closer together because of this illness/disability?" Though it may be difficult for family members to endorse completely such ideas while the patient is still in the hospital, these suggestions may provide new perspectives on how to cope more effectively with family stressors.

The family also needs to recognize and organize their personal and community resources. Because many persons tend to overlook or underestimate their coping strengths, family members need help in acknowledging these assets. Many professionals could be more effective if they directed more attention to the strengths of families. Many such strengths were identified in Chapter 1. Other resources that could be utilized by the family may include friends, support groups, and agencies that provide information on financial and legal concerns. Many family members, however, are not ready during the beginning weeks of their family member's hospitalization to become involved with self-help groups. They may need time to adjust to the impact of the disability or illness.

The family may further need additional, disability-related information. Earlier contacts may have been made with family members, and basic information about disability and treatment issues shared. But family members may still be denying the important implications of the disability to family life, such as those affecting employment or other family responsibilities. Information may then have to be provided that gradually helps the family members to face reality. The emphasis, though, is on *gradually*, for as stated earlier a certain amount of denial in the early stages of an illness or disability assists family members to gain strength and support to face disability related implications. But denial of the basic facts of the situation over an extended period of time can become destructive to both the patient and to family life. When it is appropriate, the communication of information can include highlighting the patient's residual assets and what are probably rehabilitation goals. These goals help the family to think more positively about the future (Power & Sax, 1978). Unnecessary uncertainty about a disability often inhibits the establishment of family plans that focus on adjustment.

The professional's attention to strengths can also assist family members to maintain a sense of competence as they learn to adjust to the disability situation. Many factors contribute to a lowered sense of competence among family members: the new but complicated world of medical technology, the uncertainty over the specific prognosis of the disability, and the continued involvement in the hospital atmosphere, which can be impersonal, stressful, anxiety producing, and conducive to generating the belief that "perhaps we are different and something is wrong with us because this disability or accident occurred." Also, many families experience difficulties in understanding the current, in-hospital behavior of the patient, and so they tend to feel lost and frustrated. These latter difficulties may arise because of the difference in time orientation between the patient and the family. Lilliston (1985) explains that the patient's future perspective may be only as long as the next round of medication that manages pain. The patient's preoccupation with present bodily sensations and bodily functions absorb his or her total attention. The sphere of temporal focus is predominantly upon the present. Time for most patients moves painfully slowly, and they become bored, restless, and unhappy. But other family members tend to experience a more dynamic sense of time. Even though family members are severely affected by the patient's sudden disability or illness, they frequently review the past and leap to the future (Lilliston, 1985).

When the professional is aware of this disparity in time orientation, and recognizes other concerns that appear to be eroding the family's sense of competence in handling the disability situation, the helper may suggest ways that the family can be as involved as is possible in the patient's care. The professional can also provide information that improves communication and alleviates uncertainty, and again direct the family members' attentions to their own assets and their contributions to the patient's welfare. Also, communicating how the family can control the impact of the disability on family life may promote a sense of security among family members. For example, the spouse of a newly disabled person may be quite worried about the future unemployment possibilities of the patient, and what this will mean for the family's security. However, when the professional indicates the different financial resources, as well as the possible vocational rehabilitation alternatives, then the spouse may begin to feel a little more optimistic about the family's future.

A frequent problem that occurs with many families at this time of in-hospital treatment is that one family member can overextend herself or himself in providing attention to the patient, to the detriment of adequate family functioning. Other family members may feel resentful that a mother or father is spending so much time away from home. Once this is identified, the professional can briefly suggest ways to balance the needs of the patient with the needs of other family members. Because resentment may be nurtured by a lack of communication, the helper may even encourage the parent or other family member to discuss his or her involvement with the others. Also, depending on how much the helping professional knows about a particular family's daily functioning, the helper may further provide ideas on how family life can be maintained as normally as possible for as long as possible, and how family members can take care of themselves while attending to patient and family needs.

Many problems occur in family life at this time, simply because family members did not ask the right questions, did not ask questions at all, or did not understand the helper's responses. The family needs to become aware that concerns should be identified and appropriate questions asked. Family members can be told to plan their contact with a physician, for example, and to be prepared to take notes or to bring a tape recorder so that communicated facts can be accurately and faithfully remembered. The helper can suggest to family members that such statements as, "I don't understand what you are saying, Can you repeat that in simpler words. Doctor, this is all going too fast for me, can you slow down a bit? I need more information," are appropriate and may frequently open the way to real two-way communication. Once family members learn to ask questions, it can get easier and easier. As Cohen (1987) states, "Two communication problems . . . impair patient relationships: not listening and not talking" (p. 8). Talking by family members to health professionals promotes a more effective relationship. Health care is a two-way street.

Helping by Support and Prevention

The helper's responses to the above areas of family needs and adjustment concerns is through providing information that is educational. Yet support and prevention are two additional threads in this fabric of helping. Support during the patient's hospitalization can take the form of not only listening to the questions of family members, but also showing them that what they have said makes sense and has been understood. Family members will also harbor many negative feelings because of the perceived threats to family life generated by the disability situation. The professional can reassure the family that many of their negative feelings are to be expected. Allowing family members to ventilate their feelings can reassure them that the professional is supportive of their coping efforts.

An issue that is frequently raised at this time is what kind of support to offer the family. As Nelsen (1980) states, most professionals will have already offered acceptance when taking a family assessment. Family members will often benefit from this accepting atmosphere and plan solutions to their problems. They may need no other type of support. Yet some families with many available resources to use in the resolution of a problem may lack confidence to take advantage of these resources. Nelsen believes that validation should be extended to the family, namely, feedback to family members that in using these resources they are on the right track, that they possess personal and family strengths to cope with the situation, and that they have the confidence of the helper.

Prevention is another form of intervention during this second critical period for family members. It implies that the professional will assist family members to recognize potential stressors and identify additional, needed resources to meet these demands. Such stressors may include a family member's prolonged absence from the home or a change in family duties and responsibilities. Both of these events may have occurred earlier in family life, but now, because of the different issues created by a disability, previous coping strategies may be inadequate. In handling difficult times, families frequently prefer to look to their own immediate family for any assistance. When the helping professional perceives, however, that a family member's absence, or a change in family duties, or impending caregiving responsibilities at home may cause undue stress to family members, then the helper should encourage the use of outside resources. In fact, when there are severe financial concerns or, for instance, when a home needs architectural modifications because of the person's disability, then outside resources must be promoted to family members.

The issue of architectural redesign is a troubling one for many families. Though persons with such disabilities as quadriplegia, paraplegia, and spina bifida will usually need functional changes in the home, parents of disabled children, for example, tend to delay making environmental adaptations. Exterior home changes (e.g., ramps or enlarged entranceways) may stimulate feelings of stigma among family members; in addition, the family may actually have difficulty accepting the implications of the disability for family life (Lewis, 1985).

Professionals should be aware of impending difficulties for the patient when he or she returns home, and attempt to assist the family to prepare for the necessary changes. The helper during the family contacts can encourage the goals of mobility, independence, and normalization for the disabled person, urge parents to get in touch with parent groups where other parents can explain what home improvements have been made in the past and what they have learned from these adaptations, and remind family members that a delay in removing architectural barriers can frequently lead to severe stress and continued anxiety (Lewis, 1985).

The intervention forms of education, support, and prevention, consequently, assist the family to alleviate stress, to maintain normal patterns of living, and to become aware of their strengths. All of these factors are beginning steps for family members that lead to their possible roles as resources for the disabled person's eventual rehabilitation. The groundwork for this is developed before the patient returns home.

Third Critical Point: Discharge from Hospital and Return to Available Family

For patients leaving the hospital after many weeks or months of treatment, a return to the home and available family can be a turning point for their daily adjustment and eventual rehabilitation. Unfortunately, the home can become a refuge, a place of moratorium where the disabled or chronically ill family member escapes from possible opportunities and renewed activities. On the other hand, the home can become a valuable resource, where families are viewed as not only responsible caregiving agents who provide substantial physical, emotional, and social support, but are also continued facilitators for the patient's productivity and achievement of rehabilitation goals.

Whether the family becomes this important resource, or represents a deterrent to adjustment and rehabilitation, can often be determined as the family gathers to take their disabled family member to the home residence. Effort should be made by the helping professional to have some family contact at this time. It is hoped that it is not the first time that the helper has met the patient's family members. But if it is, in many hospital settings such a meeting is a structured time when information is usually provided to the family on patient needs. Discharge planning is conducted during this meeting, and preferably the patient's family has been included in the development of plans. If the discharge plan is to be viable, the provision of an aftercare plan that includes the family's recommendations, capabilities, and resources for their relative's rehabilitation and/or treatment program should be considered (McElroy, 1987).

This discharge-planning meeting with the family provides the opportunity not only for a family assessment, as suggested in Chapter 1, but also the chance for the helper to formulate, when needed, appropriate intervention strategies. Having gathered information on who will be mainly responsible for the care of the disabled or ill family member, what the family's expectations are for the patient, and what emotions the family has about the patient's reentry, the professional can filter these issues into one main focus for intervention, namely, family needs. The identified assessment areas provide information on what the family actually needs at this time, and not what the professional believes the family needs. What professionals want and what families want from each other may be quite different. Spaniol, Zipple, and Fitzgerald (1985) believe that "assuming what families want without adequately checking out underlying assumptions usually leads to families discounted, devalued, and disenfranchised by professional intervention" (pg. 4). The family's viewpoint on needed services is extremely important, for how well the family manages the patient's adjustment and rehabilitation depends on the kinds and qualities of services designed to help them (Power & Dell Orto, 1980).

This author has learned from family members that at the time of hospital discharge their needs are varied and often include the need to express their feelings on the patient's return to the home and the need for information. The latter is especially related to how they can assist the patient at home; what are effective behavioral-management techniques; where can particular services be provided; and, when possible for the patient, what is involved in the vocational rehabilitation process. Additional family needs are: knowing how to handle caregiver fatigue and possible burn-out; maintaining a normal life; building a fulfilling life for themselves; sustaining a productive relationship with health professionals; and developing more personal skills of managing and parenting. The professional's response to all of these needs suggests the intervention forms of education, support, and prevention, with an emphasis on attention to the family's educational needs. Sharing of information by the professional must contain language that is easy for the family to understand. The use of technical language erects barriers and boundaries that can be counterproductive, and creates high anxiety and a sense of helplessness among family members (Hatfield, 1986). Providing information alone, however, is sometimes not enough. McElroy (1987) explains that few mental health professionals, for example, seriously consider the family's educational needs in ways that are meaningful to the family.

Allowing family members to discuss their feelings and problems over caring for the patient at home is a form of support provided by the professional. When issues are raised about possible difficulties in taking care of the disabled or ill family member, the family may not only be seeking answers to treatment questions, but may also be looking for validation of what they propose to do for their family member. An accepting, reassuring attitude from the professional can promote feelings of confidence within the family. When family members have more information about management concerns, the course of treatment, available resources, and the support that can be provided by helping professionals, then they frequently feel better about their home responsibilities with the patient.

Communication of relevant information that highlights the family's role in the patient's treatment and/or rehabilitation should emphasize the family's expectations for the disabled person. Family members frequently encourage the disabled individual to remain in the "sick role." The family's almost exclusive attention to what the patient cannot do, combined with the apparent availability of entitlement benefits, encourages the conviction that the patient should remain inactive at home. Expectations related to the sick role also flow from the family understanding of the disability (Power & Sax, 1978). For example, if the family incorrectly perceives that the disability or illness causes a person to be different, rather than just to act differently on occasion, then family members place the patient in a dependent role that may be unwarranted by the condition. This attitude usually prevents disabled family members from returning to many family duties, and often suggests to them that they should relinquish even satisfying social activities.

The helper, therefore, should encourage the family members to allow the disabled person to function at his or her maximum level of independence, to engage when possible in the regular performance of family duties, and to participate in leisure opportunities. The helper can also assist family members to direct their attention to the patient's capabilities, and to reinforce the patient for her or his performance of treatment duties and family responsibilities. Through all of these activities, persons with a disability can get in touch again with their strengths. This awareness, and the accompanying feelings of competence and usefulness, may be added motivating factors to reach rehabilitation goals (Power & Dell Orto, 1980). How can disabled persons participate, for example, in the vocational rehabilitation process if they have not been involved in family life and responsibilities, and if they do not feel useful?

Other facts that can be communicated at this time of hospital discharge are particular techniques for managing disability-related behaviors; these techniques are disability specific and are discussed in other chapters of this book. For example, Chapters 3 and 4 describe specific skills that parents may use at home when caring for a child. Chapter 8 suggests helping strategies that respond to the sexual needs of adolescents. Also important are what additional community resources could be utilized by family members, and what happens to someone when he or she begins the process of vocational rehabilitation. Among available resources, self-help groups are particularly valuable for family members after living with the patient for a few weeks. These groups can help the family to meet social needs, needs for hope, and be a sustaining force in the week-to-week lives of individuals who have assumed the daily burden of care (Spaniol, 1987).

Information on the vocational rehabilitation process is important to convey to family members. When this involvement is a possibility for a disabled person, an understanding of each step in the process can alleviate many frustrations and uncertainties. Family members are usually strangers to the services provided for disabled people. They may also harbor negative attitudes or misunderstandings about these opportunities. But a detailed explanation of what is available, the time usually required to receive the service, and what may be a few of the difficulties when participating in a specific resource can alleviate many concerns and even serve as a motivating factor when it is feasible for one's rehabilitation. When their fears are allayed, then family members may be more willing to endorse the lengthy process of vocational rehabilitation.

Preventing Caregiver Burn-Out

When working with families, moreover, the professional can become aware of the family's need both to handle caregiver fatigue and possible burn-out and to lead a fulfilling life. It is a relentless, demanding task to deal with the everyday family and treatment duties for someone with a severe disability or chronic illness. The demands on time and the energy required are often a tremendous drain on a family member's personal resources (Spaniol, 1987). Activities, interests, and daily routines that once were habitual are either no longer occurring or are no longer occurring in the same way. A family member can become easily fatigued and, without the frequent opportunities to pursue leisure-time activities, or simply to get away from it all, the family member can become physically, intellectually, and emotionally exhausted. Also, feelings of guilt and worry, or the nagging question: "What would happen if I were not there?" often inhibit someone from seeking temporary relief from the continued demands of caregiving.

During the discharge planning meeting, or soon thereafter, the professional can gently remind family members that if they don't take good care of themselves, then they really cannot take good care of the disabled or ill person. Families often need permission to put greater time and energy into themselves (Zipple & Spaniol, 1987). Families need frequently to refocus much of their energy on their own needs and wants. When the professional can suggest positive options for family members, which may include activities such as spending time alone or with old friends, going to the theater, getting away on weekends, and reinvolving themselves in activities that have nothing to do with disability and illness, then such suggestions may facilitate the belief that they can make their life work for themselves on a daily basis (Zipple & Spaniol, 1987).

Helping professionals can also indicate to the family that one way to alleviate possible fatigue is to alter stress-inducing behavior patterns in the home. In other words, family members need to adjust the demands on them to the limitations of their own resources. The goal of this strategy is to balance the demand-resource equation by advising families to become aware of escalating stress situations. Other dimensions of this strategy are to urge a family member to discuss her or his need for some free time with other family members, and remind families to be supportive of this need. It is also helpful to remind families to work toward what is possible in the situation rather than maintaining unrealistic expectations. Much family burn-out is caused by the unrealistic expectations a family member holds for himself or herself.

With this attention to family-member fatigue is the accompanying emphasis on the family's need to lead a fulfilling life. But a fulfilling life develops from a family member's sense of positive self-esteem. With persons facing the severe adaptational challenges that disability and chronic illness create, self-esteem must be maintained at all costs, and enhanced if at all possible (White, 1974). In other words, family members need to feel an inner assurance that they can do things necessary for a satisfactory life. Personal worth is reinforced by the care and concern exhibited by the professional, by a network of friends and relatives, and by an understanding of personal and family strengths. In recognizing these assets, family members can often begin to feel better about themselves and then take additional steps to pursue satisfying activities.

Families need to maintain a normal pattern of activities. The professional may have to indicate to family members that when possible the patient should be helped to follow the family's daily schedule, and not vice versa. The sooner the disabled person returns to a normal, family environment the better will be the patient's long-term psychosocial adjustment.

Though frequently family life may have to be reorganized to make room for the needs of the patient, efforts to follow a customary pattern of family activities can enhance family morale and promote family survival; for if family members are to be of valuable assistance for the patient's achievement of rehabilitation goals, then they must survive. Survival is facilitated by appropriate patterns of living for family members.

Family members could often use more information on particular treatment or behavior-management duties. Many of the individual chapters in this book explain specific skills needed, for example, by parents of disabled or at-risk children and the caregivers of chronically ill adults, such as Chapters 3 and 13. During the discharge planning meeting the professional could identify resources where information can be obtained on management and parenting skills.

This referral service is another way for the helping professional to continue a working relationship with family members. In turn, the family needs to sustain open communication with the professional. The patient's return to the family does not necessarily have to radically change the relationship between the professional and family members. Questions may still have to be asked because treatment plans for home care may be occasionally quite complicated; in addition, further community resources, such as those involving respite care, may have to be pursued. Professionals can provide reassurance that the family's questions will be openly received and that they are still available to family members. The family still needs the support that generates strength for caregiving tasks.

The threads of education, support, and prevention consequently form the pattern of helping at this time of the patient leaving the hospital and returning home. The intervention through education particularly responds to the many concerns and challenges that family members will face when caring for the disabled or ill person. But the family contact at hospital discharge can be perceived as a mutual interaction process between the patient, family members, and the helping professional. This contact is designed both to promote the disabled person's well being and to assist the family in their coping efforts. Developing positive expectations for the patient, providing appropriate information to all family members, facilitating the utilization of support systems, developing family competencies, and encouraging confidence among family members in their caregiving responsibilities are each intervention goals that can help the disabled or ill family member to reach an optimal level of functioning.

Fourth Critical Point: Outpatient Status and Continuation of Treatment/Rehabilitation

This stage embraces those weeks and months that the patient is recuperating at home and continuing to learn how to live with the disability or illness. It may also include that time when the chronic illness or disability has been finally stabilized, if possible, and family members are not settling into the routine of living with a disabled person. The extent of family contact with professionals who provided education, support, and prevention during the previous three critical points usually diminishes over time. Many other helping professionals may now become newly involved with the family. Some of these are rehabilitation nurses, visiting home-care nurses, selected social workers, and rehabilitation counselors. For these workers, and those others who have been involved since the beginning of treatment, there are selected interventions that could be done for the family. These include education, crisis management, and support. Education implies a reemphasis of treatment-related information, the further identification of available resources, and perhaps a restatement of the different aspects of the treatment or rehabilitation process. The author has discovered that frequently many family members have either forgotten or misunderstood the information that was communicated at discharge planning. Family anxieties at that time might have blocked the retention of important facts. The helper, therefore, may have to repeat information that was previously imparted in order to alert family members to those areas of knowledge that should be remembered for the patient's treatment.

One specific information area that may need to be reemphasized is what the family can do to involve the disabled person in family life and responsibilities. Though initially enthusiastic about urging this individual to be productive within the home, family members may diminish their efforts if the patient wants to maintain a dependent role on others, or if warranted, entitlement benefits begin, or if the caregiver becomes so fatigued that only the essential treatment duties can be provided. Unfortunately, after leaving the hospital many disabled adults never return to their former employment or level of productivity, even when it is possible. Although there are many reasons for this occurrence, such as employer attitudes, the patient's depression over lost capabilities, and few existing opportunities for retraining in a particular geographic area, the family should be aware that they have a definite role in their disabled family member's rehabilitation progress. Basic to this role are the family's positive expectations within the home for the productivity of the disabled person. The professional's viewpoints on these expectations may have to be stated again sometime during the outpatient phase.

An additional area of information that may need restating is how to balance caregiving responsibilities with the caregiver's personal needs. Over a long period of time family members may realize that the disability situation is not likely to change radically for the better, and this perspective may cause families to be drained and worn out (Spaniol, 1987). To maintain the necessary balance, a few suggestions can be offered by the professional. These include exploring meaningful work outside the home, seeking the companionship of close friends, or performing a favorite, enriching activity. These ideas may have been provided before, but their repetition may find a more receptive audience after family members have experienced the everyday burdens of caregiving.

During this outpatient phase of the disabled person's rehabilitation, however, a sudden worsening or exacerbation of the illness or disability may occur. Such a perceived trauma can represent a serious crisis for family members, and crisis-management skills may have to be utilized by the professional. Intervention directions for a family crisis can include: the identification of what really is causing the crisis; the further exploration of reality issues; assisting the family to break the assumed problems into manageable pieces; facilitating the free expression of feelings; and helping family members to have a basic trust in themselves. Yet when exacerbations occur, or the clinical course of a disability or chronic illness is uncertain, professionals should be clear with families about the complexity of the condition and the limitations of current knowledge or treatment. Families need to hear that professionals also are struggling to determine how best to help their disabled family member. This awareness will help families to come to terms with their own hopes, fears, and limitations (Zipple & Spaniol, 1987).

The provision of support should be an ever-present available resource for families as they learn to deal and live with the illness or disability at home. Those elements of support that were shared with family members from the beginning of the patient's treatment could again assist all in the family. Reinforcing feedback, listening to family concerns, identifying what is functionally possible for the disabled person, and indicating to the family that the helping professional is available when necessary to answer questions about rehabilitation, all demonstrate that someone cares abut the family's welfare. Family members can easily become discouraged when they realize that caring for their disabled or ill family member is really more than they imagined; or that the disabled person is making some progress toward improved functioning, but very, very slowly; or, that suggested community resources may prove to be quite disappointing. The family may need hope, new resources, and a sense of optimism, when appropriate, about the future. A professional who offers reassurance, acceptance, and timely information represents a source of hope.

CONCLUSION

Though helping professionals have many job-related responsibilities, any attention to a patient's family does not have to compromise these duties. Family members can make a difference in the disabled person's rehabilitation, and helping professionals, especially those working in a health setting, need to become more involved with the patient's family if they are to be effective promoters of rehabilitation and treatment. A premise of this helping approach is that involvement with families usually requires an enhancement of diagnostic, relationship, and planning skills that many professionals use regularly. Family contact invites a further application of these specific skills, with the added dimension of an understanding of family dynamics related to disability and how assistance to families involves different forms of intervention. An awareness of what a family needs at a particular time in the patient's treatment, and how family members can be valuable resources for achievement of rehabilitation goals, provides important contributions to the professional's intervention strategies.

Two issues need to be emphasized. First, for effective family intervention, the helping professional does not necessarily have to be a family counselor or therapist. The approach explained in this chapter builds on a knowledge of individuals in need of assistance, an awareness of the existence of internal and external resources available to them, a thorough understanding of referral principles and techniques, and the possession of at least a basic knowledge of crisis intervention in order to provide necessary assistance when appropriate. With this knowledge and skills, combined with the additional information on families and family intervention explained in this chapter, then one can frequently assist a family on a short-term basis.

Second, any family contact presumes that the helping professional is motivated to involve family members in the patient's care in some appropriate, feasible way, and even to take the initiative for this intervention. Yet often professionals themselves do not receive any support from within their own work environment for family contact. The implementation of any approach to assist families, therefore, implies a strong conviction about the importance of family utilization in rehabilitation and at times advocating for this conviction. For the best interests of the patient, the professional needs the family's help. Providing attention to the family enlarges one's ability to offer quality services to clients.

REFERENCES

Caroff, F., & Mailick, M. D. (1985). The patient has a family: Re-affirming social work's domain. *Social Work in Health Care, 10,* 17-34.

Christ, G., & Adams, M. A. (1984). Therapeutic strategies at psycho-social crisis points in the treatment of childhood cancer. In A. E. Christ & K. Flomenhaft (Eds.), *Childhood cancer: Impact on the family* (pp. 109-130). New York: Plenum.

Cohen, V. (1987, June 16). Dealing with a silent doctor. *Health Magazine, Washington Post,* p. 8.

Hatfield, A. B. (1986). Semantic barriers to family and professional collaboration. *Schizophrenia Bulletin, 12,* 327-332.

Lewis, B. E. (1985). *Inventors, explorers, experimenters: How parents adapt homes for children with mobility problems.* Unpublished manuscript. Humanized Environments, 14 Hillside Terrace, West Newton, MA 02165.

Lilliston, B. A. (1985). Psychosocial responses to traumatic physical disability. *Social Work in Health Care, 10,* 1-7.

Matheny, K. B., Aycock, D. W., Pugh, J. L., Curlette, W. L., & Cannella, K. A. (1986). Stress coping: A qualitative and quantitative synthesis with implication for treatment. *The Counseling Psychologist, 14,* 499-549.

McElroy, E. M. (1987). The beat of a different drummer. In Hatfield & Lefley (Eds.), *Families of the mentally ill* (pp. 225-243). New York: Guilford Press.

Mitchell, L. K., & Krumboltz, J. D. (1987). The effects of cognitive restructuring and decision-making training on career indecision. *Journal of Counseling Development, 66,* 171-174.

Nelsen, J. C. (1980, September). Support: A necessary condition for change. *Social Work,* pp. 388-392.

Okun, B. F. (1987). *Effective helping: Interviewing and counseling techniques.* Monterey, CA: Brooks/Cole.

Power, P. W., & Dell Orto, A. E. (1980). *Role of the family in the rehabilitation of the physically disabled.* Austin, TX: Pro-Ed.

Power, P. W., & Sax, D. S. (1978). The communication of information to the neurological patient: Some implications for family coping. *Journal of Chronic Disease, 31,* 57–65.

Satir, V. (1967). *Conjoint Family Therapy.* Palo Alto, CA: Science and Behavior Books.

Spaniol, L. (1987). Coping strategies of family caregivers. In A. Hatfield & H. Lefley (Eds.), *Families of the mentally ill* (pp. 208–224). New York: Guilford.

Spaniol, L. Zipple, A. M., & Fitzgerald, S. (1985). How professionals can share power with families: A practical approach to working with families of the mentally ill. *Psychosocial Rehabilitation Journal, 8,* 77–84.

White, R. (1974). Strategies of adaptation: An attempt at systematic description. In R. H. Moss (Ed.), *Human adaptation: Coping with life crises* (pp. 17–32). Lexington, MA: Heath.

Zipple, A. M., & Spaniol, L. (1987). Current educational and supportive models. In A. Hatfield & H. Lefley (Eds.), *Families of the mentally ill* (pp. 261–277). New York: Guilford Press.

Personal Statement: My Life With a Disability— Continued Opportunities

Paul Egan

For me life began very comfortably over 57 years ago, in a then affluent suburb of Greater Boston. I was the third son of a prominent up-and-coming general contractor. I also had an older sister. A month before I was born, tragedy befell the family when the firstborn son, then aged 6, died of diphtheria. So, when I arrived healthy and sound, I was a most welcome addition to a grieving mother and father. Just before I turned two another brother was born.

In September 1944, I entered the U.S. Navy and, after completing boot camp, I was initially assigned to motor-torpedo boats in the Philippines. I was then assigned to a yard minesweeper with a team of 22 officers and men. Our assignment consisted of sweeping (dragging) the shipping channels and ports of the Philippine Islands. During this time, my job performance was classified as outstanding, and I received many promotions. However, my life suddenly came apart. While I was moving a keg of concentrated ammonia across the deck, it blew up in my face. The ammonia burned my eyes, the linings of my nose and throat, and also the skin around my facial area. I was rendered unconscious, and upon regaining consciousness 3 days later, the doctor told me that my eyes were badly burned and that I would have to be patient and pray for a miracle to take place.

One year, seven hospitals, and several operations later, vision returned to my right eye to the degree of 20/70 with corneal scarring. Other complications emerged as my head and my right hand became involved in a constant tremor. This ailment was incorrectly diagnosed as a nervous anxiety reaction. So I became a psychiatric bouncing ball. In May of 1947 I was discharged with a 70% Veterans Administration (VA) compensation.

I immediately went to work for a friend, pumping gas in a gas station. But I had greater ambitions, and I enrolled at Boston Business Institute in a business administration curriculum for two years. Shortly after returning to school my mother developed cancer and passed away on December 15, 1947. This was a profound loss to all of us, as my mother was always on hand with her guidance and sense of fortitude. She was always there to listen, to encourage me to make the most of myself and to go back to school. In fact, in the initial stages of my readjustment to civilian life and to my own disability, it was Mom's positive attitude, including her expectations for me, that inspired me to move forward. Her philosophy of making one's residual assets work for the fulfillment of goals is one that I have adopted in my own life.

In June 1948 I married Marietta, a girl I had known before I entered the service. Around this time, my father went on a trip to Newfoundland, his place of birth, and came back a few months later, married. He had married his brother's housekeeper, a plain-appearing woman who was 25 years younger than he was. They immediately isolated themselves from all family and friends for years to come.

In June 1949, I graduated from business school and started experimenting with the real world. Although I was very fortunate in not being unemployed for more than a month during the next 24 years, my choice of expanding my horizons was limited greatly by an uninformed business environment. Time after time when applying for positions for which I was qualified, ignorance, fear, stigmatizations and prejudices were barriers I found most difficult to overcome.

During the next 20 years, my wife gave birth to five daughters, we moved to a larger house, and I was employed in various jobs. Shortly after the birth of our first daughter, I began a series of operations on my left eye. These operations climaxed with an unsuccessful corneal transplant, which resulted in the surgical removal of my left eyeball. Soon after the birth of our second daughter, I had a laminotomy. I understood this operation as involving the transection of the thin layers of connective tissues around the optic nerve. The pain and suffering endured were the most excruciating of my life. But I was able to get through all of this because of the support of my wife. We didn't think about the past or about my other disabilities. We focused on the present, and together we often discussed our mutual concerns. This was a tremendous help to get through my own sufferings. But in 1968 my tremors got worse, and I went into a VA hospital for a brain operation. After doing an encephalogram, the doctor thought the risks were too high. Instead of the operation, a new experimental drug was tried, but that increased the body involvement and was quickly discontinued.

Moreover, a trauma occurred in our family, when on a night in January 1970 when the temperature was 25 degrees below zero, our oil-burning furnace exploded, destroying our home and all of our possessions. All of our neighbors came to our support, and they held a fund-raising party for us that resulted in not only a substantial amount of money but also in donations of services in our efforts to rebuild. Another factor in our rebuilding effort was that after an absence of over 20 years my father reappeared and lent us the remaining necessary funds to rebuild. After we had made a few repayments he said, "You've shown good faith," tore up the note, and then chose to go back into hibernation with his wife. I tried on numerous occasions to visit with him on his 90-acre farm, but he was always "out" or had to go someplace in a hurry.

After getting settled into our new home in June 1970, our life returned to a semblance of normalcy until late in 1973 when I lost my job. My employment was not the only loss, however, for I also lost my sense of dignity and self-respect, and I drifted aimlessly in a sea of self-pity and depression for nearly 4 years. Though my family was very supportive of me during this time, I knew this was my own struggle and they themselves had to survive. My daughters were married, had their own families, but seemed to be there when I needed someone to share my feelings.

In June 1977, I was classified as blind. That November I entered the VA Blind Rehabilitation Center at West Haven, Connecticut and from that time on life took on a new perspective. After 14 weeks of intensive training and guidance, I was again doing things for and by myself. The educational-testing evaluations done at the center indicated a potential for higher education. So in September 1978 I returned to school with the goal of becoming a social worker. In May 1982 I received my B.S. from Suffolk University, and then in 1984 I earned an M.S. from Boston University. In April of that year, I began a new career as a field representative and outreach-employment specialist with the Blind Veteran's Association. Yet as I look back now on all of these years of family life, of living with my disabilities, and then finally becoming blind, I often think of my own family, with their patience and understanding. They made the difference so often during my many rehabilitation efforts. Even when I became depressed, they urged me to continue, for somehow they appreciated what I could still do. Probably I would never have gone back to school without their encouragement. Even my father, who died in 1978 and who really never got over the shock of seeing his first financial empire disintegrate, was there one time when we really needed some assistance. To all of my family, I say thank you.

PART I: Study Questions and Suggested Activities

1. After reading the personal statement by Paul Egan, at what time during the progressive deterioration of his eyesight do you think that family intervention would have been most effective?
2. After reading the intervention approach in Chapter 2, and considering your own opportunity for family contact, how do you think this proposed intervention approach could be applicable to Paul Egan's family?
3. If disability or a severe illness occurred in your own family, which suggestions in the intervention approach discussed in Chapter 2 would you be most comfortable with? Which ones would you feel least comfortable with?
4. Assuming that you have the opportunity for a meeting with Paul Egan and his wife at the time when he was discharged from the VA Blind Rehabilitation Center in 1977, design a family-assessment approach utilizing the assessment model in Chapter 1.
5. Discuss the issues related to the following statement: "I really can't have any effective contact with a family that is living with a disability situation unless I have a degree in family counseling or family therapy."

II
Child and Family Issues

Introduction

When a child is born into a family, the family constellation is transformed. Where once there was a dyad, a triad now exists. Husband and wife are now father and mother. Additional births in the family create sibling relationships. Extended families assume new roles and respond to new expectations. These family alterations represent new responsibilities and nonending challenges. As the child grows, he or she develops a unique relationship with each family member. In turn, each stage of the child's growth and development is experienced differently from the individual family member's perspective.

When a child is ill or disabled, the crisis is not confined to the child alone. Each member of the family is touched by the situation and reacts according to a complexity of factors. How successfully the family unit can adapt to the illness and disability will be determined, in part, by the ability of each member involved to participate in the provision of support. In addition, the availability and efficiency of resources outside of the family system, such as allied health professionals, will be a critical determinant in the eventual outcome for the patient and family. The degree of effectiveness of professional support will depend, to a large extent, upon the professionals' understanding of the manner in which the family functions as a system.

Unfortunately, many professionals have based their interventions on an objective understanding of the family that is challenged by the illness and disability experience. Although it is important to maintain objectivity on selected situations, is is also important to be aware of the clients' and families' subjective frames of reference.

Consequently, a major component of this book is the use of personal statements. Part II begins with a statement by Linda Pelletier, who poignantly describes how the disability experience has affected her, her family and the family's dynamics. She looks back on her life and reflects on the obstacles and strengths within her family that made a difference in her own adjustment to disability. Themes of overprotection and overcompensation, the relationship between her mother and father, and the strain on her parents because of the disability are all discussed. Yet, Linda still came to believe in herself as a whole person and as one who possesses many abilities. She writes, ''I was shaped by all my experiences and those people who cared about me, especially my family.''

In a disability or illness circumstance, family members can provide support and encouragement. They can make a difference for the disabled or ill person's treatment, adjustment, and when possible eventual rehabilitation.

The ongoing stress, uncertainty, and state of crisis for a family is presented in Chapter 3, ''Infant Life on a Monitor: Family Implications,'' which presents a portrait of the family struggling with the threat of Sudden Infant Death Syndrome (SIDS). The author, Susan R. Leibold, is a clinical nurse specialist with extensive experience in counseling these families and providing follow-up for those who have lost a child as a result of this phenomenon. She describes how living with a child on a monitor affects each member of the family. The frustration, fear, isolation and insecurity experienced by these families is described within the context of the phases of adaptation to the monitoring process. The author reveals important points that health care professionals must consider when formulating interventions to both assess the family's coping capacity and assist them in the adaptation process.

In spite of the low incidence of cancer in childhood, it remains second only to accidents as the leading cause of death in children younger than 15 years of age (American Cancer Society, 1985). Chapter 4, ''Coping with Childhood Cancer: A Family Perspective,'' illustrates how the diagnosis of cancer is experienced not only by the child, the identified patient, but is also shared by the entire family unit. The chapter is authored by Martha Blechar Gibbons, a nurse practitioner and clinical specialist who had been involved with pediatric oncology in several research and treatment centers. From diagnosis through recovery or death, she provided a framework for intervention that incorporates identified crisis points apparent in each phase of the disease. The author shares a strategy for supporting families experiencing their child's terminal illness that facilitates the child's expressions and assists the family to focus on the meaning of their lives together.

The number-one health care priority demanding the nation's concern at this time is Acquired Immunodeficiency Syndrome (AIDS). In Chapter 5, Dorothy Ward-Wimmer, the Nurse Coordinator for the AIDS care team at the Children's Hospital National Medical Center in Washington, DC, addresses this issue. ''Children of Hope: Learning to live with HIV Infection'' presents a picture not reflected in many other publications regarding this topic. The author portrays the child carrying the Human Immunodeficiency Virus (HIV) as infected and infectious; yet the child may well be free of symptoms, or minimally symptomatic. Therefore, in children HIV infection can be viewed as a *chronic* process with acute exacerbations. The fact that no one yet knows how long the child might live reflects the crucial need for a philosophy that encompasses rehabilitation and hope for the child and the family.

Chapter 6, "Deafness and Family Impact," is a comprehensive overview of how deafness creates a variety of needs in the family system. A unique aspect of deafness is that it is typically unanticipated, because most deaf children are born to hearing parents. The author, Marita Danek, Professor at Gallaudet University, has worked with the deaf population for many years. She discusses the myths and misinformation about deafness that are present in our culture and that are sometimes unwittingly reinforced by those well-meaning professionals who intend to provide support. The chapter discusses the impact on the family system of early-onset or congenital deafness in a child. The role of the involved professional is examined in terms of specific techniques and strategies for intervention.

A personal statement by Janet Miller, a mother of a handicapped child, is titled, "Mechanisms for Coping with the Disability of a Child: A Mother's Perspective." The author identifies the ongoing family challenges and needs and documents the stresses that are experienced by the family unit as it strives to incorporate disability into its system. In this illustration of family life through crisis, transition, and rehabilitation, Mrs. Miller relates how each member (father, mother, patient, and sibling) attempt to incorporate the disability into the self-concept and the changing image of the total family unit.

The chapters in Part II are a reflection of the personal and professional challenges experienced by children, their families, and the professionals involved in providing support. In responding to the demands resulting from illness and disability, each person gains insight into the complexities of living with a situation that permanently alters and challenges the family system. Part II concludes with Study Questions and Suggested Activities. These are designed to stimulate individual awareness or to be used as approaches to discussion in classroom or professional training sessions.

REFERENCE

American Cancer Society. (1985). *Cancer facts and figures: 1984*. New York: Author.

Personal Statement: The Challenge of Cerebral Palsy: Familial Adaptation and Change

Linda Pelletier

The contribution of family dynamics to what a person actually becomes cannot be overstressed. Such familial shaping is even more significant when the individual in question is physically disabled. At present, I am a 32-year-old woman who is severely disabled with cerebral palsy. I cannot walk, use my arms or legs with any degree of coordination, or speak with perfect clarity. I have, however, been able to live independently for the past 6 years. What factors in my childhood and adolescence enable me to overcome the obstacles posed by my disability and to achieve what I have so far accomplished? A great deal of the answer lies in a comprehensive analysis of the role played by my family in my childhood years.

My childhood was unique, different from that of other children. From my earliest memories, I can recall being aware that there was something different about me that caused me to be the focal point of much attention and solicitude. I was an only child and had no brothers or sisters to relate to, or to use as standards by which I could measure my normality or lack of it. Every waking moment of my parents' lives was devoted to me and to my care. I naturally came to regard myself as the center of the universe because everything revolved around me.

I first became aware that my situation imposed a burden when I overheard arguments between my mother and father. In attempting to find a reason for my congenital disability, they would blame each other for the difficulties that had occurred at my birth. For example, my mother would blame my father for allowing her to carry laundry up the cellar stairs during the final stages of her pregnancy. In turn, my father would accuse my mother of not knowing how to have a baby because her water broke before her labor, and she did not know what to do. After reading the literature on congenital disability and its impact on the parents of the disabled child, I can look back in retrospect and recognize the guilt and self-blame that each of my parents experienced as a result of my disabling condition.

Research indicates that mothers of congenitally disabled children exhibit a tendency of being afraid to become close to their children due to the fear that they will die. My mother was never afraid to become attached to me. In fact, one could say that she became too attached and overly possessive. In retrospect, I can recognize her fear of losing me as a result of my sickness. At my birth, I had respiratory problems that prevented me from getting a sufficient amount of oxygen to keep all my brain cells alive. The brain damage that resulted in my cerebral palsy was caused by my not being able to breathe for one-half hour. One of the complications of this birth trauma was that I was more susceptible to respiratory infection. From reading about the reactions of other parents, I can now see that my mother was desperately afraid of losing me. Her acute anxiety in this regard greatly complicated my life in childhood and adolescence. She was afraid to allow me to go outdoors for fear of my getting a chill. Whenever I did go out, I would be bundled up so much that I would become overheated and drenched with perspiration within a matter of minutes. One of my most vivid recollections is going to see fireworks on the Fourth of July. I was sitting in a car with the windows rolled up, wearing ski pants, thermal underwear, and a winter coat. I became nauseous and almost fainted before the fireworks were even over. Another of my mother's phobias related to overprotection was her dread of germs. She was so afraid that I would contract an infection that she went to extreme means to protect me from contamination. This would include giving nasty looks to people who happened to sneeze near me in public and requiring two of my girlfriends to wear surgical masks when they would come into the house to visit me. This latter circumstance stands out in my mind as a source of embarrassment that still bothers me to this day.

The relationship between my mother and father deserves special consideration because it highlights some of the essential elements of family dynamics and congenital disability. My parents had tried to have a baby without success for 5 years before I was born. Having a family was extremely important to them because it represented the conventional lifestyle. After I was born, they were unaware that anything was wrong with me for almost a year. It was only when I could not perform the expected developmental activities—such as rolling over by myself, reaching for objects, and beginning to crawl—that they began to realize that there was a problem. I was not quite a year old when my pediatrician informed them of his diagnosis of cerebral palsy. As time went on, they sought out specialized medical treatment for me at Children's Hospital in Boston. I underwent a battery of tests, was seen by a variety of specialists, and was fitted for casts and braces. All of this extra treatment consumed much time and energy for my parents, who regularly traveled to the medical appointments and were involved in the prescribed therapeutic regimens such as putting on my night cast and my walking with braces. I am not sure at what point they decided not to have any more children. I am not even sure whether this was a conscious choice or that it merely happened that way. There is evidence for the latter possibility, because my mother had a miscarriage when I was 11 eleven years old.

The relationship between my parents was strained to a great degree by my disability. My mother was always a highly nervous person, so my condition naturally heightened her anxiety level. My father was a very calm, quiet, introspective individual who was able to maintain his equanimity in the face of my mother's emotional imbalance and continued states of turmoil. As time went on, she attempted to assume my total care and to leave him more out of the picture. She was almost always upset, and this precluded any meaningful communication between them. My reaction was to obtain my emotional and psychological support from my father while being aware that my mother was the primary source of my physical care. Without my father's intervention in our unique and difficult family triad, I would not have been able to make anything faintly resembling a normal psychological and emotional development.

I could always sense the tension that existed at home between my parents. Usually my father would accept my mother's endless tirades, and he seldomly involved himself in any arguments. Although I was young, I was cognizant that he wanted to maintain as much equilibrium in the house as possible for my sake. When I grew older, he openly admitted to me that he stayed with my mother and did not leave because he knew how much I needed him to remain there. The only thing that eventually separated him from the family that he struggled so much to keep together was the terminal cancer that took his life at the age of 61 when I was 25.

The concept of overcompensation is a major element in individuals with congenital disabilities. What is lacking in physical abilities is often made up for in other ways. What transpired in my family in this regard is a perfect example of these dynamics.

My parents were acutely aware that I was of above average intelligence from my earliest years. When the time came to enroll in school, my mother made every possible effort to see that I would obtain a quality education. I was not able to attend school physically because of the architectual barriers in the school building at that time, so I was forced to go to school at home by means of home tutors provided by the public school system. I will never forget the determination and drive exhibited by my mother to initiate these educational services. My father assumed a more passive role in this instance because he was not sure if it would be worth all the effort. My feeling is that he could not foresee what benefit I would receive from going to school because I was severely disabled. After several years of receiving tutoring at home, I started to utilize a home-to-school telephone system in the fifth grade. This system had been advertised in *Time* magazine, and my mother had read about it. She showed the advertisement to my teacher, who was reluctant to have the system installed because it was innovative and would create much extra work for her in acting as a liaison. After constant harassment from my mother, she agreed to let me try it. Once it was installed, my educational career began to blossom. For the first time, I could hear everything that was said in the classroom, and I was able to answer questions, which I did frequently. Since there were no distractions, I was able to concentrate on my schoolwork to such an extent that I earned outstanding grades. I continued to utilize this unique system throughout elementary and high school. Much of my motivation and determination to achieve could be directly attributed to my mother's influence. Although she could never fully accept my physical limitations, she was driven by the ambition to see me compensate for my disabilities by gaining outstanding academic recognition. The countless hours she devoted to taking notes, assisting me with my homework, and typing my written assignments can never be measured.

My mother's preoccupation with my educational development became almost neurotic at times. When I was in high school I received the best marks in almost all of my classes. Nothing less than an A would satisfy her because she knew what my intellectual capabilities were. This neurotic tendency also had a positive dimension to it. Although I came to place too much emphasis upon high grades, my excellent record was a tremendous assistance in getting me accepted into college. At this point, my father expressed reservations about my going on to college because he could recognize the strain that all of this academia placed upon my mother and me. While she devoted most of her day to assisting me with my school work, my father assumed the role of homemaker by performing most of the household chores and grocery shopping. My mother was more interested in helping me with my latest project than in assuming the conventional role of housewife. My father was often neglected by my mother, whose total attention was focused on me. This role imbalance contributed to the emotional conflicts that characterized my parents' relationship. In order for me to be accepted into college, I was convinced that it was necessary for me to prove myself academically superior to the other students in my high school class. As a result, I studied for my college board examination on my own for 4 months. This constant cramming became an obsession with me. At this time, in the late 60s, the idea of giving courses to prepare students for their college boards had not yet come into vogue. I even amazed myself when my scores came back—they were all in the high 700s, far above any of my other classmates. After this example, my high school initiated a college board preparation course that became a popular elective. I went on to attend college by means of the same home-to-school telephone system.

My mother's overprotection was also a destructive element in my development. She assumed complete care of all of my physical needs. This meant
that I was lifted in and out of bed, onto the toilet, and in and out of our
car. I was bathed, dressed, groomed and fed without my lifting a finger to
help myself. I realize now that it would have been extremely difficult for her
to sit by passively and watch me struggle to perform these basic activities
of daily living. Although my mother meant well by catering to me in this
way, it retarded my physical development because I was never given the opportunity to work on doing these essential tasks. Such a relationship caused me
to be completely dependent upon my parents. When I was young, I often
wondered what would become of me without them and if I would die without their care.

It was precisely these anxieties that motivated me at the age of 25 to admit
myself to a rehabilitation hospital to begin to achieve the vital independence
of which I had been so long deprived. Over a time frame of approximately
3 months, I learned to transfer myself, to partially dress myself, and to begin
feeding myself for the first time. The self-esteem and pride this new sense
of independence gave me turned my whole life around in a matter of months.
What eventually transpired from this metamorphosis was that I moved away
from home at the age of 26, established myself in my own apartment, and
obtained a full-time position as a rehabilitation counselor. It is almost impossible to describe my mother's reaction to this drastic change. Because my father
had already died and my leaving would mean she would be alone, she was
extremely upset and hurt when I decided to move away from home. Her intentions were to keep me home all my life so she could take care of me. She
was completely at a loss because I was the center of her world. My independence has been the source of much conflict between us over the course of the
more than 6 years that I have been gone. I don't think that her anger and
hurt will ever be fully resolved.

I cannot fully account for all that happened to me over the years, or why
things occurred as they did. I am certain, however, that much of what I was
as a child and became as an adult is the direct outgrowth of the variety of
unique influences of my family. To say that my family dynamics were a mix-
ture of positive and negative elements is an understatement. The conflicts
between my parents were balanced by the positive impact that their love and
care had upon me. The pain, anguish, and anxiety that I experienced
throughout my life undoubtedly made me a stronger person who was better
equipped to cope with the challenges and frustrations posed by my disability.

Because my parents loved me so deeply and sacrificed so much for my
advancement, I was able to come to believe in myself as a whole person and
to capitalize on what I perceived as my abilities. Would I have done anything
differently? It goes without saying that if I could have been born able-bodied

I would have opted for that state. One never achieves complete acceptance—only adjustment to what one has. I would not change the way that I am now or my outlook on life, because for the first time I am beginning to like myself for who I really am.

In summary, I often think of a plaque I have on my bedroom wall. It says, "We are shaped and fashioned by what we love." I was shaped by all my experiences and those people who cared about me—especially my family.

3 Infant Life on a Monitor: Family Implications

Susan R. Leibold

Sudden Infant Death Syndrome (Sids) is "the sudden death of an infant or young child which is unexpected by history, and in which a thorough post-mortem examination fails to demonstrate an adequate cause of death" (Beckwith, 1970). Sids is the leading cause of death in infants between the ages of 1 month and 1 year. Currently in the U.S., 2 out of 1000 births will end in Sids. This phenomenon occurs without warning, and to date there is no known etiology. Both of these factors provide a great frustration to parents and researchers. Monitoring infants' breathing and heart rate (apnea monitoring) is an attempt to prevent deaths from Sids, and therefore, the use of cardiorespiratory monitors has been increasing over the past decade.

This chapter discusses the history of Sids, the relationship between Sids and apnea, problems with research, types of children monitored, the purpose and function of the monitors, the needs of the family and how they adjust, and knowledge and skills needed by the helping professional.

SIDS/APNEA: THEORY AND TREATMENT

Sids and Apnea Relationship

Sids is an entity that has plagued parents and physicians for centuries. The first documented evidence is found in the First Book of Kings, Chapter 13. Incidence of Sids has increased relatively as other causes of infant death have receded with the advent of antibiotics, intensive care nurseries, and improved nutrition.

Typically in cases of Sids, a parent or caretaker who has put an infant to bed returns later to awaken him, and finds the infant dead. No sign of a struggle is evident, the infant's color is pale to blue, usually with mucus in the mouth. The infant has been essentially healthy and the event is always unexpected.

Apnea, like Sids, occurs unexpectedly. It is "an unexplained and frightening episode of cessation of breathing for 20 seconds or longer, or a shorter respiratory pause associated with bradycardia, cyanosis or pallor" (Brooks, 1982, p. 1012). The major research focus has gravitated to apnea as the mechanism causing Sids because there are similar factors leading to both events, namely healthy infants, unexpectedness, pale to blue color, and occurrence during sleep.

Characteristics of Sids

Over the years, multiple theories about the causes of Sids have attempted to implicate many body organs, such as the thymus gland, adrenals, heart, lungs, and brain. Other theories have included infanticide, suffocation, aspiration of stomach contents, nutritional problems with vitamins or minerals, infectious theories, anaphylaxis, and neurologic-conduction deficits such as chronic hypoxia. The majority of these theories cannot be substantiated by the usual course of experimentation because there is no animal besides humans that has exhibited the characteristics of Sids. Examination of the infant autopsies has yielded no cause for the cessation of breathing and subsequent death. However, researchers have identified a profile of the typical Sids victim:

1. The infant's age is between 1 month and 1 year, with the highest incidence occurring between 2 and 4 months of age.
2. Death occurs during sleep.
3. Sids occurs more in the cold-weather months.
4. 60% of Sids deaths are males, versus 40% females.
5. Preterm, low-birth-weight infants are at greater risk to die of Sids.
6. Evidence of a mild respiratory infection not requiring treatment with medication is present on autopsy.
7. There is a greater prevalence among the offspring of adolescent mothers.
8. A surviving twin of a Sids death is at a 10% greater risk than is the average population.
9. Subsequent siblings are at a 2% greater risk for dying of Sids than the average population (Spitzer & Fox, 1986).

Due to the broad range of similar characteristics, researchers feel there must be a "final common pathway" that represents a similar mechanism of death shared by many conditions. The current theory is that there is a triggering stressor predisposing a sleeping infant to a prolonged cessation of breathing (apnea), from which the infant is unable to recover, subsequently dying. Because at this stage in research Sids cannot be treated, the goal is to prevent this tragic and unexpected ending.

Types of Infants Monitored

Currently the mechanism for attempting to accomplish prevention is twofold. The first part of the task is to identify the infants who are at risk for a Sids event. This is done by matching the profile of Sids victims to the general infant population and identifying a high-risk group. The second part is to examine these infants for other disease entities (i.e., seizures or gastroesophageal reflux). If nothing else is diagnosed, the infant is placed on an infant-apnea monitor. Three groups of infants typically match the profile of Sids victims:

1. Siblings of infants that have died of Sids.
2. Preterm, low-birth-weight infants experiencing apnea or bradycardia in the nursery.
3. Full-term infants experiencing an apneic spell requiring stimulation. The parents are instructed in the use of the monitor and in cardiopulmonary resuscitation (CPR), and the infant, monitor, and family are sent home.

Purpose and Function of Monitors

The monitor's sole purpose is to act as an alarm system while the infant sleeps. This allows the parents to attend to other household functions, to other siblings, and to get rest themselves, instead of maintaining a 24-hour vigil beside the infant. The monitor operates by sensing chest movement and interpreting the chest movement as breathing. It also registers the heartbeat. The monitor sounds an intermittent beeping alarm if no chest movement is sensed (apnea) or if the heartbeat drops to a dangerous level for the infant (bradycardia). The heart rate alarm also acts as a backup in the rare instance that the apnea alarm does not sound. It is important to note that the monitor is only a piece of equipment and can overalarm when there is nothing wrong with the infant. The most common causes of this are loose or faulty sensing devices (electrodes). The monitor is only as effective as the training the parents received in operating and troubleshooting the monitor, as well as in assessing the infant and providing resuscitation if needed.

FAMILY ADAPTATION

The goal for the family is to incorporate the monitor into the routine of the infant and not to create a *special-child syndrome*. Parents have reported that there are three phases they have experienced in adapting to the monitor. The first phase is overcoming fear, the second phase is lifestyle adjustment, and the third phase is feeling secure (Barr, 1980).

Initial Phase

The initial phase is overcoming the fear associated with every monitor alarm. Parents report that when the monitor's beeping alarm is heard, the first thought is, "Will I have to do CPR?" The second thought is, "Will I do it right?"

Another fear parents have expressed is, "Will I awaken when the monitor alarms?" These fears and anxieties produce a variety of responses from parents that may include insomnia, projection of fears and anxieties onto older siblings, and crying. The length of the initial phase is directly related to the cause of monitoring. Many parents of preterm infants are more relaxed with initial alarms, due to time spent observing the nursery nurses as they respond to the multiple false alarms calmly and confidently. Parents of infants experiencing an apneic spell, predictably, are more anxious with initial alarms, due to the memory of the emergency they experienced with their infant. Parents who have lost a child to Sids vary in the intensity of their response to the initial phase.

In general, the initial phase of adjustment takes up to 2 weeks. Few families report problems sleeping after this period. An important aspect in the adjustment process is experiencing alarms and not having to do CPR. In fact, the fewer alarms and the mildness of the required response greatly aided the adjustment to the second phase (Barr, 1980; Black, Hersher, & Steinschneider, 1978).

Second Phase

The second phase, adjustment, is characterized by parents' developing safe and creative solutions to the restrictiveness of the monitor. Parents express feeling a decrease of fears and an increase in confidence.

Feelings of isolation arise as reality sets in during the first few days at home, namely, dealing with the restrictiveness of the monitor. Many household routines must be readjusted because of an inability to hear the monitor (e.g., washing clothes or taking a shower) (Barr, 1980; Black et al., 1978). The restrictions placed by having to have someone willing to assume the responsibility of babysitting an infant on an apnea monitor increase the isolation experienced by parents, especially mothers. Most apnea-monitor programs encourage having more than one family member trained in CPR, monitor function, and troubleshooting. This at least allows the mother a chance to take a shower or to get other household chores accomplished.

Isolation seems to inspire parents to be creative problem solvers. Parents may have identified where in the home the monitor can be heard, and how long it takes to get to the baby. They begin to realize that the baby is fine while awake and they begin to disconnect the monitor during feeding, playing, and bath time. Parents have developed a plan or schedule for certain family tasks and activities, such as:

1. When to take a shower.
2. When to vacuum, wash clothes, and perform other noisy household chores.
3. How to drive alone in an emergency.
4. What to do about babysitting; baby-sitters must be trained in CPR, know how to operate the monitor, and be willing to accept the responsibility (Barr, 1980; Hersher et al., 1978).

Receiving adequate training in CPR and monitor functioning prior to the parents' first night alone with the infant contributes to effective problem solving. Additional information that aids parents' success includes:

1. Assessing the infant's breathing status (learning to tell the difference between shallow breathing and true apnea by placing their hand lightly over the infant's back to feel for breathing while also looking at the infant's color).
2. Troubleshooting false alarms by checking the electrode wires and connecting cable.
3. Having a plan to drive alone with the infant and monitor if necessary.
4. Knowing when to call the doctor versus the monitor company.
5. Anticipating problems and having a ready list of potential solutions; this facilitates problem solving and may ease confusion elicited by the stress (Black et al., 1978; Dimaggio & Sheetz, 1983).

If the mother has to return to work, another stressor parents face in this phase is day babysitting. The availability of extended family members who can help in this situation is often limited, due to the mobility of the nuclear family. Many parents need encouragement in utilizing other family members and friends for assistance with general household and family tasks. This support is invaluable, but many parents believe it is an imposition to ask friends for help—or even to accept help when it is offered.

Parents also need encouragement to call on health care providers for more information and/or help. Parents seem more inclined to call health care professionals if it is provided in structured guidelines regarding the infant's care.

Guidelines given about driving a motor vehicle almost universally include: *Do not drive alone with an infant on the monitor.* The reality is that most parents do at one time or another have to drive alone. It is important to help parents to do this as safely as possible. The infant and monitor should be placed where the parent can glance at both. Interstate highways should be avoided, and parents should use roads on which the parent can stop the vehicle to assess the infant if necessary. Some parents have dealt with this problem by requesting that a teenager ride with them, to keep an eye on the monitor to identify which alarm is sounding and what the infant is doing. Car seats also need to be evaluated by the parent. Some car seats do not.allow quick entry and exit. Parents should be encouraged to make practice runs of "car emergencies" prior to assuming that responsibility alone.

An added support system involves utilizing other parents who have experience in infant monitoring. This provides an invaluable link with another parent who is experiencing similar stressors. It helps to bridge the gap of isolation and the feeling of "I'm the only one going through this." A few communities have started support groups that meet monthly to share trials and successes. This has been found to be very beneficial to some parents. Others are too uncomfortable with groups and are content to talk with another parent over the phone. Sometimes parents will offer to babysit one another's infants. This does pose the problem of two monitors in the home. Parents of twins cope with this daily, but some parents may be unnerved or not have adequate strategies for dealing with the rare occurrence of two monitors alarming at once. Many parents are willing to help other parents once their infant no longer requires monitoring. The importance of social support cannot be underestimated. This is an essential factor contributing to the mental health of each family member.

Mothers should be encouraged to have some time alone, unburdened by the care of the infant. Couples must plan time for just themselves. This can be difficult if babysitting is a problem, but the importance of ongoing communication and time away from the monitor cannot be stressed enough.

Siblings always pose concerns, ranging from the possibility that they will play with the monitor, to how they will deal with the stress of the alarms. Most siblings respond by seeming unconcerned about the alarms. Parents have related that, surprisingly, the most common problem is normal sibling rivalry, but that if, for example, siblings are included in helping mother identify which color light is illuminated, as well as participating in other infant-care activities, the rivalry response diminishes. Older school-aged siblings may require reassurance from parents regarding the decision that monitoring is no longer required (Black et al., 1978). As these issues minimize, the adjustment phase merges into the third phase.

Third Phase

The third phase, feeling secure, is characterized by the parents' description of the monitor as a security blanket. They feel the monitor is an additional set of eyes and ears, allowing them freedom from worry. There are usually fewer alarms during this time, and parents relate family functioning to be as optimal as is possible with an infant in their lives. The family focus is the infant and the stresses that imposes—not the monitor (Barr, 1980).

Preparation for discontinuing the monitor begins during this phase. Stopping the monitor can be a relief to some families and a nightmare to other parents. Parents should be given an anticipated date at which the monitor may no longer be required, and the criteria to assess this. The criteria differ depending upon each infant-apnea monitor program. As the infant approaches the anticipated date of monitor discharge, the parents need to wean themselves from their dependence on the green blinking lights, which have provided assurance that the infant is breathing. Parents will position the monitor so they can see the lights from the hallway, or so that they can see a reflection of the green light on their bedroom wall. Encouraging a parent to cover the green blinking light, but not the red alarm light, is important. As one mother described it, "Getting off the green lights was like quitting smoking." Most parents feel that once they are no longer dependent on the green lights and their infant is not triggering alarms, the monitor can be stopped. Reaching that point is a significant step.

Most parents need to stop using the monitor gradually. They find that stopping the monitor during naps is the first step. The first day, parents may need to check the infant frequently; as the days progress, the parent builds confidence that the infant is breathing well. The next step is encouraging parents to identify a night on which to stop the monitor. Most parents pick a night when one parent can sleep and the other parent can check the infant frequently, sleeping the next day. The first night is difficult for many parents, but as the nights go by they begin to relax. Some parents can stop monitoring by the "cold turkey" method (boxing up the monitor as soon as the doctor discharges the infant, without any weaning time). This method is also perfectly acceptable for parents who demonstrate the ability to do this successfully.

KNOWLEDGE AND SKILLS OF THE HELPING PROFESSIONAL

Professionals should be aware that apnea monitoring is stressful and can test any family's coping abilities. Any person working with a family that is using a monitor should have a working knowledge both of the monitor and of how to assess the infant if an alarm occurs. Role modeling a calm approach to the infant conveys reassurance to the family. This implies that their training has prepared them adequately, and that the professional (if needed) knows how and when to intervene.

Monitoring encompasses many factors that have been identified as predictors for threatening situations leading to crises. The result is a potential for coping difficulties within the family unit. Factors that should be considered include:

1. *Surprise*: Discovering that an infant requires an apnea monitor can be a shock. Such knowledge may imply the infant could die at any minute or has a life-threatening condition.
2. *Experience*: Families who have never worked with a monitor before usually imagine the television version of a monitor, which often is being used with bleeps, blips, and beeps in an emergency room or intensive care unit. Families with premature infants usually have a more realistic view of the monitor usage and response if they have spent time in the nursery observing their infant.
3. *Confusion*: This can occur if the instruction regarding the monitor, response to the monitor, and cardiopulmonary resuscitation (CPR) is provided in a hasty manner without providing the parents with enough practice time prior to discharge.
4. *Perceived effectiveness*: This is the most common feeling the majority of families experience during the first 1 to 2 weeks at home. There are fears such as of not awakening to an alarm, of not responding to the alarm appropriately, and that CPR will be required.
5. *Perceived allies*: It is important to identify those persons who can help relieve the parent, whom the parent can call with questions regarding the baby or the monitor, and who are available to share one's concerns.
6. *Perceived uniqueness of threat*: Many parents have never known any other family that has used an apnea monitor, and therefore they feel isolated.
7. *Overload*: This occurs easily with multiple alarms and exhausted parents (MacElveen-Hoehn & Eyres, 1984).

These factors identify the potential threat that apnea monitoring can impose on families. Providing anticipatory and ongoing support throughout the monitoring course assists families in mastering this potentially threatening situation. Support has been defined as "augmenting a person's strengths to facilitate mastery of the environment" (Caplan, 1974, p. 129). It is felt that a support system is an enduring pattern of continuous or intermittent ties that plays a significant part in maintaining emotional and physical integrity of the individual over time. It can act as a buffer protecting the person experiencing the stress by delaying the impact of the stress until the person is strong enough to begin to deal with it (Caplan, 1974).

The Concept of Support

Many authors have attempted to categorize the actions that constitute supportive actions. It is this author's experience that support consists of promoting coping, providing empathy, and nurturance.

1. Coping consists of confronting a change or problem that defies familiar ways of behaving. It also requires the production of new behavior, and gives rise to uncomfortable affects such as anxiety, despair, guilt, shame, or grief. To promote coping, three factors should be assessed:
   a. *Information*: Does the person or family have enough information to understand the situation and to problem solve if necessary?
   b. *Autonomy*: Does the person or family have enough control or options within the confines of the situation?
   c. *Maintenance of an internal organization*: Does the individual or family feel competent to handle the situation satisfactorily?

By assessing the family members both individually and as a unit, the type of intervention leading to effective family coping is identified.

2. Empathy occurs "when one individual is hearing or understanding another . . . It involves experiencing another person's world as if you were he" (Carkhuff, 1978, p. 119). This may be very difficult; as families like to point out, "If you have never done this, how can you know?" To provide empathy involves active listening, an open body posture, and a gentle voice that reflects feelings.
3. Nurturance is providing or encouraging another to eat properly, rest adequately, stock supplies for monitoring, seek funds for monitor rental and supplies, obtain comfort, and guidance in learning new activities (i.e., adjusting to the monitor).

Recognizing the stress factors impacting on monitoring, and utilizing a framework for supporting the family, professionals can better assess the family's adjustment to the monitoring experience.

Initial Family Assessment

Family assessment based on the predictors of threatening situations provides an excellent framework and assists in planning appropriate supportive interventions. Families adjust at different rates and to different levels. A home visit is an excellent means of beginning the family assessment focusing on the predictors of confusion and surprise. In a home evaluation, the type of monitor setup that is evident indicates the parent's compliance to the guidelines for using the monitor and precautions for a potential emergency. The assessment should focus on the following areas:

1. *Confusion*: The parents demonstrate that they remember and understand the guidelines for monitor usage, versus exhibiting confusion regarding the instructions given. This part of the assessment would include:
   a. Ascertaining if the monitor is on the baby if the baby is asleep, or plainly visible if the baby is awake. A monitor that is kept under the bed or in a box is probably not being used.
   b. Finding out if there are adequate supplies (electrodes, wires, alarm records) and that the family knows how to obtain more.
   c. Seeing if forms for recording the alarms are available by the monitor and that the parent can explain how and when to complete them.
2. *Surprise*: The parents are prepared for an emergency by:
   a. Visibly posting CPR instructions and readily explaining all the steps.
   b. Locating a list of emergency telephone numbers by the phone or phones, including the home address and nearest cross street.
   c. Identifying in which rooms in the home the monitor is audible and that traveling time to the monitor is within 10 seconds (alarm drills).
3. *Overload*: The initial monitor alarms have been infrequent, allowing the family some rest.
4. *Perceived allies*: The parents are able to identify whom they can call with questions, concerns, or for assistance.

A relatively small number of families have difficulty trusting the monitor, even after positively completing the first assessment. For example, a parent should be able to leave the side of the sleeping infant with the monitor on, and not simply sit and stare at the green blinking lights. The following example illustrates the tremendous stress the use of a monitor can impose on a family that has few support systems, as well as the need for assistance in moving through the initial phase of adjustment.

A single mother of four, with three older children aged 17, 12, 5, was having a great deal of trouble leaving her 5-month-old infant alone on the monitor while she prepared meals. The infant was monitored for a blue spell requiring stimulation. The mother would sit by the infant and watch the green blinking lights. She insisted that the 5-year-old sibling sit and watch the green blinking lights while she prepared a meal. The mother complained to the apnea clinic nurse that she was having behavior problems with the 5-year-old. He was exhibiting attention-getting behavior, and the mother was responding to him with anger. The mother was encouraged to cover the green blinking lights so no one could see them, and then take the opportunity to spend time with the 5-year-old while the infant slept. The mother needed a great deal of encouragement, but promised to comply. She later reported that she had been successful: Her 5-year-old's behavior had improved significantly, and she was more relaxed.

If the assessment indicates the family is not confused by monitoring guidelines, is prepared for a potential surprise, is not experiencing overload, and can identify allies, the initial phase is moving toward completion and adjustment is being achieved.

Subsequent Family Assessments

The assessment of second and third phases of adjustment focus on the threatening-situation predictors of perceived effectiveness, experience, perceived allies, and perceived uniqueness of the threat.

Assessment of a family's perceived effectiveness in adjusting to life with a monitor begins with a discussion of alarm response. Alarms should be intercepted within 10 seconds (10 beeps of the monitor). Also, it is important for the family to be aware that they should first assess the infant to ascertain what action is required, rather than stimulating the infant unnecessarily.

A mother reported to the apnea clinic that her infant's monitor was alarming during the night. The baby was monitored following a witnessed blue spell requiring stimulation. When asked by the nurse what the status of the infant was (breathing pattern, color, etc.) the mother replied that she did not check the infant, but would lie in bed and tell herself that the alarm was not real and the baby was fine. She wanted the nurse, without considering any clinical data about the infant's condition, to reassure her that the alarm was not real.

This mother was not complying with the guidelines and was experiencing difficulty in dealing with the stress of a potential life-threatening situation. Breathing assessments were reviewed with the mother. The leader of the county parent-support group was requested to help reinforce the mother's ability to perform a good assessment of her infant's condition. The next time the mother called with alarms to report, she was able to give an adequate description of the infant's breathing.

The perception of having allies remains an ongoing need throughout the monitoring period. Adjustments for families include taking a break from the constant responsibility of caring for a monitored infant. Finding adequate baby-sitting remains one of the greatest problems families encounter. The easiest solution is for the spouses to relieve one another. The hardest solution is to find a baby-sitter so spouses can spend some time together. Parents frequently express their readiness for an outing away from the baby, but they may need assistance in finding an adequate solution.

> The parents of a preterm baby had not left the baby alone since discharge from the hospital four months earlier. They were feeling a great need to spend some time together alone, but also felt guilty about leaving the baby with a baby-sitter. When they finally decided to go out, they could not find a sitter who knew CPR. They called nursing agencies, but found the prices prohibitive. A friend expressed interest in helping them, but did not know CPR. Arrangements were made to teach the friend CPR, assessment of the infant, and monitor operation. The mother requested that the friend practice by staying with the infant while the mother was at the home. The friend felt comfortable, and the parents went out the next night. The mother called home one-half hour after she left, and then again one hour later. After reassuring herself, she relaxed and enjoyed her dinner.

Utilizing support systems to deal with a stressor is an indicator of a family's healthy adjustment. Another positive indicator is the family's use of creative problem solving when allies were not available. For example:

> One mother wanted to take a night class. Her husband never believed the infant needed the monitor, and would not adjust his work schedule to be at home to watch the infant. The mother received permission from her instructor to bring the infant to class with the monitor. The infant slept through the classes. However, the mother did not enjoy the time out of the house because the stress accompanied her.

Monitor alarms greatly increase the stress on the family, and tax their coping resources if they occur frequently. While conducting an assessment of the alarms and the family's knowledge of the infant's breathing pattern, assessment of the parent's ability to deal with the alarms effectively becomes apparent.

> The mother of a preterm infant called to report an increase in alarms following an outing to the pediatrician's office the day before. The infant was healthy, but there had been an increase in the number of alarms throughout the night. The mother was quite concerned because the infant had required mild stimulation

for the first time. Review with the mother of alarms over the past several weeks identified an increase in the alarm rate following a change in the infant's routine. The parents decided to limit the baby's changes in routine to no more than once a week—and then only when the parents were rested. For several weeks, alarms did occur after a change in routine, but as the baby grew the alarms diminished. The parents felt they could deal with the alarms because they were somewhat predictable. A sense of autonomy was achieved, which aided in their adjustment.

The stress of failing to identify the triggering event for alarms can be overwhelming for families. Parents not only are sleep deprived, but they begin also to mistrust their assessments and thus may begin to overreact to alarms. It may be necessary to request that the monitor company evaluate the equipment. The infant's breathing pattern may need to be assessed by a pneumogram, a process that requires a physician referral. In addition, having other parents who have experienced similar stresses contact the family helps the family realize they are not in a unique situation and can survive the stresses.

CONCLUSION

Apnea monitoring will be used as a method of preventing Sids until the cause of Sids is learned. With the advent of improved newborn intensive-care units, more preterm infants will be living and requiring apnea monitoring. Professionals should be familiar with the need for monitoring, and with the stress that parents face. The goal for all professionals involved should be to help the family live as normal a life as possible during the time period when monitoring is ongoing. This can be accomplished by acquiring familiarity with the monitoring process, by assessment of the infant, and by providing ongoing support through the adjustment process.

Families encountering supportive help in adjusting to life with a monitor can successfully cope with the situation, developing a strength that may see them through family crises in the future.

RESOURCES

National Sids Foundation
2 Metro Plaza, Suite 205
8240 Professional Place
Landover, MD 20785
1-800-221-Sids

REFERENCES

Barr. A. (1980). *At home with a monitor: A guide for parents.* Chicago: National Sudden Infant Death Syndrome Foundation.

Beckwith, J. B. (1970). Discussion of terminology and definition of Sudden Infant Death Syndrome. In A. B. Bergman, J. B. Beckwith, & C.G. Ray (Eds.), *Proceedings of the Second International Conference on Causes of Sudden Death in Infants.* Seattle: University of Washington Press.

Black, L. Hersher, L., & Steinschneider, A. (1978). Impact of the apnea monitor of family life. *Pediatrics, 62*(5), 681–685.

Brooks, J. (1982). Apnea of infancy and sudden infant death syndrome. *American Journal of the Diseases of Children, 136,* 1012–1023.

Caplan, G. (1974). *Social support systems & community mental health,* New York: Behavioral Publications.

Carkhuff, R. (1975). *The art of helping,* Amherst, MA: Human Resource Development Press.

Dimaggio, G., & Sheetz, A. (1983). The concerns of mothers caring for an infant on an apnea monitor. *Journal of Maternal/Child Nursing, 8,* 294–297.

MacElveen-Hoehn, P., & Eyres, S. (1984). Social support and vulnerability: State of the art in relation to families and children. B. Raff, P. Carroll (Eds.), *Birth Defects,* (5), 11–43.

Spitzer, A., & Fox, W. (1986). Infant apnea, *Pediatric Clinics of North America, 33*(3), 561–581.

4 Coping with Childhood Cancer: A Family Perspective

Martha Blechar Gibbons

THE IMPACT OF CANCER

When the diagnosis of cancer is made in childhood, the illness reverberates throughout the family system. The impact on each family member is significant and individualized. The child's own emotional response to the illness and treatment is directly related to the family's reaction (Levine & Hersh, 1982). It has been suggested that the total psychosocial and familial setting, characterized by calm or by stress, has major effects on the response to the treatment of disease (Caplan, 1981).

Although cancer in children is rare, it remains the leading cause of death due to disease between the ages of 3 and 14 years (Pizzo, Miser, Cassady, & Filler, 1985). The American Cancer Society estimates that 6000 new cases of cancer occur in children under 15 years of age in the United States each year, with approximately 1600 deaths annually (American Cancer Society, 1984).

The many recent advances in the treatment of cancer have resulted in the fact that what had been previously seen as a short-term fatal illness is now more commonly regarded as a chronic disorder with a fatal outcome. Approximately 50% of all children with malignancies can expect to be cured of their disease (Klopovich & Trueworthy, 1985). As increasing numbers of children experience longer survival, new problems arise for patients and families. Issues surface regarding improvement of the quality of life, and how the risk of relapse impairs a child and family's involvement with life in general (Koocher & O'Malley, 1981). There is growing recognition that both chemotherapy and radiotherapy may have adverse effects upon normal body tissue that may not be manifested until months, or even years after completion of treatment. Such late effects are both physiologic and psychologic, ranging in severity from scanty hair growth to the life-threatening complications of a second malignancy (McCalla, 1985).

Treatment of the child with cancer necessitates multiple hospitalizations and frequent clinic visits. Regardless of the length of hospital stay or the number of outpatient visits, these hours and days away from home are anxiety producing. The child is not only faced with a serious illness, but also experiences separation from family, friends, and school. The child must endure intrusive procedures, and side effects from medications that often seem more stressful than the disease itself. This period is characterized by high levels of patient and family stress. The child and family must strive to develop and maintain adequate coping skills to adapt to the sudden alteration in lifestyle.

Within this chapter, major issues are addressed that pertain to each member of the family system coping with cancer. Guidelines for intervention for health care professionals are presented for each stage of the disease process.

PORTRAIT OF THE PATIENT AND FAMILY

When a child has cancer, the goals are: (1) to eradicate the disease, (2) to return to as normal a life as possible, and (3) to live as well as possible (van Eyes, 1977). Cancer occurring in the first year of life can alter the normal process of a child's development, for it can interfere with his growing ability to differentiate himself from a significant other. This interference is due to physiologic and psychologic changes the child experiences, and the psychologic effects of the disease on the family system (Illingworth, 1975).

The Infant With Cancer

The infant may suffer separation from the mother, pain from intrusive procedures, and forced alterations in diet and sleeping habits during treatment. The infant's inability to comprehend cognitively the disease contributes to the parent's despair, for they are unable to offer explanations and reassurance to the child. Whenever possible, parents should be allowed and encouraged to remain with the infant. It is essential to foster normal growth and development through visual and auditory stimulation. If possible, the parents may continue to bathe the infant. Mobiles can be created, and musical toys can be brought from home. Black-and-white contrasts are particularly alluring visually to the infant. Glossy black-and-white photographs of family members provide provide needed visual stimulation, as well as a sense of comforting familiarity. These can be pasted on or near the infant's crib, and staff involved can make use of such stimuli while caring for the infant.

The Toddler With Cancer

The toddler is striving to accomplish the task of autonomy (Erikson, 1963). The stresses imposed on the child by the diagnosis of cancer may lead to psychological and developmental regression. Unable to comprehend the disease, the child may seek refuge in a "safer," more dependent stage; the danger lies in the child's continued dependency on those around him or her, and inability to progress normally developmentally.

Normal growth and development should be facilitated through stimulation of gross motor skills (pushing, pulling, walking, running) and fine motor skills (touching, holding, drawing), with the object of mastery of body skills. Encouragement should be provided for the toddler to participate in feeding, dressing, and other daily care activities. Activities in which the toddler can interact with other children will facilitate socialization needs. It is important for parents and professionals involved to explain procedures to the child, focusing on the child's own level of comprehension. The child's ability to conceptualize at this stage is limited, and language is egocentric, decreasing the capacity to consider others' points of view (Thomas, 1985). Toddlers benefit from preparation for intrusive procedures, and it is important that the parents be present during the child's preparation (Gordon & Cotanch, 1986). Some parents do not wish to be with their children during the actual procedures, and these wishes should be respected, for this will directly affect their ability to support the child. For parents who remain, it is most helpful for them to assume a comforting, supportive role, and for staff to restrain the child, if needed. It is best if parents decide ahead of time what they will do during the procedure (explain what is happening, or distract the child). It should be explained to parents that continued discipline is a necessary element of the child's life during treatment, serving to normalize the environment. Too often, parents feel uncomfortable setting limits, fearing that they will further "traumatize" the child.

The Preschooler and Cancer

Cancer interrupts the preschooler's developing sense of initiative. Due to his inability to think concretely, the child cannot yet understand the meaning of disease. Intense anger and aggressive behavior may be manifested. Parents may find their children refuse to acknowledge their presence after an intrusive procedure has been performed. The child may ventilate tension and frustration by biting, hitting, throwing, and screaming. Some children react by becoming quiet, withdrawn, and by regressing. A preschool child is particularly vulnerable to fears associated with cancer, due to her or his developing sense of good and bad. The child may interpret the disease as punishment for something that he or she has done (Hockenberry, 1986).

It is important to provide the preschooler with reassurance that she or he is a "good" person, in no way responsible for the disease. The child needs opportunities to express fears and feelings. Such expression may be encouraged through the use of clay, puppets, games, drawings, and bibliotherapy, in which the child may work out feelings "in concert" with characters in a story (Gibbons, 1986). As with younger children, staff and parental participation in preparing the preschooler for procedures is essential (Gordon & Cotanch, 1986).

The School-Age Child

The school-age child is becoming increasingly independent; cancer may alter this process and significantly affect the child's self-image (Selekam, 1983). Most children of this age have experienced an illness in their lifetime. Thus, their exposure to what an illness such as cancer is is increased, yet their awareness of why it happens is limited. The child has the capacity to conceptualize concretely, but has no ability to generalize beyond actual experiences (Thomas, 1985). At this age the child may still view the disease as punishment for acts and thoughts (Geist, 1979). As the child questions why the disease has occurred, he or she may begin to distrust those around him or her. Initially, the child may withdraw, refusing to discuss fears and concerns associated with the illness.

Parents of school-age children may be more actively involved in the child's care and preparation for treatment. For some, there is more of a feeling that such involvement is beneficial, in that they believe they can help their child to better comprehend. The professional involved should take advantage of parental involvement, using parents as a resource to determine the pace and style of preparation required for the child (Gordon & Cotanch, 1986). Following procedures, school-age children may choose to work through their feelings through drawing, story writing, or the use of dolls on which they repeat procedures they have experienced. The helping professional can facilitate such expression by responding to the child's verbalizations with empathy. It is important to assist the child by attempting to clarify the meaning of and reasons for procedures, and to provide reassurance that the child is not to blame for the disease.

Studies of children with cancer of all ages have noted immature behavior, alterations in self-concept, and increased anxiety and apprehension (Spinetta, Rigler, & Karon, 1973). Some children react by living each day to the fullest; they are able to look forward to the future, and not dwell on the illness. Others are angry, even hostile, and some withdraw from family and friends. The chronically ill child must learn to live with varying degrees of constant or frequent life disruption, and to develop heightened stress tolerance. Many children learn to live with their disabilities, and to develop effective coping mechanisms.

Children may ask specific questions beyond what is explained (e.g., as in bone marrow aspirations) in an attempt to cope more effectively. Posing questions may be an example of assertiveness behavior that serves to mediate anxiety and may be related to the child's personality or to a previous pattern of reinforcement or curiosity. Children who express inquisitiveness about procedures tend to exhibit fewer anxious behaviors than do children who do not ask questions (Katz et al., 1980). Questioning by the school-age child and adolescent can be an indication that positive defenses, such as intellectualization, are being mobilized. This can be encouraged by providing appropriate information at the time that it is requested (Kellerman, Zeltzer, Ellenberg, & Rigler, 1980). Patients and family members who actively question various aspects of the treatment, and who demonstrate an ability to follow through with instructions, are considered in general to be adapting well to the disease (Christ & Adams, 1984).

The Adolescent with Cancer

One of the major goals for the adolescent with cancer is to mitigate the side effects of treatment with medical and behavioral therapy. This is a worthy endeavor, considering that the treatment may be viewed by the adolescent as worse than the disease itself (Zeltzer, Kellerman, Ellenberg, & Rigler, 1980). The psychological impact of cancer can be more devastating during adolescence than at other stages, because of the additional stresses associated with achieving independence and consolidating identity (Goldberg & Tull, 1983). At a time when a child normally rebels against parents, the adolescent with cancer must be dependent upon them. The word *cancer* (which can become a label) can traumatize the family acutely, and disrupt previous interactional patterns (Zeltzer, Kellerman, Ellenberg, & Rigler, 1980). A continuing concern for the adolescent patient is the uncertainty of remission, a period creating hope as well as continual stress (Pfefferbaum & Levinson, 1982). The adolescent's developmental stage places such a patient in a precarious position: mature enough to realize the implications of the diagnosis and prognosis, but not equipped with the range of coping mechanisms characteristic of the older adult (Goldberg & Tull, 1983).

Adolescence is a period during which multiple and rapid changes are experienced; therefore, additional change due to disease can be particularly anxiety provoking (Kellerman, Zeltzer, Ellenberg, & Rigler, 1980). *Normal* teenage concerns include body image, sexuality, and self-esteem. The malignant tumor affects all these things. The adolescent is in the process of trying to *develop* control; the diagnosis of cancer halts this process. Even the adolescent with a positive self-image suffers greatly with the dramatic change in body image resulting from cancer treatments. Chemotherapy, radiation therapy, and surgery may significantly alter the individual that "once was." Rejection by friends and social isolation may follow such treatments. It is not uncommon for a teenager with cancer to say, "I'd rather *die* than lose my hair!" This statement reflects how the adolescent sincerely feels during this period. Loss of hair is one of the single greatest concerns expressed by adolescents afflicted with a malignant disease, reported by some to be more difficult than the loss of a limb (Wilbur, 1980).

Physical changes may affect some female adolescents with cancer more than they do males. Females tend to believe that physical attributes are strongly related to social acceptance. Males tend to believe they may gain approval for other attributes, such as physical strength or mechanical abilities (Zeltzer, Kellerman, Ellenberg, & Rigler, 1980). Through medical management of the disease, there is often interference with the adolescent's ability to develop sexually, which affects emotional development. Teenagers hesitate to engage in relationships, for fear others will discover the cancer and reject them. Patients may limit themselves, due to lack of confidence resulting from hair loss, weight loss or weight gain, and other alterations in body image. Such self-induced limitations may include their limiting dating and any contact potentially leading to intimacy. The professional involved can make an important and helpful suggestion that may help such adolescents to avoid social isolation— for them to try double-dating with other teenagers who have cancer. These adolescents will understand one another's concerns, for example, those related to nausea from chemotherapy, hair loss, and body-image fears.

Chronically ill adolescents who are under medical surveillance for serious diseases may tend to underplay any but the most major illness as a disruption. This deemphasis of illness may lead to denial of the disease (Zeltzer, Kellerman, Ellenberg, & Rigler, 1980). Even seriously ill adolescents may be able to deny their disease in order to function adaptively and with hope. Denial to a certain degree may be considered maladaptive, but in individual situations, the helpful nature of denial should not be overlooked (Zeltzer, 1980). Adolescents may cope by displacing their anger regarding their illness onto their treatments. They may view decisions to enter or continue with treatments as potentially controllable (Wilbur, 1980). Displaced anger may be a factor in problems of noncompliance, which are common in adolescent patients (Zeltzer, Kellerman, Ellenburg, & Rigler, 1980).

Parents are often the ones who may interfere most with the adolescent's normal growth and development. They assume that, because the child has cancer, he or she cannot continue to engage in activities shared by peers. This is a common reaction that must be dealt with by the professionals involved early on. It is essential to assist the parents to understand the concept that the child who is sick is still a normal individual; illness is not an abnormality (van Eyes, 1979). The professional working with the family can help them to sort out what is best for the child, and what can be done to alleviate their own anxiety. Home, school, clinic, and hospital environment must be such that the child can live a full life, not one that primarily focuses on disease and treatment (Deasy-Spinetta, 1981).

It is crucial, when dealing with teenagers, to acknowledge their important role in the treatment plan. The adolescent must be provided with knowledge about the disease and therapy. Some treatment centers achieve this by allowing their patients to read their own medical records (Zeltzer, 1980). The fact that teenagers are risk takers should be considered when encouraging them to become actively involved in their own treatment plans. When adolescents are treated as passive recipients, they will not readily cooperate. When explanation is provided as to why therapy is valuable and what the risks are, there is better chance of involvement. It is often effective to encourage the adolescent's natural sense of humor to stimulate the involvement. Some teenagers will find creative ways to cope with treatment, such as painting a flower on an abdominal scar, thus starting a fad (Wilbur, 1980).

The helping professional must frequently assess the adolescents' recognition of their own physical limitations and emotional capabilities. Parents and staff involved can be supportive by suggesting alternative activities or goals that might be more consistent with the individual's abilities. For example, a high school track star might become a coach, or a jogger might switch to a less strenuous bicycle. Despite the diagnosis of cancer, it is important to the achievement of autonomy that young people continue to develop increasingly greater levels of control over themselves and their environment (Goldberg & Tull, 1983).

Although an adolescent with cancer may have significant problems with social and peer activity, is is essential that peer relationships be maintained. Through this contact, the objective is to promote self-esteem and to diminish fears of rejection and abandonment. For some, involvement in peer groups will provide the socialization that might otherwise be missed. The strategy of such group programs is to increase long-term adjustment for the patient through better interpersonal relationships (Goldberg & Tull, 1983).

An important consideration for professionals involved is to acquaint adolescents with *therapeutic life-oriented programs*. These diverse programs are offered in a variety of settings and forms, such as patient discussion groups, music therapy, creative writing, relaxation training, video production, self-help groups, and individual counseling. Such programs can provide the foundation for a milieu in which adolescents can ventilate and work through their anxieties. They can reaffirm group acceptance through social and recreational interaction, and resume independence and control through achievements in selected activities (Goldberg & Tull, 1983).

Relaxation and desensitization techniques can be employed successfully by the adolescent to help deal with such intrusions as painful procedures. Relaxation exercises can help provide awareness of body tension, as well as skills to reduce it. Another activity, the production of videotapes, has resulted from the need expressed by some adolescents with cancer to discuss their feelings related to the disease. The purpose of such tapes is to act as a catalyst for discussion and open nonjudgmental exploration of issues. It is hoped that such discussions encourage greater acceptance of the complexity of feelings that accompany the diagnosis of a life-threatening illness (Goldberg & Tull, 1983).

For the adolescent with cancer, the treatment itself can become the arena for power struggles and confrontations. Fewer such problems will occur if these patients are offered, whenever possible, a range of options, such as choices in treatment schedules. Making such choices available will help foster a spirit of independence by investing the patient with responsibility in the control of the disease.

In assisting parents, the professional involved can stress the importance of their conscious attempts to refrain from being overprotective and intrusive. Adolescents with cancer are subject to scrutiny, and sometimes to cruel and inconsiderate remarks from peers. Parents can be assisted in responding to this by explaining to the patient that their peers may feel threatened by the disease, and are reacting that way because the concept of cancer confronts each individual with his or her own vulnerability to disease and to potential disability. Parents can thus reassure the adolescent patient that they (the patient and family) know more about the hopeful nature of the disease than do the young person's peers (Goldberg & Tull, 1983).

The Parents

The parents of the child with cancer are frequently displaced from home to hospital. In this setting, parents and children alike often have difficulty articulating their needs. Lack of communication can result in frustration and solitude; some families withdraw from staff who are providing care. Intense involvement with the management of the child's care can be an isolating experience in itself. Many parents are not prepared to care for the child who is not well, and when the child has a chronic illness, this situation is exacerbated. There may be inconsistency in parenting style; parents may be overindulgent one moment, and overprotective another. The child may experience difficulty with this inconsistency, and confusion and increased anxiety may result.

Families of children who have cancer often express concerns that the child is being treated as an experimental "object," exposed to a barrage of intrusive procedures, and treatments. This is particularly true when the child is treated in a setting where research is being conducted. When the child is hospitalized for an extended period of time, the family may become overwhelmed. The parents may be ineffective in providing support, often at a time when it is critical for the child. Some parents complain that when they believe their child is seriously ill and they feel in need of support themselves, friends and extended family members, as well as staff, appear to avoid them (Gibbons & Boren, 1985).

The professional providing support for the child and family should consistently attempt to involve the parents in activities that return some of the sense of control they believe they have lost. It is known that early knowledge of the cancer diagnosis is related to positive psychosocial adjustment among long-term survivors of childhood cancer. Many parents who initially did not share the diagnosis with their child identify this lack of candor as a source of stress both during and after treatment (Koocher & O'Malley, 1981). Thus, the facilitation of ongoing, open communication is an essential element of the plan of intervention formulated by the involved professional.

CRISIS POINTS

Awareness of periods in which families may experience particular difficulty in adapting to the demands resulting from the child's illness will enable the professional to plan therapeutic interventions more effectively. It has been found that there is a significant relationship between the degree of support families receive and their psychosocial adjustment to the child's illness (O'Malley, Koocher, Foster, & Slavin, 1979). Crisis points in the course of cancer and its treatment have been identified. These include: (1) diagnosis; (2) induction of treatment; (3) remission; (4) termination of the treatment protocol; (5) reentry into school, family, and social life; (6) recurrence or metastasis of the disease (relapse); (7) initiation of research treatment; (8) termination of active treatment and terminal disease; (9) other stress points such as anniversary phenomena; (10) symptom consciousness; (11) developmental marker events; (12) experiencing societal prejudices; and (13) the period continuing for several months after the death of a pediatric cancer patient (Christ & Adams, 1984; Koocher, 1985). These crisis points, as well as supportive interventions appropriate during that period, will be discussed within the framework of the disease process as experienced by the patient and family, from diagnosis through bereavement.

Diagnosis

The diagnosis of cancer in a child has repercussions for everyone in the family, and the response of each family member will affect the adjustment of the others. A prediagnostic phase is experienced by some families. During this period, the family may realize that the child has not been well, yet they refuse to accept the gravity of the situation (Hughes, 1976). The child's problem may go undiagnosed for weeks, even months. Initial diagnostic tests may not immediately reveal the answer. During this time the parents may project their anxiety onto professionals involved, becoming angry and bitter.

Once the diagnosis is confirmed, parents commonly manifest symptoms of shock, which may be accompanied by a deep sense of mourning and grief (Katz et al., 1980). They may feel stunned, numb, and paralyzed with fear. Parents may express feelings of guilt, stemming from concerns associated with believing they have in some way caused the illness, or had failed to recognize symptoms early enough (Katz et al., 1980). Parenting a child with a malignant disease may lead to emotional stress in a variety of ways, some resulting in psychological problems. One study reported that in more than one half the families observed, at least one member required psychiatric hospitalization after the diagnosis of cancer in the child was made (Binger et al., 1969).

When the child is initially hospitalized with cancer, many parents relate feeling a "loss of control." Some state that they "never really know what is going on" (McQuown, 1981). The cancer diagnosis represents immediate losses to parents. Future goals must be postponed, and sometimes forsaken entirely. Families express anxiety, sadness, depression, and concern for the child. In the initial phase, many families are too focused on the beginning of treatment to have the opportunity to reflect on what is happening to them. Anger and somatic concerns may come later, when the family has had time to settle into a routine of treatment. Vacillation of mood may often be observed in family members.

In the initial stages, there may be a cognitive, but not emotional, acceptance of the illness (Christ & Adams, 1984). What is actually discussed—the amount of illness-related communication—varies from family to family. Some families are more open in sharing with each other than is evident in other family systems. As the disease process continues, a variety of reactions have been documented, ranging from fairly rapid mobilization by parents to act on their child's behalf, to denial. Some research suggests that parents progress from initial numbness to a split between emotional acceptance of the diagnosis and prognosis, and then to intellectual acceptance of the reality (Koocher & O'Malley, 1981).

The stress of illness and hospitalization may result in communication problems within the family system. Both parents and child may understand the severity of the illness, but not communicate fears and apprehensions to each other. The child may want to "protect" the parents from realizing what he or she knows. The parents may believe the child does not know the diagnosis and its implications, and hesitate to discuss the illness. At a time when the need for mutual support is most crucial, family members often cope separately, in silence.

Initial Intervention

The professional assisting the child and family will need to consider that all initial information shared with them will need to be repeated later, once the initial shock has subsided. Some families are so distressed that postponement of the initial discussion is warranted, allowing them time to regain control (Adams, 1976). After the diagnosis has been made, families strive to comprehend the meaning of what they have been told. The most important message that can be conveyed to them is hope for their child. Even the family whose child has a poor prognosis needs to know that those providing care have hope. It is essential for health care professionals to maintain this hope, and to reassure the child and family that everything possible will be done.

Parents who have been interviewed after the period of diagnosis share that there are certain interventions that have been helpful in the initial stages of the disease. Some have stated that it is important that at first they have conferences alone with those providing care for the child. This allows them time to absorb the information, and to prepare the child. Parents who have been given information related to diagnosis at the same time that the facts are first shared with their child state that it is impossible to conceal their shock. They believe this hinders their ability to support the child effectively and to problem solve as a family unit (McQuown, 1981).

Families report that it is important not to dwell on the illness. Many have said that as soon as they are able to acknowledge the facts, it is most helpful to attempt to return to as normal a schedule as possible, in order to preserve family unity. It is important for professionals involved during this period to encourage reinvolvement with the activities the family engaged in prior to diagnosis. This maintenance of structure (to the extent that it is possible) provides a sense of security for the children, who may be bewildered by the sudden changes in their lives.

Early intervention has been made more comprehensive by the emergence of the multicisciplinary team in pediatric oncology. Team members are composed of physicians representing all specialties involved in the child's care: psychologists, nurses, counselors, social workers, art and play therapists, rehabilitation and occupational therapists, chaplains, dieticians, and other patients and families who have dealt with cancer (Hammond, 1978; Hersh,

1978). The team strives to promote adaptive behavior, recognizing that, in order to accomplish this goal, the child and his or her family must be considered members of the team (Levine & Hersh, 1982). The historical medical model of care, with an almost exclusive focus on biologic factors, has been found inadequate because of the complex interaction of medical, psychologic, ethical, and social issues that must be confronted in childhood cancer (van Eyes, 1977).

One of the most important ongoing interventions to be considered by the helping professional is the facilitation of consistent communication among the child, family, and those providing care. Family members may need to feel sanction to express ambivalent feelings about the sick child. At some level, there is always resentment at the disruption in their lives, complicated by feelings of guilt and anger, caused by the perceived potential loss. It is important to acknowledge that, even though parents are often aware of their right to be informed of the treatment plan, they may feel uncomfortable exercising this right, asking for further explanation and clarification. Encouraging this type of verbalization—perhaps even identifying someone who can assist them in formulating questions—will help decrease anxiety. If one becomes an astute observer of the family's behavior, much information can be obtained as to how they are coping with the illness. Communication is enhanced by careful, attentive listening, focusing on what family members are sharing, clarifying to avoid misconceptions, and assisting them to integrate information shared in discussions.

Family members will experience psychologic changes as a result of having a child who is seriously ill. A depressed or anxious parent will be unable to conceal feelings from the child, and will be less available to support the child emotionally. In some families, the need for psychosocial intervention may focus on the symptomatic parent or sibling, rather than on the diagnosed child (Koocher, 1985). Parents are at risk of losing confidence in their parenting skills when the child is hospitalized for treatment. Confused and bewildered by the diagnosis and therapy—perhaps by themselves for not having recognized the symptoms, or feeling that in some other way they have failed— parents may wait helplessly for the outcome. It is crucial to assist parents to regain a sense of confidence in themselves as caregivers for their children.

Once past the initial shock, it is imperative to help the family move from a fear of death to a life focus. A useful technique for facilitating this movement is to enlist the child and family's participation in predicting how they will cope, identifying their strengths as well as areas with which they may need assistance, and inquiring how this may best be provided for them. Such exploration gives permission for, and models, a self-monitoring process (Christ & Adams, 1984).

A family that is coping well during the early stage following diagnosis will probably make visible progress in dealing realistically with the information provided by the end of the first week. The family should have begun the process of planning and making appropriate modifications in their lives to prepare for the next stage, the induction of treatment. At this point, the family who is coping effectively will realistically review and evaluate plans they made before the child's diagnosis (Christ & Adams, 1984).

Induction of Treatment

Although the treatment may be rigorous, once it is initiated, the child and family often experience a lift in mood. The feeling is that now something is actively being done to fight the disease. Cancer therapy has evolved from providing merely comfort to delivering aggressive regimens in hope of cure (Sutow, Vietti, & Fernbach, 1983). Thus, there is a return of some sense of control through active efforts to eradicate the illness. Treatment protocols vary in intensity and frequency, and are designed to treat the specific types of cancer. It had been found that the more complex and intense the treatment, the more difficult are the phases of the family's rehabilitation and reintegration (Spinetta & Deasy-Spinetta, 1981).

The cost of care may become a major concern and stress factor for the family. Treatment requires commuting, time away from work, additional child care for siblings at home, and countless other hidden costs. It is essential that the professional involved investigate all available programs providing financial assistance to families in such a situation. It should be anticipated that another anxiety-provoking issue will be the first discharge home from the hospital. The family and child may feel dependent on the treatment team and unsure of their own ability to function at home. Time should be spent preparing them for discharge each day, as soon as they have demonstrated ability to progress cognitively and emotionally beyond the initial diagnosis.

At this point, psychosocial interventions should focus on: (1) clarifying information about the treatment and side effects; (2) providing practical assistance to the family in order to help meet the emotional, social, and economic demands they are experiencing; (3) assisting the family to motivate the child to become actively involved in the treatment; and (4) encouraging the family to integrate the cancer patient and treatment regimen into normal family living patterns while attending to the needs of all family members (Christ & Adams, 1984). Gradually over time, the family will redefine normal patterns.

Families who can pose questions and follow through with directions during this period may be viewed as adapting well. Families having difficulty may ask the same questions repeatedly without being able to follow directions, may demonstrate a distressed mood incongruent with the patient's physical status, and may demonstrate an inability to problem solve (Christ & Adams, 1984). These families may be unable to grasp anything beyond the presentation of the diagnosis.

Group Interaction as a Supportive Intervention

It is important to consider that for many children the diagnosis of cancer may be the first time they experience a serious illness. This diagnosis results in major changes in daily living, altering patterns that previously have been a source of security for the child.

For the very young child, support may be offered by providing the opportunity to play with real equipment that is ordinarily seen as threatening. The child can master anxiety regarding stressful situations by hands-on experiences with tools and supplies, gradually becoming familiar with these objects and viewing them as less "toxic." Such supervised play may take place in sessions either with other children or alone, as the need indicates.

Children with cancer experience altered relationships with peers. Obvious changes in body image may be frightening to other children. There is frequently the myth that cancer is contagious. Some children isolate themselves due to fear of peer rejection. Family and friends may refrain from visiting, or alternately overindulge the child, both of which are confusing.

For children aged 3 to 11, a therapeutic play group provides a safe environment in which to express their feelings. It offers each child an opportunity to "play out" anxiety, interact with peers, achieve and demonstrate mastery of treatment-related procedures, gain emotional support, and become educated about the disease in a nonthreatening setting (McEvoy, Duchon, & Schafer, 1985).

A therapeutic play group serves as a diagnostic tool to identify underlying conflicts that a child might otherwise be unable to express. As the child becomes more open within the group, he or she may be better able to cope with changes resulting from the illness. Group play enhances feelings of belonging and socialization that cannot be attained in individual play (Adams, 1976).

If space is provided, adolescents form peer groups naturally. They may relate situations to others in groups, deriving support from one another. The group enables a facilitator to assess the needs of each participant, and to identify specific problems that might require attention beyond the group setting. As the individual need arises, a child or adolescent may be referred for individual counseling.

Parents congregate in natural group settings outside the pediatric oncology unit, in waiting rooms and in clinics, in cafeterias, and wherever space permits. This natural group formation can be developed into an organized, goal-oriented setting for the benefit of parents of children with cancer. As a stress-reducing intervention, the group lends itself to the use of a variety of strategies.

The following group interventions are designed specifically to reduce stresses identified by parents in a pediatric oncology setting (Gibbons & Boren, 1985).

TABLE 4.1 Stress-Reducing Interventions and Outcomes

Stress-reducing strategies	Outcome
Identification of personal, institutional, and community resources available for family assistance.	Decreased sense of isolation.
Identification of individual strengths and realistic self-expectations.	Increased self-confidence and sense of competency as a parent.
Sharing of information related to the disease process and treatment provided.	Decreased confusion; increased sense of mastery of the environment.
Opportunity to express feelings in peer-supported sessions: interaction with others sharing similar experiences in an atmosphere of acceptance and commonality.	Development of personal insight; increased sense of worth, resulting from opportunity to support others.
Opportunity to learn about and associate with others who are successful in dealing with similar problems.	Development of a positive self-image as a socially competent and productive individual.

Parents and their ill children who cope effectively with the crisis of cancer may use intellectual processes to master the distressing emotions elicited by the illness. By learning about all aspects of the disease and becoming familiar with the likely course, they can decrease their anxiety. The group provides the environment necessary to facilitate this process. When families realize that they are not alone in their feelings of frustration, confusion, apprehension, and isolation, they are better able to pool their knowledge collectively and become better resources for each other.

Remission

Many children with cancer experience a period of relatively good health, or remission of the disease, during treatment. The pattern of remission and relapse in some forms of cancer can cause emotional difficulty for the family. There may be renewed hope, or doubt that the original diagnosis was correct.

As the child returns to normal health and vigor, the parents begin to hope that somehow *their* child will be the one who is cured. The longer the child remains in remission, the longer the parent can foster this hope. Although the treatment team may endeavor to help the family to maintain a realistic outlook, parents hear about others who have survived for many years. They inquire into new and more sensational discoveries in cancer research (Goldberg & Tull, 1983).

Periods of remission of diseases are often associated with widely opposing emotions. Some families experience an enhanced sense of confidence, diminished expression of doubt, and hope of misdiagnosis (Stolberg & Cunningham, 1980). Many parents are more aware and troubled than are their children by the potential terminal nature of the illness. After having come to believe that death is likely or inevitable, with the lengthening of the time of remission they become increasingly hopeful for a cure. Yet the threat of relapse is an ever-present reality. Many parents continue to have difficulty discussing the illness with each other and with their children during this period. Some continue to have periods of anguish, depression, and intense need for support from family and friends (Obetz, Swenson, & McCarthy, 1980).

In remission there is often a search for meaning, to understand how the child's illness fits into a broader perspective of life. As the remission lengthens, the family moves toward reinvestment in life. Yet the threat of relapse is always present. The health care professional involved with the family at this time should be aware of these contradictory feelings, and provide opportunities for such expression. While hope is maintained, it is important to continue to assist the family to consider that a cure has not yet been achieved; however, that is indeed the goal.

Termination of the Treatment Protocol

Long-term survivors of cancer recall the termination of treatment as a time of particular stress. There is relief that therapy is completed, but there are also the concerns of being "unprotected," and of separation from medical and nursing staff (Koocher & O'Malley, 1981). Treatment becomes a way of life, with the necessary clinic visits and chemotherapy cycles. Most families adapt to the change in lifestyle. They learn to manage the child's disease, becoming effective decision makers regarding this aspect of their lives (Krouse & Krouse, 1982). The treatment itself becomes a means of security, providing the family with the sense that their child can be cured (van Eyes, 1977). When therapy is discontinued, the security it provided is removed. There is a feeling that nothing now actively protects the child from disease. It is essential to prepare the family for the termination of therapy, allowing for the fact that it takes months for families to adapt to this change (Ross, 1979).

Families may be uncertain as to how they should treat the child after therapy is terminated (Koocher, 1985). Restrictions and concerns that related to the child's previous therapy are no longer a reality, but such a sudden change in attitude is not easily achieved. A "weaning" process may need to be provided, in which the number of clinic visits and routine procedures, such as blood counts, are gradually lessened, rather than discontinued abruptly. This allows the family time to adapt. As the parents become more confident, this attitude may be shared with the child, and it provides a more stable support system once the child has returned home (Koocher & O'Malley, 1981).

It must be considered that the child may fear the cessation of therapy as much as the parents (Koocher & O'Malley, 1981). Such fears may be expressed verbally, or may be evident in alterations in the child's behavior. It is important for the helping professional to support the child in identifying and expressing such anxieties in an age-appropriate manner. Such interventions as play therapy, group interaction, or individual counseling may help to elicit the child's concerns and to decrease anxiety.

At this time, it is important to provide a review of the course of treatment for the family, emphasizing the normalcy of feelings of ambivalence regarding the loss of consistent professional monitoring. During the discussion, ways in which the family has succeeded in coping with earlier stress points can be acknowledged and affirmed, encouraging the formulation of new goals for the future. When families can begin to become involved in long-range planning, there is indication that they are effectively managing the treatment-termination phase (Christ & Adams, 1984).

Reentry into School, Family, and Social Life

The preparation for reentry into school, family, and community life should be completed by the time treatment is terminated. The process of reentry occurs not once, but rather each time there is a remission (Christ & Adams, 1984). Children with cancer have not lost the potential for growth and development. While in school, they have the opportunity to grow, to develop, and to prepare for the future, as do their healthy classmates (Deasy-Spinetta, 1981). If the health care team places priority on the psychologic, social, and education preparation of patients for cure, then school attendance is particularly significant as a normalizing factor in the life of the child with cancer (van Eyes, 1979). It has been demonstrated that chronically ill and even seriously ill children derive much satisfaction from school (Kaplan, Smith, Grobstein, & Fischman, 1974). The child needs the stimulation and peer association of school in order to feel a sense of accomplishment and social acceptance (Herman, 1986).

Patients and families who are particularly vulnerable during this phase include: (1) those of low socioeconomic status, implying less accommodating schools for children with disabilities; (2) those with a passive attitude; (3) those with the tendency to withdraw; (4) those demonstrating cultural differences with school personnel, which often results in poorer communication; and (5) those families with closed communication patterns, limiting their ability to resolve conflictual feelings (Christ & Adams, 1984).

The child with cancer who is denied school participation is actually being denied a major opportunity to engage in age-appropriate, goal-oriented behavior. If normal activity such as this is not encouraged, increased frustration, reinforced feelings of hopelessness, and despair may result. Such feelings can prevent the child from effectively coping with his illness, and impinge on the rehabilitation process in general. School experience can be important in providing a sense of emotional well-being, even for the child who is facing imminent death (Katz et al., 1980).

Interventions designed to support the child and family at this point require that the helping professional become involved with school personnel and other community agencies. It is necessary to provide school personnel with factual information to assist them in understanding the disease process, treatment, and how this affects the child and family. A knowledge of available community resources for individual family needs, such as transportation, financial aid, medical equipment, and support groups, can be of valuable assistance at this time.

The health care team must be committed to doing everything possible to assist the child and family in living as normal a life as possible. School is an integral part of a child's life. Parents who perceive that the health care professional shares this attitude will interpret the question of school reentry to be not "if," but "when" the child returns to school (Deasy-Spinetta, 1981). When the child or adolescent is able to return to the school, family, or vocational environment with renewed enthusiasm and enjoyment, there is indication of optimal coping during this phase (Christ & Adams, 1984).

Relapse

Relapse is a word that is feared by all families who have experienced cancer. There is never complete confidence that the disease will not return, regardless of the length of time that has passed since diagnosis. Relapse often comes without warning; disease may be discovered on a routine clinic visit. Relapse confirms the initial diagnosis, and shatters illusions, particularly about the extent of the healing powers of the medical team. Many families experience this period as being worse than the crisis of diagnosis (Christ & Adams, 1984). There is recapitulation of earlier stress, accompanied with diminished hope for long-term survival. The family is challenged by the task of confronting their despair and helplessness "in the face of destruction of the destructive power of the disease and yet restore hope for a prolonged remission, and reinvest in a rigorous treatment protocol" (Christ & Adams, 1984, p. 109).

The initial reaction to relapse may be denial that the cancer has returned. There may be expression of grief, rage, and continued heightened anxiety. Parents may be unable to believe or understand why the cancer has returned (Ahmed, 1981). They should be told of the relapse in private, without the child present, to allow them to express emotions, regain control, and prepare together to inform the child. Parents may request that health care professionals involved inform the child in their presence, if they believe they are incapable of doing this themselves. The news of relapse may be more shocking to families who believe that the treatment has been successful, reinforced by the child's positive response; they may have assumed that the disease would never return (Kellerman, 1980).

Children should be informed honestly about the recurrence of disease. A child experiencing relapse is aware of the seriousness of the situation (Ahmed, 1981). Often, the child has observed other children who have relapsed, and understands that it is a bad sign. The child may experience fears related to the next treatment, and question whether this means that he or she will die (Spinetta & Deasy-Spinetta, 1981).

Psychosocial intervention at this time should focus on facilitation of the family's processing of information and communication about the patient's new situation by all family members. The patient and siblings may require more updated, age-appropriate information, because they may have reached different developmental stages from the time of diagnosis. It is important at this time to assist the family to regain a life focus with a time perspective reflective of the altered prognosis. Parents may express hopelessness, anger, guilt, and self-blame at this point, believing that in some way they should have prevented the disease from returning. Reaffirmation of family strengths and abilities to cope with earlier crisis points is essential. There may be practical problems related to reinduction of treatment, with which the family will require assistance.

Families who are vulnerable at this stage are those who are unrealistically optimistic or excessively pessimistic about the disease process, wishing that it were "all over." It is crucial for the health care professional to be consistently available at this point to avoid withdrawal of the family's involvement with the child (Christ & Adams, 1984). A family who is coping effectively at this stage is likely to respond emotionally to the change in prognosis, but be able to reinvest in the next treatment, and future plans.

Initiation of Research Treatment

The need for research treatment indicates that the disease is uncontrolled. This is a particularly stressful time for families. Home life may become chaotic, and the child's condition may require frequent and unpredictable hospitalizations. Facilitation of the communication among the child, family and the staff providing care is even more critical at this time. The health care professional may need to intervene at this point to prevent or minimize alienation between parents and staff. Staff may feel out of control, helpless, and even guilty regarding the failure of the previous treatment. The family may displace their own anger and guilt onto the staff.

Families who have coped well during other crisis points may begin to experience difficulties during this period (Christ & Adams, 1984). Problems may result from the stress experienced in relation to the rapid changes in the child's condition, which negates efforts to maintain a normal schedule. It is important at this point to provide respite care for the family, and to encourage ventilation of feelings, rather than blame. It is likely that families are coping effectively during this period when they can articulate their feelings, and can tolerate behavioral changes in the staff, interpreting this as a reflection of the staff's sensitivity to the situation (Christ & Adams, 1984).

Termination of Treatment

It may be better for the family if the decision to terminate active treatment is initiated by the medical staff. For all families, guilt needs to be relieved by helping them to acknowledge that they have done everything possible for the child. It is essential to assist them to recognize that it is the *treatment* that has failed, not the patient, parent, or the hospital staff (Christ & Adams, 1984).

If the child is old enough to understand the disease process and the meaning of end-stage disease, the child may request that the treatment be terminated. The child may be unable to bear more stress from painful procedures, and hospitalizations. His or her desires should be considered by the family and the treatment team.

The length of end-stage disease is unpredictable; it may last from weeks to months. Families who are striving to cope with the intensity of this phase of the disease may find that all previous successful strategies now fail. Fatigue often sets in, rendering parents ineffective in providing support at a time when the child needs them most. Extended families and friends, previously involved, may not be emotionally capable of moving beyond their own grief to support the family. The health care professional at this time is challenged with the task of sustaining family members, and identifying significant others to provide essential support.

Stress Points

There are additional stress points related to the psychologic aspects of surviving childhood cancer. These include events that trigger reminders of the residual risks, and therefore precipitate recurring concerns about the illness (Koocher, 1985). Examples are anniversaries, such as in the case of the child whose cancer was diagnosed at the start of the school year. The child may become increasingly anxious each September, without consciously realizing why. The return of symptoms similar to those that preceded the diagnosis of cancer, or *symptom consciousness,* is a crisis point. This may generate intense anxiety, which may persist despite the reassurance that such symptoms are not a sign of malignancy (Koocher, 1985).

Developmental marker events constitute other stress points. These are social or achievement events that emphasize progress or growth, reminding the patient and family of the future, and recalling feelings of uncertainty. (Koocher, 1985). Patients diagnosed with cancer encounter societal prejudices, another crisis point. These include the wide range of reactions displayed when others learn that someone has cancer. Nonsupportive reactions include avoidance, fantasies of contagion, ostracism, or actual denial of employment to a childhood cancer survivor who reaches healthy adulthood. (Koocher, 1985).

Another event that can trigger anxiety for the child and family is the recent diagnosis of another person with cancer known to them. In addition, media coverage of cancer reminds these children that they are different from others; they have something to worry about. This voids the use of adaptive denial as a defense (Koocher, 1985).

It is essential that staff working with the child and family be sensitive to these events and issues as potential stressors of adverse emotional reactions. It is helpful to assist the patient and family to anticipate the stress that may be experienced in relation to these occurrences; this may decrease anxiety. In addition, it is often effective to assist the child and family in identifying the particular stressor responsible for such apprehension. In such discussions it is possible to normalize the family's reactions to these stressors.

THE CHILD'S AWARENESS OF DEATH

One of the dilemmas most frequently encountered by parents and staff is how to communicate with the child who is terminally ill. Should the prognosis be shared with the child? If not, does the child sense that she or he is seriously ill, even when this is not explained? It has been found that, even when the family does not discuss death, children display death anxiety. The affects of children associated with death are often unhappiness, loneliness, or sadness, suggesting reference to early life stages, when fears of separation and abandonment are paramount (Obetz, Swenson, & McCarthy, 1980).

Studies have demonstrated that a child's conception of death matures developmentally. Children under 5 years of age appear to view death as something that is reversible like departure or separation. Death is conceptualized from approximately ages 6 to 10 years as an inevitable, external process often resulting from the actions of others, or from purposeful forces. God is viewed as such a force. Death is interpreted by children at this age as punishment for evil thoughts or deeds. Past the age of 10, children begin to conceptualize death as an internal process, and universal to all forms of life (Gartley & Bernasconi, 1964; Goldberg & Tull, 1983).

It is generally accepted that the older child with a fatal prognosis, especially an adolescent, can be aware of the seriousness of his or her illness. Yet some authorities contend that the fatally ill child under 10 lacks the intellectual capacity to formulate a concept of death, and is therefore not aware of his or her prognosis. They theorize that if the adult does not discuss the illness and prognosis with the child, the child will experience little or no anxiety related to this subject (Debuskey, 1971; Ingalls & Salermo, 1971). Others contest this approach, favoring open communication with the dying child and family. They maintain that the normal development of the ability to conceptualize death is accelerated when the child is terminally ill at an early age. They state that the awareness of impending death becomes stronger as the child progresses through terminal illness (Bluebond-Langner, 1977). The theory of communication that has been referred to as the *open approach* provides an environment that is supportive of the child's questions and concerns, from diagnosis on, as the illness progresses (Spinetta & Deasy-Spinetta, 1981). Some authorities have stated that telling the child is not the most important issue. What should be emphasized is providing a climate of openness and support for dealing with the child's concerns (McQuown, 1981; Spinetta & Deasy-Spinetta, 1981).

If professionals working with the child do not acknowledge that the disease is serious, the child may perceive it as an obvious contradiction to the fact that another child may have died in the same ward, with a similar diagnosis. Such denial may not lend credibility to further statements made by the professional. Acknowledgment that the illness is serious does not mean eliminating hope, which, for many, becomes a lifeline throughout the progression of the disease (Gibbons, 1986; Hockenberry, 1986).

When cure and remission are beyond the capacity of the available treatment, intervention focuses on palliative care. The goals at this point are to achieve a state in which the patient is as symptom-free as possible, alert, comfortable, and free of pain (International Work Group on Death, Dying and Bereavement, 1979). Psychosocial interventions during this period should focus on assisting the family to anticipate what lies ahead, exploring with them their desires for their child, and alternate methods of achieving these goals (Christ & Adams, 1984). Taking the needs of the patient and all family members into consideration, the parents must decide whether the child should die at home, in the hospital, or in hospice care.

The communication within the family unit can decrease in extent and effectiveness as the child faces death. It is crucial for the helping professional involved at this time to consider the following guidelines for intervention, which can significantly enhance family communication (Gibbons, 1986).

1. *Explore and accept personal feelings regarding death.* One must come to terms with the emotional process that, in grieving for the child who is dying, the caregiver is also grieving for her or his own death (Charles-Edwards, 1983). The professional who has not dealt with personal feelings about mortality will have difficulty coping with emotions related to the child's imminent death. Such emotions are difficult if not impossible to conceal, and may interfere with effective communication. The extent to which the helping professional sincerely reflects on personal feelings and reactions related to death directly influences the ability to assist others in the process.

2. *Maintain availability and consistent involvement.* Involvement of trusted professionals involved in the care of the child may be actively sought by the family during terminal illness. At other times, the helping professional will need to take cues from the family and respond appropriately; they may *need* support, but not request it. Although family communication patterns differ and may alter during terminal illness, it is important to consider that it is most likely that the family will actually *require* support during this critical time. Energy is required to establish a relationship and to invest trust in an individual. The family does not have the emotional energy to reinvest during this period. Therefore, those individuals who have been important to the family may now be even more essential to them. Families during this time are vulnerable, and sensitive to changes. If at all possible, familiar, trusted caregivers should remain consistently available to the child and family.

3. *Promote open communication.* Open communication must take place first among the professionals who provide care for those experiencing terminal illness. Staff must take time to acknowledge the emotional investment required to care for the terminally ill child and his family, and the stresses encountered while providing such care (Gibbons, 1986). This is not only essential for medical and nursing staff, but for all professionals involved during this period. The sharing of feelings and experiences aroused by caring for seriously ill patients is considered by many health professionals to be essential to cope effectively with emotional pressures resulting from such involvement (Beardslee and DeMaso, 1982).

4. *Support the family as a unit*. Illness and death may require a change in the roles that family members previously assumed. If the child who is dying maintained a vital role, someone else may be required to substitute in the child's absence, However, in some families, there may be no substitute available. The illness and death of a child will change the family system dramatically and affect each member. It is essential to determine how this crisis affects each individual and, in turn, the functioning of the family as a system. As decisions are made for the child, the effect of such determinations should be considered in relation to each family member.

In the final stages of the disease process, the author has found one intervention to be valuable to both the patient and the family. It must be stressed, however, that each family will have different needs in terminal illness, which must be assessed by the health care professional in determining what intervention, if any, is indicated.

Life Review

The literature describes the use of *life review*, with adults as patients, to facilitate reminiscence and the completion of unfinished business in life (de Ramon, 1983; Wysocki, 1983). Expansion of this concept to include interventions in periods when the dying patient is a child allows for parental reflection. It allows the child and family to examine past experiences and present feelings (Gibbons, 1986).

The tools for life review are often pictures, which are excellent props for stirring memories (Wysocki, 1983). The desire to engage in a review of the child's life may be indicated by the patient, by the family, or both. Verbalized cues, indicating readiness, may include statements about what the child "used to look like," "used to be able to do," or "used to enjoy." The individual expressing such statements may refer to a picture while speaking. It is important for the professional supporting the family unit to assist the individual(s) involved to achieve self-expression. In general, the goal of life review is to assist the family or patient in acknowledging the significance of the child's life and the time they have shared together. If possible, it is important to allow for private, uninterrupted time during the process to achieve this goal.

Life Review for the Child

The child can benefit greatly from reliving past experiences with assistance from someone who personally knows and cares about him or her. The younger child, who views death more as separation from loved ones, experiences fears related to this concept. With support, the child can be reassured that those whom he depends upon will not abandon her or him when they are needed. Photographs placed near the child, illustrating the child's important position in the family, can confirm this. Discussions, led by the helping professional, can focus on the importance of the child's role to each member of the family.

The school-age child is striving to achieve a sense of industry; terminal illness arrests that process. Feelings and fears related to loss of this need, and the impending losses perceived by the child, can be expressed through the process of life review. The professional can assist the child, with the aid of pictures depicting favorite activities, to acknowledge his or her own accomplishments. The child who is mourning the loss of such activities, due to the debilitating disease of cancer, may be encouraged to ventilate such feelings. A knowledgeable professional may be able to use past photographs of the child to elicit present concerns (Gibbons, 1986).

Life Review for the Adolescent

The terminally ill adolescent may be questioning the meaning of his or her life, and seeking some understanding of the process that is ending it prematurely. Life review can assist the individual in such an evaluation. The professional who is supporting the adolescent may help to emphasize positive live experiences, while acknowledging the difficulties encountered with change in body image and loss of independence. For some, this is a method of resolving disturbing conflicts, and focusing on life work that one still desires to complete.

Life Review for the Family

Parents and siblings of a terminally ill child frequently experience the need to share special memories with a helping professional. In verbalizing memories, the family is initiating important tasks. They are evaluating, understanding, and finding new meaning in the roles they have played, and in the life they have shared with the patient. In addition, the family is beginning to engage in the process of anticipatory grief, working toward an acceptance of the child's impending death, and beginning to "let go."

It has been advocated that during terminal illness, whenever possible, the family should be encouraged to express their feelings about the patient's impending death, before the actual occurrence. This expression serves to mitigate the pain that is experienced after the loved one has died (Kubler-Ross, 1969). Life review is one method for initiating and completing that task.

The Period of Bereavement

A final crisis point is the period several months after the death of a pediatric cancer patient. Support is often well provided to the family in the first week after the child's death. Yet often by 5 or 6 months thereafter, such support is withdrawn—when friends and relatives beyond the immediate family do not understand why there is not "full recovery" from the loss. The advent of the deceased's birth date, a family holiday, or some similar event, may result in renewed mourning or grief reaction among the survivors (Koocher, 1985).

There is a period of critical need when contact with former advocates for the family (nurses, physicians, psychosocial professionals) might be most helpful; however, this is the time when such support is often unavailable. The inclusion of a plan for follow-up during the period of bereavement, especially throughout the first year following the child's death, is an essential element in the support provided by health care professionals. An additional important time for outreach to the family is at the 1-year anniversary of the child's death (Koocher, 1985). The professional who has been involved in supporting the child must realize that, although it is a painful process for a child to die and leave the family, the most difficult period is for the survivors. They must learn to live without the child.

CONCLUSION

When a child or adolescent has cancer, the disease is experienced by all members of the family unit. Knowledge by health care personnel that there are *crisis points,* particularly stressful periods encountered by the family system, is vital in planning therapeutic interventions. An awareness and understanding of the psychologic implications inherent in each stage of the disease process provides involved professionals with a realistic overview. This better enables them to fulfill optimal short- and long-range planning for the patient and the family.

RESOURCES

Children's Hospice International
1101 King Street, Suit 131
Alexandria, VA 22314
(703) 684-0330

The Compassionate Friends, Inc.
National Headquarters
P.O. Box 1347
Oak Brook, IL 60521
(312) 323-5010

A non-profit, self-help organization of bereaved parents and siblings.

National Cancer Institute
Pediatric Cancer Information
All states except Maryland:
1-800-638-6694
Maryland: 1-800-492-6600

Starlight Foundation
9021 Melrose Avenue, Suite 204
Los Angeles, CA 90069
(210) 205-0631 or (213) 208-8636

A non-profit charity organization dedicated to fulfilling wishes of chronically and terminally ill children.

REFERENCES

Adams, M. (1976) A hospital play program: Helping children with serious illness. *American Journal of Orthopsychiatry, 46*, 416–424.

Ahmed, P. (1981). *Living and dying with cancer.* New York: Elsevier.

American Cancer Society. (1984). *Cancer facts and figures,* New York: Author.

Beardslee, W., & DeMaso, M. (1982). Staff groups in a pediatric hospital: Content and coping. *American Journal of Orthopsychiatry, 52*, 712–718.

Binger, C., Ablin, A., Feuerstein, R., Kushner, J., Zoger, S., & Mikkelson, C. (1969). Childhood leukemia: Emotional impact on child and family. *New England Journal of Medicine, 280*, 414–418.

Bluebond-Langner, M. (1977). Meanings of death to children. In H. Feifel (Ed.), *New meanings of death* (pp. 50–67). New York: McGraw-Hill.

Bowen, M. (1978). Theory in the practice of psychotherapy. In M. Bowen (Ed.), *Family therapy in clinical practice* (pp. 337–389). New York: Aronson.

Caplan, G. (1981). Mastery of stress: Psychosocial aspects. *American Journal of Psychiatry, 138*, 413–420.

Charles-Edwards, A. (1983). *The nursing care of the dying patient.* Bucks, England: Beaconfield.

Christ, G., & Adams, M. (1984). Therapeutic strategies at psychosocial crisis points in the treatment of childhood cancer. In A. Christ & K. Flomenhaft (Eds.), *Childhood cancer* (pp. 99–115). New York: Plenum.

Deasy-Spinetta, P. (1981). The school and the child with cancer. In J. Spinetta & P. Deasy-Spinetta (Eds.), *Living with childhood cancer* (pp. 153–168). St. Louis: Mosby.

Debuskey, M. (1971). Orchestration of care. In M. Debuskey (Ed.), *The chronically ill child.* Springfield, IL: Charles Thomas.

de Ramon, P. (1983). Life review for the dying patient. *Nursing '83, 13*, 46–48.

Erikson, E. (1963). *Childhood and society* (2nd ed.), New York: Norton.

Fenichel, O. (1945). The psychoanalytic theory of neurosis. New York: Norton.

Gartley, W., & Bernasconi, M. (1964). A study in relationships between the life and death concepts in childhood. *Journal of Genetic Psychology, 105,* 283-294.

Geist, R. (1979). Onset of chronic illness in children and adolescents. *American Journal of Orthopsychiatry, 49,* 4-23.

Gibbons, M. (1986). When the dying patient is a child: A challenge for the living. In M. Hockenberry & D. Coody (Eds.), *Pediatric oncology and hematology: Perspectives on care* (pp. 493-508). St. Louis: Mosby.

Gibbons, M., & Boren, H. (1985). Stress reduction: A spectrum of strategies in pediatric oncology nursing. *Nursing Clinics of North America, 20,* 83-103.

Goldberg, R., & Tull, R. (1983). *The psychosocial dimensions of cancer.* New York: Free Press.

Gordon, A., & Cotanch, P. (1986). Coping strategies for children with cancer. In M. Hockenberry & D. Coody (Eds.), *Pediatric oncology and hematology: Perspectives on care* (pp. 450-463). St. Louis: Mosby.

Hammond, G. (1978). The team approach to the management of pediatric cancer. *Cancer, 41,* 29-35.

Herman, S. (1986). School re-entry following a diagnosis of cancer. In M. Hockenberry & D. Coody (Eds.), *Pediatric oncology and hematology: Perspectives on care* (pp. 463-468). St. Louis: Mosby.

Hersh, S. (1978). Meeting the psychosocial needs of children and adolescents with cancer. In *Proceedings of the Second National American Cancer Society Conference on Human Values and Cancer* (Vol. V, pp. 16-25). Philadelphia: George F. Stickley.

Hockenberry, M. J. (1986). Crisis points in cancer. In M. Hockenberry & D. Coody (Eds.), *Pediatric oncology and hematology: Perspectives on care* (pp. 432-449). St. Louis: Mosby.

Hughes, J. (1976). The emotional impact of chronic disease. *American Journal of Diseases of Children, 130,* 1199-1203.

Illingworth, R. (1975). *The development of the infant and young child, normal and abnormal.* New York: Churchill Livingstone.

Ingalls, A., & Salermo, M. (1971). *Maternal and child health.* St. Louis: Mosby.

International Work Group on Death, Dying, and Bereavement (1979). Assumptions and principles underlying standards for terminal care. *American Journal of Nursing, 79,* 296-297.

Kaplan, D., Smith, A., & Grobstein, R. (1974). School management of the seriously ill child. *Journal of School Health, 44,* 250-261.

Kaplan, D., Smith, A., Grobstein, R., & Fischman, S. (1973). Family mediation of stress. *Social Work, 18,* 60-69.

Katz, E., Kellerman, I., & Siegel, S. (1980). Behavioral distress in children undergoing medical procedures: Developmental considerations. *Journal of Consulting and Clinical Psychology, 48,* 356-363.

Kellerman, J. (1980). *Psychological aspects of childhood cancer.* Springfield, IL: Charles C. Thomas.

Kellerman, J., Zeltzer, L., Ellenberg, L., & Rigler, D. (1980). Psychological effects of illness in adolescence. Part I. Anxiety, self esteem, and perception of control. *Journal of Pediatrics, 97,* 126–131.

Klopovich, P., & Trueworthy, R. (1985). Adherence to chemotherapy regimen among children with cancer. *Topics in Clinical Nursing, 7,* 19–38.

Koocher, G. (1985). Psychosocial care of the child cured of cancer. *Pediatric Nursing 11,* 91–93.

Koocher, G., & O'Malley, J. (1981). The special problems of the survivors. In G. Koocher & J. O'Malley (Eds.), *The Damocles syndrome.* New York: McGraw-Hill.

Krouse, H., & Krouse, J. (1982). Cancer as a crisis: The critical elements of adjustment. *Nursing Research, 31,* 96–101.

Kubler-Ross, E. (1969). *On death and dying.* New York: Macmillan.

McCalla, J. (1985). A multidisciplinary approach to identification and remedial intervention for adverse later effects of cancer therapy. *Nursing Clinics of North America, 20,* 117–130.

McEvoy, M., Duchon, D., & Schaefer, D. (1985). Therapeutic play groups for patients and siblings in a pediatric oncology ambulatory care unit. *Topics in Clinical Nursing: Psychological Aspects of Oncologic Care, 7,* 10–18.

McQuown, L. (1981). The parents of the child with cancer: A view from those who suffer most. In J. Spinetta & P. Deasy-Spinetta (Eds.), *Living with childhood cancer.* St. Louis: Mosby.

Obetz, S., Swenson, W., & McCarthy, C. (1980). Children who survive malignant disease: Emotional adaptation of the children and their families. In J. Schulman & M. Kupst (Eds.), *The child with cancer* (pp. 43–60). Springfield, IL: Charles C. Thomas.

O'Malley, J., Koocher, G., Foster, D., & Slavin, L. (1979). Psychiatric sequelae of surviving childhood cancer. *American Journal of Orthopsychiatry, 49,* 608–616.

Pffefferbaum, B., & Levinson, P. (1982). Adolescent cancer patient and physician response to a questionnaire on patient concerns. *American Journal of Psychiatry, 139,* 348–351.

Pizzo, P., Miser, J., Cassady, T., & Filler, R. (1985). Solid tumors of childhood. In V. Devita, S. Hellman, & S. Rosenberg (Eds.), *Cancer: Principles and practice of oncology* (2nd ed., pp. 1511–1590). Philadelphia: Lippincott.

Ross, J. (1979). Coping with childhood cancer: Group intervention as an aid to parents in crisis. *Social Work in Health Care, 4,* 381–391.

Selekam, J. (1983). The development of body image in the child: A learned response. *Topics in Clinical Nursing, 5,* 12–28.

Spinetta, J. (1981). Psychosocial issues in childhood cancer: How the professional can help. In P. Ahmed (Ed.), *Living and dying with cancer.* New York: Elsevier.

Spinetta, J., & Deasy-Spinetta, P. (1981). Talking with children who have a life-threatening illness. In J. Spinetta & P. Deasy-Spinetta (Eds.), *Living with childhood cancer.* St. Louis: Mosby.

Spinetta, J., Rigler, D., & Karon, M. (1973). Anxiety in the dying child. *Pediatrics, 52,* 841–845.

Stolberg, A., & Cunningham, J. (1980). Support groups for parents of leukemic children: Evaluation of current programs and enumeration of participants' emotional needs. In J. Schulman & Kupst (Eds.), *The child with cancer* (pp. 72–83). Springfield, IL: Charles C. Thomas.

Sutow, W., Vietti, T., & Fernbach, D. (1983). *Clinical pediatric oncology.* St. Louis: Mosby.

Thomas, R. (1985). *Comparing theories of child development* (2nd ed.). Belmont, CA: Wadsworth.

van Eyes, J. (1977). *The truly cured child: The new challenge in pediatric cancer care.* Baltimore: University Park Press.

van Eyes, J. (1979). *The normally sick child.* Baltimore: University Park Press.

Wilbur, J. (1980). Sexual development and body image in the teenager with cancer. *Frontiers of Radiation Therapy and Oncology, 14,* 108–115.

Wortman, C. & Silver, R. (1979). Coping with undesirable life events. In M. Seligman & J. Garber (Eds.), *Human development: Theory and applications* (pp. 122–140). New York: Academic Press.

Wysocki, M. (1983). Life review for the elderly patient. *Nursing '83, 46,* 46–47.

Zeltzer, L. (1980). The adolescent with cancer. In J. Kellerman (Ed.), *Psychological aspects of childhood cancer.* Springfield, IL: Charles C. Thomas.

Zeltzer, L., Kellerman, J., Ellenberg, L., & Rigler, D. (1980). Psychologic effects of illness in adolescence. Part II. Impact of illness in adolescents; crucial issues and coping styles. *Journal of Pediatrics, 97,* 132–137.

5 Children of Hope: Learning to Live With HIV Infection

Dorothy Ward-Wimmer

This chapter considers the child carrying the Human Immunodeficiency Virus (HIV). Regardless of the clinical staging, the child is infected and infectious throughout the course of the disease (Rogers, 1985). No one yet knows how long a child might live in an asymptomatic or minimally symptomatic state. It is within this context, therefore, that HIV infection can clearly be viewed as a chronic process with acute exacerbations and secondary infections. Care must be philosophically rehabilitative, that is, aimed at maximization of strengths, and hope is seen as an integral part of planning for both the patient and family.

AIDS

Definition

Acquired Immune Deficiency Syndrome (AIDS) is characterized by an inability to ward off opportunistic infections, that is, those caused by microbes ubiquitous in our environment and usually destroyed by the normal immune response. The disease is caused by a retrovirus now named HIV for Human Immunodeficiency Virus (it was originally known as HTLV-III/LAV). The virus has a particular affinity for certain cells, especially T4 lymphocytes and glial cells, which harbor it indefinitely (Bennett, 1986). By specifically impairing and ultimately destroying the T4 helper cells, the virus effectively cripples the immune system, the person falls prey to usually innocuous diseases, and the classical syndrome emerges. Eventually the body is overwhelmed, and the person dies.

Transmission

The virus is known to be transmitted sexually, through blood, and in utero. One case involving transmission via human breast milk has been reported (Ziegler, Cooper, Johnson, & Gold, 1985). Although viral particles have been cultured from tears, urine, and saliva, no evidence has yet been found to prove transmission from these sources. Studies have shown that casual (i.e., nonsexual) household contact including kissing, hugging, and sharing common kitchen and toilet facilities does not transmit the infection (Fischi, Dickinson, Scott, Klunas, Fletcher, & Parks, 1987).

Diagnosis

Viral culture is not generally available, therefore the diagnosis of infection is usually based on the presence of antibodies to HIV. Diagnosis of AIDS is made when there is evidence of infection with HIV, absence of any other reason for immune suppression, and a confirmed diagnosis of opportunistic infection, certain malignancies, or, in children, lymphoid interstitial pneumonitis (Centers for Disease Control, 1987). Diseases that may confirm a diagnosis include:

Cancers
  • primary lymphomas of the brain
  • Kaposi's sarcoma in persons under 60 years of age
  • B-cell non-Hodgkin's lymphoma
Protozoal infections
  • toxoplasmosis
  • *Pneumocystis carinii* pneumonia
  • cryptosporidiosis
Bacterial infections
  • atypical mycobacterium
Fungal infections
  • candidiasis
  • cryptococcosis
Viral infections
  • cytomegalovirus
  • herpes simplex

In between asymptomatic infection and full-blown AIDS lie the lesser degrees of illness known as ARC or AIDS-Related Complex and shown in Table 5.1.

TABLE 5.1 General Course of Pediatric HIV Infection

Diagnosis	Clinical signs	Treatment
Infected	Usually none Remains asymptomatic	Prevent infections; no live immunizations; prevent transmission
ARC	Any or all of the following: failure to thrive, parotid swelling, organomegaly, lymphadenopathy, and neurologic abnormalities; also, recurrent: otitis media, thrush (oral/genital), diarrhea, respiratory infections, and fever.	As above, with the addition of aggressive treatment for all infections, use of prophylactic antibiotics, regular administration of gammaglobulin, and special attention to good nutrition.
AIDS	Primary immune deficiencies In the absence of primary immune deficiencies, presence of chronic interstitial pneumonitis, and/or clearly diagnosed opportunistic infection(s), and/or certain malignancies.	As above; in addition, shift treatment goals from acute to palliative when appropriate.

Diagnosis in the newborn is complicated because the immune system is immature and there is no way of distinguishing whether the antibodies to HIV present in neonates' blood are their own or maternal. Therefore all infants found to be HIV-positive must be regularly assessed until a positive or negative status can be confirmed (usually by 12 to 18 months of age). Recently the Centers for Disease Control (CDC) has recommended a new method for classifying pediatric AIDS infection (see Table 5.2) in its varying presentations.

There are many contingencies and complexities in establishing a diagnosis. The course of the infection, once established, is erratic and uncertain, and its full manifestation is always fatal. Given all of these issues laced throughout with misunderstanding, blatant fear, and discrimination, it is clear to see why these children and their families require an absolute commitment from caring professionals. Those involved must provide comprehensive, coordinated, consistent, and, most importantly, loving programs of care. These programs need to be geared not only to treating medical issues, but also to realistically integrating the child into his or her own community.

As with any chronic pediatric illness, the parent is both the primary care person and part of the primary unit of care. It is essential to be ever mindful of this. The professional's role is to teach, support, counsel, and provide direct

TABLE 5.2 Center for Disease Control (CDC) Recommendation for the Classification of HIV Infection in Children Under 13 Years of Age.

Class P-0. Indeterminate infection, including newborns who may have been exposed.
Class P-1. Asymptomatic/confirmed infection
    Subclass A. Normal immune function
    Subclass B. Abnormal immune function
    Subclass C. Immune function not tested
Class P-2. Symptomatic/confirmed infection
    Subclass A. Nonspecific findings
    Subclass B. Progressive neurologic disease
    Subclass C. Lymphoid interstitial pneumonitis
    Subclass D. Secondary infectious diseases
        Category D-1. Specified secondary infectious diseases listed in the CDC surveillance definition for AIDS
        Category D-2. Recurrent serious bacterial infections
        Category D-3. Other specified secondary infectious diseases
    Subclass E. Secondary cancers
        Category E-1. Specified secondary cancers listed in the CDC surveillance definition for AIDS
        Category E-2. Other cancers possibly secondary to HIV infection
    Subclass F. Other diseases possibly due to HIV infection

service in the context of a team that includes the parent (note: *parent* refers here to the caregiver, be it foster parent or extended family member). It must also be remembered that because of the awesome isolation experienced by these families, the act of simply being consistently "present" for them becomes an exquisitely valuable therapeutic tool.

PARAMETERS FOR CARE

A three-pronged approach to care is discussed here, an outline of which is found in Table 5.4.

Physical (Physiologic, Clinical)

Physical presentations will vary, as previously mentioned. The child who carries the virus but is not symptomatic from the virus, does *not* have AIDS. It is not yet known how long a child may remain in this state, but cases of up to 7 years have been reported (Oleski, 1987), and that span may be ever longer.

Medical Management

As the disease progresses, specific illnesses will require specific medical management. What remains constant throughout is that the child is infectious and is especially prone to developing secondary infections. A basic care strategy that protects the child and prevents the spread of the HIV infection can be taught easily to caregivers. Unless the child develops another type of secondary infection that mandates augmenting care with more elaborate isolation, these rules are generally effective even the child with a full AIDS diagnosis. This basic list includes:

- Avoid crowds and sick people; report exposure to chicken pox immediately to physician.
- Live immunizations (oral polio and measles, mumps, and rubella) may need to be avoided.
- Wash hands before and after care.
- Don't share personal items such as toothbrushes, razors, or pierced earrings.
- Wash dishes in hot, soapy water, rinse well, and air dry.
- Launder soiled items in hot water with bleach or Lysol; dry thoroughly.
- Wear disposable gloves if changing messy diapers or cleaning blood spills.
- Dispose of soiled diapers in plastic garbage bag; if bags are not available, wrap the soiled diaper in enough newspaper to stop all leakage before throwing it away.
- Clean soiled surfaces first with soap and water, then rinse with a fresh solution of bleach and water (mix ½ cup of chlorine bleach in half a bucket of water); keep a separate bucket and sponge just for this and flush unused solution down the toilet.

Nutrition

Another constant is the need for optimal nutrition. These children are often troubled with intermittent bouts of chronic oral candidiasis and diarrhea. During this time, it is especially difficult to maintain even adequate caloric intake. Supplementing the basic food groups with small, frequent feedings of high-caloric foods such as a rich pasta dish, eggnog, and ice cream may be helpful. Sometimes, when diarrhea is persistent, lactose-free diets, which eliminate milk products, are required. If thrush or oral herpes makes chewing or swallowing difficult, offer bland pureed foods served at room temperature. Be sure to rinse the mouth after eating with cool (not cold) water.

When an infant eats poorly, consistency becomes very important. Having the same person(s) feed the child regularly has been shown to have a positive correlation with intake and weight gain (Krener, 1987).

Dental Care

The dentist also plays an important role in keeping the child healthy. Good teeth are essential to good nutrition and, given the frailty of the developing immune system, cavities can serve as the entry point for a potentially lethal infection. The parents may need to be reminded to inform the dentist that the child requires blood precautions (because most dental procedures result in some bleeding of the gums, the dentist should be told that the child's blood might be infectious and that rubber gloves are appropriate). It must be remembered that the decision of who to tell is one made repeatedly throughout the child's life. It is the parent's responsibility (unless reporting is mandated by local law), and their right to confidentiality must be judiciously guarded.

Advanced Disease

Throughout the course of infection, it is the parent who, seeing the child daily, is most in tune with the subtleties of behavior and intangible clues that something may be amiss. Health care givers are well advised to listen to those parents if life-threatening infections are to be identified and treated early.

Those children who do go on to develop full-blown AIDS eventually may experience pain as a result of mucousal ulcerations or neurologic pathology. It is essential to respect the child's right to comfort and not assume that because it is an infant or young toddler he "really doesn't know." Hospice professionals are often the best persons to turn to for expertise in the management of pain if consultation is needed by the health care team. Pain management is often complex and may be frustrating. It is important, however, that the objective efficacy of "touching" and "soothing" he stressed. Children are physically comforted best by those who love and know them. Reminding a parent of that not only helps the child, but also offers positive balance to persons usually overwhelmed with guilt.

Sexual Transmission

One final point on physical issues concerns the parents (and if the patient is himself or herself approaching adolescence, it includes the patient also). That point is safe sexual techniques. Infants most frequently acquire the disease perinatally, which means the mother (and often the father) is infected with the virus. It therefore becomes an absolutely essential component of prevention (1) to assist parents in determining their own status; (2) to discuss with them the need to use a condom during all oral, anal, and genital sexual activity; and (3) if the mother is antibody-positive, to delay future pregnancies. This is an exquisitely difficult area in which to intervene, because sexuality is interwoven with personal, social, cultural, and religious issues. Nonetheless, it must not be ignored but rather must be addressed repeatedly, respectfully acknowledging all of the many implications.

Social (Concrete, Extrinsic Factors)

Isolation

The primary social problem is that of isolation. This begins when the parent is first told that the child is infected, and continues throughout the course of the disease. Much of this isolation exists as rejection or discrimination by friends and family as well as by professional caregivers. Usually, it is based on fear of contagion and/or on underlying value judgments that label certain "types" of people as undeserving of care. Isolation and the patient's parent's response must be addressed directly, right from the start.

It is here that the old adage "actions speak louder than words" holds especially true. Body language is far more important than verbiage. A simple pat on the arm or a hug for both parent and child goes a long way toward letting them both know that they are accepted and not feared. The establishment of a trusting acceptance is vital as the basis for the ongoing support of these families.

Confidentiality

At the time of diagnosis or soon after, the subject of who and how to tell must be discussed. Giving the patient and parent control of this is essential (within, of course, existing legal requirements). At present, most jurisdictions require only the reporting of confirmed full-blown AIDS cases. It is important to let the parents know about existing laws. Then, decisions can be made concerning who needs to know. Role play is often a useful technique for practicing how to tell someone about the diagnosis of HIV infection. Whenever possible, the health care team should be available to confer with other family members at the patient's or parent's request. Respect for privacy cannot be overemphasized. Casual discussion of a patient's diagnosis by medical personnel outside the care setting is absolutely unacceptable.

Case Management

A case management/advocacy approach is most useful for dealing with the multiple, complex issues that these families face. Without such supportive coordination of services, the child may very well get lost in the system. The case manager must know the available resources both quantitatively and qualitatively.

It is incumbent upon that person to have done the legwork necessary to insure that resource personnel (i.e., dentists, physical therapists, home-health organizers) are educated about HIV and are willing to serve persons with the infection. This is not always easy to do and may require that the caseworkers themselves establish, nurture, and maintain active networks of appropriate service providers.

Attention to detail is an important part of case management. How does the local first-aid squad feel about HIV infection? Is housing available? Which pediatricians and dentists will provide care? What are local school and day care policies; reporting regulations; medicaid, welfare and SSI requirements? Will the child be accepted in Sunday school? What support groups exist for parents? How do they get there? And who baby-sits so they can attend?

Personal Rights

Patient and family rights must be considered in all aspects of planning. This infection carries with it an unusually heavy social and psychological burden. It is important, therefore, to review on an ongoing basis definitions and care options. This is necessary to assure that the patient and family fully understand the facts and choices. Including the patient and parent as part of the team right from the start will have a positive impact on compliance and also makes it easier to address more difficult issues later on, such as if and when to stop treatment.

Personal/Spiritual (Subtle, Intrinsic Factors)

It is within this parameter that perhaps the most devastating potential exists. Psychic trauma can be difficult if not impossible to fully appreciate. Too often it is assumed that children "don't really understand" what is happening. It is a wrong assumption; they can understand.

The following example clearly shows how sensitive a child can be. A 5-year-old boy with AIDS had been hospitalized several times with severe infections. He knows he has "bad pneumonia" and has been allowed to talk about his fears. At his parents request, however, he had never been told his exact diagnosis. His awareness and interpretation of the subtle actions and attitudes of his frightened though well-intentioned caregivers became clear in one of his drawings. It looked, simply enough, like a picture of a house (note: there were no figures at all in the drawing). As he talked about it, he stated that he was a part of the picture. "But," he said, "I'm so far in you can't see me." He had learned, without ever being told, that he was untouchable, and so removed that he could not even be seen. Fortunately he lived for several months after that, allowing time to overcome his awesome sense of separation. The point is that both our attitudes and our clinical skills have equal impact, and both must be continually addressed.

Wherever possible, trained social workers should be available to assist staff as well as patients and families. Communication on all levels must be consistent, ongoing, nonjudgmental, and accepting.

Coping

Supportive counseling should be aimed at facilitating the venting of feelings, then identifying issues and positive coping skills, and formulating focused, realistic plans. This is not usually the time for psychotherapeutic strategies aimed at major behavior change.

Denial, guilt, and anger are frequently seen. All are appropriate responses at various times. They will recur throughout the course of the illness, yet are not problematic unless they get in the way and cannot be worked through.

Denial, for example, can be a useful means for a family to experience periods of emotional respite. Parents can be encouraged to put the illness aside at times in order to deal with other issues or just relax. That very same defense mechanism, however, can become an issue if, for example, the parent consistently denies his or her own infectivity. Parents may refuse to practice safe sex or to tell their partners. Intervention by a skilled social worker or mental health professional is essential here.

Guilt is almost unavoidable, especially in those cases of perinatal transmission. It cannot be circumvented, but rather must be acknowledged and openly discussed. Blame is not the issue. It is better to simply acknowledge that the infection was passed on unknowingly. It is no one's fault. Then the focus can be shifted from the past to present and future issues of care. It is especially important, at this time, for the caregiver or counselor to be absolutely nonjudgmental. Unless that is so, nonverbal messages will be clearly perceived by the parent, and the counseling process will not be totally effective.

Anger may be expressed overtly as rage at the partner, at God, or at whomever or whatever is seen as the cause. It may also be present as depression. In either case, it will require ventilation and clarification. Frequently, the child or parent may need permission to express anger. This is not a casual process and often requires intervention by a trained counselor or social worker.

Grieving

Lastly, it is important to recognize the role of the grieving process. This begins when the diagnosis is first made, because it is then that the family loses a "healthy child." Throughout the course of the infection, other losses occur.

It may be the tangible loss of a spouse, friends, support networks, or, eventually, the death of the child. It may be the intrinsic loss of self-esteem or dreams of future healthy children. Whatever the loss, real or perceived, the reactions may include periods of denial, anger, depression, sleep disturbances, and a general sense of being disconnected or being unable to concentrate (Pine, 1974). It is important to recognize the process and continually work it through. Tranquilizers and avoidance are rarely the best choice.

THE CAREGIVER

Finally, we must look at the caregiver. How does one prepare to work with these little ones and their families? What does one need to know? Table 5.3 is a self-evaluation questionnaire for caregivers, and Table 5.4 outlines a care plan for HIV-infected children. Together these Tables provide a guide to clinical as well as personal areas for consideration. These are not meant as checklists for specialists but rather as starting points for all caregivers.

TABLE 5.3 Self-evaluation Tool for Caregivers of HIV-Infected Persons

Professional/Clinical: Do I: No-Yes-Enough to teach
1. Understand how the immune system works?
2. Know what HIV is and how it is transmitted?
3. Know appropriate precautions (including rationale) to use when caring for an HIV-infected child?
4. Know what resources exist in my hospital and/or community for patients, families, and myself?
5. Know how to contact and utilize those resources?
6. Know how to listen to persons in crisis?
7. Know how to teach children?
8. Understand a variety of sexual-pleasuring techniques?
9. Know how to care for Broviac catheters
10. Know which vaccines are live?

Personal: Am I: No-Yes-Sometimes
1. Comfortable hugging a person infected with HIV?
2. Angry with mothers who have infected their children?
3. Aware of my own attitudes toward sex and drugs?
4. Comfortable discussing sexuality with:
   a. someone of the same sex?
   b. someone of the opposite sex?
   c. someone with a sexual preference different from mine?
5. Willing to "take on the establishment"?
6. Able to cope with the death of a child?
7. Able to deal with parents' anticipatory grieving?
8. Comfortable with street language?

TABLE 5.4 Care Plan for Children Infected with HIV

I. Physical parameter
   A. Problem: positive blood test for HIV antibodies
      1. Goal: to maintain optimal health by
         a. avoiding exposure to communicable diseases; teach
            caregivers to report immediately any such exposure,
            especially to chicken pox
         b. regular follow-up visits to physician and dentist
         c. withholding live immunizations
         d. maintaining healthy environment (adequate food/shelter)

      2. Goal: to prevent transmission of infection by
         a. teaching parents/caregivers
           • to wash hands before and after care
           • not to share toothbrushes, razors, personal-care items
           • to wash dishes in *hot, soapy* water, rinse well and air dry
           • to launder items soiled with blood or body fluids in hot
             water with bleach/Lysol and dry thoroughly
           • to wear disposable gloves if changing diarrheic diapers
           • to dispose of diapers or soiled items in plastic garbage
             bags (if bags are not available, wrap soiled items in
             sufficient newspaper to stop any leakage)
           • to clean soiled surfaces first with soap and water, then
             rinse with *fresh* bleach solution (1/2 cup for each 1/2
             bucket of water; keep separate bucket and sponge for
             only this purpose)
         b. teaching *safe sex* as appropriate
         c. encouraging testing of parents and siblings
         d. maintaining blood and body-fluid precautions during health
            care visits and hospitalizations
         e. encouraging parents to inform health care providers of need
            for precautions

   B. Problem: failure to thrive
      1. Goal: To maximize potential by
         a. monitoring physical and developmental parameters
         b. evaluating and addressing identified problem areas
            (nutrition, occupational therapy/intake and output consults)
         c. using ancillary personnel such as volunteers and
            grandparents to enhance infant stimulation

   C. Problem: Poor nutrition
      1. Goal: to maintain adequate intake and eletrolyte balance by
         a. monitoring I & O, weight, and electrolyte status
         b. treating identified causes
         c. nutritional consults based on family's reality
         d. emphasis on use of *consistent* feeder
         e. social work referral
         f. hyperalimentation

(continued)

TABLE 5.4 *(continued)*

D. Problem: Ineffective immune response
  1. Goal: To prevent recurrent bacterial infections by
     a. maintaining wellness
     b. regular administration of Gammaglobulin
  2. Goal: To prevent opportunistic infections by
     a. administering prophylactic antibiotics
     b. avoiding exposure

E. Problem: Infection
  1. Goal: To eliminate or control secondary infections by
     a. teaching caretaker(s) to monitor regularly and report
        • temperature elevation
        • decreased food intake, vomiting, or diarrhea
        • irritability
        • breathing changes
        • appearance of white patches or rash in mouth or on skin
        • changes in usual bahavior patterns
     b. treating specifically and monitoring adminstration of medication
  2. Goal: To avoid or minimize untoward reactions to medication by
     a. monitoring parameters specific to medication(s) being used (e.g., kidney or liver function)

F. Problem: Neurologic abnormalities
  1. Goal: To identify etiology and minimize deterioration by
     a. regularly assessing neurostatus
     b. treating specifically where possible
     c. enhancing developmental stimulation as appropriate

G. Problem: Pain
  1. Goal: To maintain a state of responsive comfort by
     a. assessing character, intensity, and rhythm or pain
     b. determining etiology and treating cause
     c. administering medication regularly, assessing efficacy and side effects, and titrating dosage as needed
     d. utilizing creative noninvasive, nonpharmacologic adjuvent
     e. *documenting*

II. Social parameter

  A. Problem: Physical abandonment of child or parent/child
    1. Goal: To maintain adequate housing by
       a. providing *supportive* education at time of diagnosis
       b. social work referrals
       c. knowing and utilizing appropriate resources
       d. providing education to foster parents and other personnel as needed (respite facilities, landlords, churches, etc.)

  B. Problem: Absence or unwillingness of caregivers to provide services
    1. Goal: To locate a physician and dentist to provide care by

(continued)

TABLE 5.4 *(continued)*

---

    a. formal and informal contact with physicians, dentists, agencies and school programs to determine
       • their willingness to accept the child
       • any constraints that should be imposed
  2. Goal: To locate agencies to provide needed services by
    a. referring to known personnel or agencies (specific contacts)
    b. appropriately sharing information with parental consent
  3. Goal: To integrate child into appropriate day care or educational program by
    a. participating in specific and/or general advocacy activities

 C. Problem: Inadequate financial resources
  1. Goal: To identify specific needs and provide maximal assistance by
    a. monitoring compliance with
       • keeping scheduled appointments
       • appropriate nutritional intake and appropriate clothing
       • following precautions
    b. conferring with other agencies to assess fiscal needs
    c. social work referrals
    d. adjusting schedule to maximize use of visit

III. Personal/spiritual parameter

 A. Problem: Fear of isolation
  1. Goal: To maintain an accepting atmosphere by
    a. consistent communication (emphasis on team concept)
    b. providing opportunities for ventilating feelings
    c. establishing and maintaining strict protocols for the sharing of information
    d. referral for individual conseling as appropriate

 B. Problem: Inappropriate use of denial, guilt and/or anger
  1. Goal: To accept the diagnosis to a degree that allows for consistent follow-up care and prevention of HIV transmission by
    a. consistent and repetitive sharing of information
    b. allowing parents to ventilate and "own" their feelings
    c. focusing on concrete issues and specific positives, maintaining realistic hope where possible

 C. Problem: Inability or unwillingness to practice safe sex
  1. Goal: To practice safe sex regularly by
    a. assessing understanding of safe sex, being sure to clarify language
    b. role playing ways of talking about it
    c. discussing erotic or fun use of condoms
    d. offering to discuss subject with the couple
    e. providing written information
    f. referral as appropriate

(continued)

TABLE 5.4 *(continued)*

D. Problem: Complicated or pathologic grieving
   1. Goal: Parents will be able to work through and complete their grief by
      a. encouraging verbalization of feelings during anticipatory grief
      b. providing for inclusion of parent at time of child's death
      c. providing follow-up contact during first year of bereavement
      d. referral as appropriate for individual counseling or self-help group
      e. including support for siblings throughout the bereavement process

---

The reality is that most of us will, in time to come if we have not already, be caring for HIV-infected children. We have a responsibility to them and to ourselves. We must know and acknowledge our attitudes, strengths, and limitations. In that way we will best use our own talents and refer appropriately to those with expertise in other areas.

We also have a responsibility to take care of ourselves. Professional networks that offer mutual support are essential. Memorial services for patients will allow us to attend to our own grief and need for closure. Flexible hours may be useful when they can be arranged. Creative self-care, even occasional pampering, need to be part and parcel of the caregiver's routine.

CONCLUSION

Clearly, children infected with HIV are not an imminent danger to others. It is our responsibility to continue to learn, to search for a cure, to maintain hope, and to advocate on their behalf. We must not only address their physical needs, but offer comprehensive programs of care to their families as well. Lastly, we must work to build within our communities acceptance and gentle welcoming environments in which we may all grow.

ACKNOWLEDGMENTS

The author wishes to express her gratitude to Charlotte Carneiro R.N., M.S., and to Shelby Josephs, M.D., for critical review of the draft, and to Barbara Cady for preparation of the manuscript.

RESOURCES

National

AIDS Action Council
729 8th St., SE, Room 200
Washington, DC 20003
(202) 547-3101

American Red Cross—National
AIDS Public Information Program
17th and D Streets, NW
Washington, DC 20003
(202) 737-8300

Centers for Disease Control
AIDS Activity
Building 6, Room 292
1600 Gliftin Rd.
Atlanta, GA 30333
(404) 329-3479

Hemophilia Foundation—National
AIDS Activity Coordinator
Soho Building, Room 406
110 Green St.
New York, NY 10012
(212) 219-8180

National Gay Task Force
80 Fifth Ave.
New York, NY 10011
(212) 741-5800

San Francisco AIDS Foundation
333 Valencia St., 4th Floor
San Francisco, CA 94103
(415) 864-4376

Local

Contact your local:
   Department of Human Services
   Health Department
   Alcohol and drug abuse services
   AIDS hotlines

REFERENCES

Barbour, S. (1987). Acquired immunodeficiency syndrome of childhood. In J. P. Prlowski (Ed.), *Pediatric Clinics of North America: Vol. 34. Intensive Care* (pp. 247-268). Philadelphia: Saunders.

Bennett, J. (1986). AIDS: Beyond the hospital. *American Journal of Nursing, 9*, 1016-1028.

Boland, M., & Rizz, D. (1986). *The child with aids (human immunodeficiency virus): A guide for the family.* Newark, NJ: United Hospitals Medical Center Children's Hospital of New Jersey.

Centers for Disease Control. (1987). Classification system for human immunodeficiency virus (HIV) infection in children under 13 years of age. *Morbidity and Mortality Weekly, 38*, 225-235.

Conte, J. (1986). Infection with HIV in the hospital; epidemiology, infection control and biosafety considerations. *Annals of Internal Medicine, 105*, 703-736.

Fischi, M. A., Dickinson, G. M., Scott, G. B., Kilmas, N., Fletcher, M.D., & Parks,

W. (1987). Evaluation of heterosexual partners, children and household contacts of adults with AIDS. *The Journal of the American Medical Association, 257*, 640–644.

Iazetti, L. (1986). Nursing management of the pediatric AIDS patient. *Issues In Comprehensive Pediatric Nursing, 9*, 119–129.

Klug, R. M. (1986). AIDS beyond the hospital. Children with AIDS. *American Journal of Nursing, 10*, 1126–1132.

Krener, P. (1987). Impact of the diagnosis of AIDS on hospital care of an infant. *Clinical Pediatrics, 26*, 30–34.

Oleski, J. (1987, April). Statement made during presentation at the Surgeon General's Conference on Pediatric AIDS, Philadephia, PA.

Pine, V. (1974). Dying, death, and social behavior. In B. Schoenberg, A. C. Carr, A. Kutscher, D. Peretz, & I. K. Goldberg (Eds.), *Anticipatory Grief* (pp. 31–47). New York: Columbia University Press.

Rogers, M. F. (1985). AIDS in children: A review of the clinical, epidemiologic and public health aspects. *Pediatric Infectious Disease, 4*(3), 230–236.

Rubinstein, A. (1986). Pediatric AIDS. *Current Problems in Pediatrics, 7*, 365–409.

Ziegler, J. B., Cooper, D. A., Johnson, R. O., and Gold, J. (1985). Postnatal transmission of AIDS-associated retrovirus from mother to infant. *Lancet*, April 20; 1 (8434): 896–898.

6　Deafness and Family Impact

Marita Danek

Deafness is different. Deaf adults and professionals who work with deaf people feel compelled to reiterate this point to outsiders (Higgins, 1980). Deafness is much more than the inability to hear. Rather, the condition of being deaf from birth or from an early age (which includes approximately 70% of all deaf persons) reshapes and frames the entirety of a child's developmental experiences.

Most (91.7%) deaf children have hearing parents (Rawlings & Jensema, 1977; Schein & Delk, 1974), and because deafness is a low-incidence disability their deaf child is usually their first exposure to deafness. As parents of a deaf child, they will be required to assimilate new information, master their oftentimes overwhelming emotional responses, make major decisions, and in general, deal with life demands that place them apart from other parents.

This chapter discusses the impact on the family system of early onset (pre-lingual) deafness in a child. It reviews the stages of a family's response to the birth of a deaf child and those factors that appear to mitigate for or against the integration of this child into the family. Intervention strategies and professional roles will be examined, and the chapter concludes with a listing of resources for families with a deaf member.

DIAGNOSIS OF DEAFNESS

Deafness in a child is usually discovered slowly, and the uncovering of this diagnosis is itself a painful process, often fraught with parental denial, which is sometimes reinforced by professional wait-and-see attitudes. Deafness is an invisible as well as a low-incidence disability; these two factors may contribute to the delay in diagnosis, particularly when there is no reason to suspect a hearing loss. During the time of gradual awareness, the concerned parent might suspect other disabilities (such as a learning disability or mental retardation), because of the child's seeming lack of responsiveness to external stimuli (Luterman, 1979).

Although it may seem on the surface inconceivable that parents would lack an awareness of their child's deafness—indeed, may appear to deny the deafness—this is understandable. The inconsistent responses the child makes to noise places the parents on a roller coaster of alternating elation and despair. Lack of parental self-confidence in the recognition (intuition?) of the "soft signs" of deafness, of a sense that something is not quite right, is frequently operative (Becker, 1981; Williams & Darbyshire, 1982).

To some extent, the rapidity with which the diagnosis is reached is contingent upon several external factors related to the marital relationship, family and kinship system, the existence of other children in the family, and other social and cultural factors. Mindel and Vernon (1971) note that communicating one's suspicions to one's spouse involves great risk. Cohesive couples who are mutually supportive and have open communication are more apt to take such a risk. Firstborn children are less likely to be detected early, in part due to parental inexperience with developmental milestones, and in part due to the greater attachment of parents to firstborn children (Becker, 1981).

Becker proposes that early detection of deafness is related to parents' (usually the mother's) confidence in their ability to express and receive love. When verbal expressions of love are ignored by the child, a mother who is confident of her ability to love will assume that there is something amiss in the child, not her. The intriguing but empirically unestablished implication from all this (and one that is perhaps also true for other developmental disabilities) is that the parent's ability to make an early detection of hearing loss is a reflection of both personal and marital strengths. These strengths will later be utilized to help parents deal with the implications of deafness and to make necessary accommodations as the child develops.

Unfortunately, a conclusive diagnosis of hearing impairment often appears to be hindered, not helped, by consultation with the family physician or pediatrician. Because deafness is seldom total, the child may actually respond to a noise that is above her or his hearing threshold.

Regrettably, it takes an average of 4 to 6 months (Becker, 1981; Williams & Darbyshire, 1982) between the time of the first *medical consultation* and the ultimate diagnosis. Williams and Darbyshire (1982) note a delay of 14 months between the parent's first suspicions and the final diagnosis of deafness.

STAGES OF REACTION TO THE DIAGNOSIS

Most prelingually deaf individuals have a sensorineural hearing loss, for which there is no known cure, although there are technological devices (hearing aids, telecommunication devices, etc.) that can compensate for the loss to varying

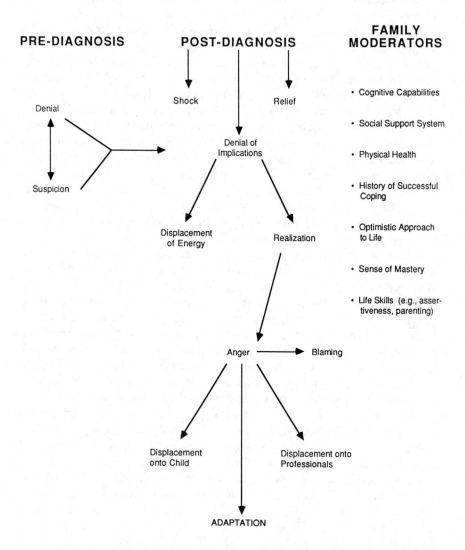

FIGURE 6.1 Reaction of the family to the diagnosis of deafness in a child.

degrees. Unlike other childhood disabilities that involve medical conditions or a threat to life (e.g., diabetes, carcinoma, or cystic fibrosis), deafness is usually irreversible and its course is stable.

Whereas the prediagnosis parental reaction to the deaf child is usually varying degrees of denial, the sequence of reactions to the diagnosis itself is similar to the response to any irreversible disability in a family. This sequence may include shock or relief, more denial, realization, anger, depression, guilt and/or adaptation (Kübler-Ross, 1969; Luterman 1979; Mindel & Vernon, 1971; Shontz, 1965; Wentworth, 1974).

Shock functions defensively to distance the parents from the diagnosis; it protects them temporarily from becoming overwhelmed by the information. Mindel and Vernon (1971) characterize shock as a combination of disbelief, grief, and helplessness, which sets the parent apart from the rest of the world.

Relief is another possible reaction (Luterman, 1979) and is perhaps unique to the diagnosis of deafness. During the long months that parental suspicions are brewing, a much "worse" diagnosis may be feared and, therefore, the diagnosis of deafness is greeted with relief.

Denial will occur again periodically after the diagnosis. Sometimes denial functions to give the parent "time out," while consolidating the personal resources necessary to confront the overwhelming implications of having a deaf child. Just as it is possible prior to the diagnosis to deny the deafness, it is possible after the diagnosis to overlook or ignore the *extent* of the hearing loss, its permanence, and its functional limitations. Denial can also be manifested through a diversion of parental energies into initiating programs for deaf children or for modifying current educational policies. Because there is no best way to educate every deaf child, parents will frequently become enamored of new unproven methods for teaching the deaf child or developing communication skills. Such procedures, by their very newness, can offer the kind of hope that older programs, with realistic but limited results, cannot offer.

Some parents will devote their lives to the cause of a new system or procedure while the child's needs go wanting. I am reminded of contact made by a father whose 2-year-old son had recently become profoundly deaf as a result of meningitis. My first response was to listen and communicate that I understood his pain, confusion, and anger. I then advised that he develop an ability to communicate through sign language so that the child would not be isolated from his family, would learn incidentally and naturally, and would benefit from parental involvement in his schoolwork (how do you help a child with his social studies, math, or whatever homework when you can't communicate?). We spent some time discussing educational options; regrettably, there were few in his rural geographic region. I sensed an incipient need on this father's part to fight the system and warned him about diverting his energies into this arena. It would be a short-term gratification during the years when his child needed direct parental involvement and language development the most. I heard nothing from him again until about a year later when he requested a letter from me supporting his right to determine the most appropriate education for his child; he was embroiled in a battle with the local school system. As this case illustrates, parents can become enmeshed in peripheral issues and never deal directly with their deaf child's specific needs.

Realization is the point where active mourning and very strong reactions to the diagnosis occur. During this time parents may often be overwhelmed by new information and technical terminology presented in too short a period of time.

Anger may then result as the parent copes with confusion and a sense of personal inadequacy and of the unfairness of it all. Many times this anger will be displaced onto professionals, particularly those involved in making the diagnosis or treatment recommendations.

Adaptation comes when the parents confront the reality of their child's deafness. This is the time when parents work together to seek solutions— short-term solutions, but solutions to problems as they evolve naturally during different stages of the child's development. They acknowledge that changes in their lives must occur and gather the strength to face them. Unfortunately, not all parents reach this stage; some may accept the deafness while never totally accepting the functional limitations of deafness.

FAMILY ADAPTATION

The impact of the deaf child on the family varies greatly depending on the family structure and its crisis-meeting resources. This section elaborates more fully on some ways families differ in their response to raising a deaf child.

Resources act as buffers to the demands of a crisis (Matheny, Aycock, Pugh, Curlett, & Canella, 1986). Crucial resources would include: (1) adequate cognitive ability to appraise the event; (2) social support from family and friends; (3) physical health sufficient to yield high energy levels; (4) a history of coping successfully with stressful events; (5) a basically optimistic approach to life; (6) a sense of personal control over life's multiple demands; (7) self-esteem; and (8) life skills such as assertiveness and parenting skills. Although empirical evidence is lacking, the buffer effect of family resources offers an intriguing explanatory possibility as to why some families perform well and others fall apart when dealing with a crisis such as deafness.

Problem-solving ability would appear to be a critical variable. In studies of effectively functioning families, it was found that such families did not have fewer problems, but that they use their existing problem-solving skills to cope more effectively (Epstein, Bishop, & Baldwin, 1982). When parents of deaf children can problem solve, it appears that both parents and children cope more effectively. For example, Bodner-Johnson (1985) found that parents of high-achieving deaf children were more likely to have made plans and have expectations for the child's future educational and occupational aspiration (e.g., had engaged actively in problem-solving behavior regarding the child's future).

Effectively functioning families have a strong social network or kinship system that buffers against stress, provides a source of practical assistance, and provides a validation of values and behavior. These support systems can provide respite for the parents of a deaf child and from the fatigue and diminished self-confidence that comes with impaired communication, demanding schedules, and constant decision making.

Adequate parental physical health appears to be an obvious ingredient in the family's overall ability to cope. A deaf child can be exhausting to live with; communication is so essential to family living that the extra demands of communicating with a deaf child are continuous and surely result in periodic fatigue.

Families that have proved themselves successful in coping with stressful events are usually adaptable. Bodner-Johnson (1985) noted that parents of high-achieving deaf children were more apt to adapt the family schedule to meet the special needs of deaf children and to use simultaneous communication (e.g., adapt to the child's communication mode and needs).

A history of successful coping would predispose a parent toward an optimistic outlook on life's challenges. Families who approach life optimistically would then tend to be able to counter a negative response to deafness (e.g., catstrophizing, blaming, externalizing) with more positive attributions and expectations.

A sense of confidence and control refers to a faith in the family's ability to manage a stressful event. Although related conceptually to optimism and a history of successful coping, this characteristic revolves around the core ability of marital partners to apply appropriate and consistent strategies to the stressful event. For example, this would include using acceptable methods of discipline with the deaf child (e.g., being neither overprotective nor too permissive).

Self-esteem is another characteristic that tends to boost the family's overall coping ability. Partners who value themselves and each other and have a strong, satisfying marital relationship are able to value the child as a person in his or her own right (e.g., the child would not be thought of as a *deaf* child, but as a child who happened to be deaf). Adequate life skills in the parents, such as assertiveness and parenting skills, combine to assist the deaf child and also help cope with the environment in a positive, forthright, and reasonable manner.

THE IMPACT OF THE FAMILY ON THE CHILD

It is obvious that just as the presence of a deaf child affects the family system, so, too, family life affects the way the child develops. Family relationships have a significant impact on the development of the deaf child's self-esteem (as they do on the self-esteem of all children). Some research indicates that hearing mothers of deaf children are less likely to be encouraging and approving toward their children (Schlesinger & Meadow, 1972). Guterman (1983) postulates that this is due to some hearing parents' unrealistic scholastic and occupational aspirations and the perceived failure of the deaf child to communicate orally—with resultant parental frustration. The impact of the family on the child will, of course, be a highly individual matter that will be shaped by the family's ability to negotiate the diagnosis and by its own crisis-meeting resources, as discussed previously.

SIBLING ISSUES

The impact of the deaf child on siblings is difficult to assess, at least empirically, due to the difficulty in separating out factors attributable to the child from factors attributable to the family's overall level of functioning (Seligman, 1983). Schwirian (1976) found that a deaf child had little impact on siblings relative to child care and household responsibilities, their level of independence and social activities, and thus concluded that there was little disruption to sibling relationships. Murphy (1979) noted that the sibling closest in age to the deaf child often has the most difficulty with overall adjustment. Luterman (1979) observed that an attention-getting pseudosensory deficit, school failures, tantrums, or overly "good" behavior that hides deep resentment can often occur among siblings. At this time, little is definitively known about sibling relationships in the family of the deaf child, and this is certainly a potentially fruitful area for future research.

FAMILY DECISION POINTS

As the deaf child grows and matures, the family will become involved in many important decisions related to or as a result of rearing a deaf child. These include the following:

Choice of Communication Strategy

To overcome the barrier of deafness, parents must use alternative communication strategies. Because the deaf child cannot depend upon sound to learn, receive, and express language, reliance must be placed on sight. Educators and early-childhood specialists have engaged in philosophical disagreements on exactly how the deaf child should use the sense of sight. Until recently, most intervention attempts used one or more variants of the oral method of communication.

A shift away from a strictly oral approach has occurred over the past two decades. Oral methods seem to work best with postlingually deafened children who already have the structure of language, have heard speech, and are capable of reproducing it; they are less effective with prelingually deafened children. In addition, a growing body of literature points to the importance of American Sign Language (ASL) in the deaf person's overall development. ASL is the basis of personal identity, membership in the deaf community, and a sense of group cohesiveness (Baker & Cokely, 1980; Kannapell, 1985).

The use of ASL or, more frequently, total communication (speech and sign) in early childhood and parent-infant programs is a relatively recent phenomenon. Empirical studies supporting the use of total communication fall into two types: (1) those documenting the social and educational superiority of deaf children of deaf parents, for example, children who were exposed to ASL as their first language from an early age (Balow & Brill, 1975; Schlesinger & Meadow, 1972); and (2) those documenting the positive effects of the early use of total communication with deaf children of hearing parents (Greenberg, 1980). These studies are not longitudinal but seem to point toward improved social competence in the deaf children studied, more positive attitudes among their parents, and more reciprocal and positive interaction between parent and child.

Educational Decisions

Before the deaf child enters a preschool program, the parents must evaluate various educational philosophies and find a school situation that most closely parallels their philosophy. This is a formidable task.

Mendolsohn & Mendolsohn (1986) refer to "trigger points" in the life of a disabled child that precipitate a reexperiencing of the grieving process in parents. The choice of a communication modality and educational program certainly are emotion-laden events that can be considered trigger points.

An added complication is that there are usually few local educational options available to parents—programs for deaf children are not always available in every community. The recent emphasis on mainstreaming means that the deaf child is frequently the only deaf student in her or his class and might have special academic or social needs that are not met.

Given the lack of local options, many parents have in the past enrolled their deaf child in a residential program. Residential schools provided good academic programming, but living away from home tended to attenuate the affective relationships between family and child.

The trend now is away from residential programming and toward community-based mainstreamed or day programs. In these programs, the child usually remains with his or her family; however, adequate local academic programming remains problematical.

INTERVENTION STRATEGIES

This chapter has already alluded to difficulties encountered by the parent in working with professionals at various times during the deaf child's development. Parental confusion and frustration tends to be additive. Meadow-Orlans (1985) reports that parents of older deaf children trust professionals much less than do parents of younger deaf children. Many times the initial problem of obtaining a diagnosis is just the beginning of years of coping with contradictory perspectives provided by educators, audiologists, counselors, and other professionals. Intervention strategies, therefore, must be on multiple levels and target the community, the family, and the child. An examination of these strategies is summarized in Table 6.1.

Community Intervention

At a community level, intervention actually means primary prevention. The family of the deaf child will encounter physicians, audiologists, hearing-aid dealers, educators, counselors, parental groups, and others involved in some way with some aspect of the child's development. These professionals vary in their training, philosophy, and intervention style. It is critical that they respond to the total needs of the child rather than to only the part that has been the focus of their training.

The problem here resides in who does what and to whom. Pediatricians are usually the initial point of contact but are sometimes at a loss to deal with the more complex issues surrounding deafness, such as long-term ramifications and parental emotional needs. Pediatricians should be trained to consider a diagnosis of deafness in any child with a family history of deafness or delayed language development and, most importantly, to take parental concerns seriously.

TABLE 6.1 Intervention Approaches

	Strategies	Outcomes
Community	Outreach Education/information Advocacy	Primary prevention Awareness Coordination of efforts
Family	Education/information Counseling/therapy Support groups Communication training Parenting training	Understanding Adaptation Healthy family relationships
Child	Parent-child communication Emphasis on language development Family involvement in child's schooling Supportive and realistic aspirations and expectations	Educational/vocational achievement consistent with potential Communication competency Mastery of developmental tasks Personal/social adjustment Identify as a deaf person Integration into family and into the hearing world

Outreach efforts by teams of audiologists, educators, psychologists, and counselors can provide information to pediatricians regarding community resources and can identify appropriate further steps for the parents to take. The recent passage of amendments to P.L. 94-142 (Education for All Handicapped Children Act of 1975) has made possible early special education and intervention efforts by the states for children with handicapping conditions from age 3 to 5. Ideally, these intervention efforts could include an outreach informational component to appropriate medical professionals.

A family's needs cannot be compartmentalized. Audiologists and educators are often called upon to provide counseling (along with assessment, information, and training). Counselors, psychologists, and social workers must provide information as well as respond to family emotional needs. Although audiologists and educators are not counselors, they should be trained to use supportive counseling skills and to identify when a parent or family needs more intensive counseling or mental health services. Conversely, counselors, psychologists, and social workers must recognize the boundaries of their roles, have a basic understanding of audiological and educational principles, and refer when necessary to allied professionals or teams of professionals.

Parents will encounter many different professionals during the child's maturation process. A crucial individual at a later stage is the state-agency rehabilitation counselor who can assist in planning and implementing the transition from high school to work or to postsecondary training. Coordinated efforts on the part of the school and parents is needed to insure contact with the appropriate rehabilitation counselor (usually an RCD, a rehabilitation counselor with a specialty in deafness) is made and maintained (Danek, 1983).

Family Intervention

The family (parents and siblings) of a deaf child will need varying degrees of assistance, depending on the family structure, resources, needs, and values. Some families will need help resolving their feelings of denial, anger, or rejection. Others will need information and emotional support. And still others will need formal programs involving communication training, peer-group involvement, and genetic counseling.

Assistance in Understanding the Hearing Loss

Families need, at a minimum, to be taught about hearing loss and be provided counseling around their feelings about this loss. Information must be provided using terminology parents understand, without reliance on jargon.

Assistance in Adapting to the Hearing Loss

Unless the initial strong negative response of denial followed by anger is resolved by the parents, the child's social growth and adaptation may be compromised (Mindel & Vernon, 1971; Moores, 1976; Schlesinger & Meadow, 1972). Counseling should begin immediately after the diagnosis and should be thereafter offered to the family on an as-needed basis. At a minimum, counseling should permit parents to express their feelings and develop reasonable expectations for their deaf child's development (Moores, 1976).

Parent-counseling groups can provide ongoing support throughout the school year. Greenberg (1980) indicates that parents of deaf children report the need for such groups and frequently feel abandoned after early intensive efforts are phased out.

Assistance in Nurturing Healthy Family Relationships

The bond between parent and child is fostered by communication. The mother-child bond is particularly important, because the mother is usually the primary caregiver (even in two-career families). Mindel and Vernon (1971) contend that, due to impaired communication with the external environment, the hearing-impaired child is dependent upon the mother for longer periods of time. The mother, in turn, may experience this dependence as a burden,

or may become overly involved with the child to the exclusion of other relationships. Counseling may be needed to assist the parents in maintaining a
balance in their lives, and in attending to their own individual needs as well
as the needs of other family members.

The deaf child might master certain developmental tasks later than the hearing child. Particularly during adolescence, parents sometimes do not permit
the deaf child to complete preadult rites of passage (e.g., a driver's license,
part-time jobs, or dating). I recall a young deaf woman in her early 20s who
had worked successfully for several years as a data-entry clerk. I was asked
by her employer to work with her when her productivity dropped and she
was in danger of losing her job. The young woman (an only child) still lived
with her parents, who did not permit her to participate in after-work social
activities because she might "meet someone and want to get married." As
an alternative to normal social outlets, this young woman was meeting her
relationship needs through fantasy and socializing at work. Considerable
parental resistance needed to be overcome before she was permitted a social
life commensurate with her chronological and emotional age.

Assistance in Maintaining Consistent Discipline

Most parents discipline by communicating their values and expectations to
the child and then providing feedback (positive or negative) when the child
attempts to comply with these expectations. For parents of a deaf child, expectations may be too high or too low. Gregory (1976) observed that parents frequently believe that their deaf child must be better behaved in order to be
accepted. This may lead to harsh child-rearing practices and too-frequent
reliance on physical punishment. Conversely, some parents may compensate
for their guilt at having a deaf child or may deal with repressed resentment
of the child by giving up and making no behavioral demands on the child.
The counselor's nonjudgmental attitude, acceptance of parental frustrations
at raising a deaf child, and suggestions for alternative ways of disciplining
the child can permit the parent to try different approaches.

The Child

The deaf child must achieve language proficiency in both English and ASL
so that ultimately the child can become identified with the deaf community
while mastering the developmental tasks necessary to achieve in a hearing
world. Parent-child communication is integral to the child's mastery of the
environment and to self-esteem (Guterman 1983).

Intervention, therefore, must focus on providing communication competency in the child and between parent and child. A parent-infant specialist

can assist with this process of language acquisition and communicative competency through regular home visits.

Bodner-Johnson (1982) notes that home and school environments must be consistently and mutually supportive of the child. Educational achievement can be optimized by (1) appropriate expectations and aspirations for educational and vocational attainment; (2) family emphasis on the use of language; (3) family interest in educational and cultural activities; (4) active parental involvement in and support of the child's schoolwork; (5) structured family work/school habits; (6) parental integration of the hearing-impaired child into the home through the knowledge of and adaptation to child's hearing loss, interest in deaf culture, and communication emphasis.

SUMMARY

In conclusion, early-onset childhood deafness presents unique challenges for the family. This chapter reviews existing issues in deafness and suggests a model for early intervention based on multiple levels of intervention. The ultimate goal is to maximize competence in every area of the deaf child's development so that the child identifies with the deaf community while maintaining an integrated existence in the larger, hearing world.

RESOURCES

Numerous resources, associations, organizations, and periodicals are available for parental and professional use. A partial listing follows.

Alexander Graham Bell Association for the Deaf
3417 Volta Place, N.W.
Washington, DC 20007

American Deafness and Rehabilitation Association
206 Steven Drive
Little Rock, AR 72205

American Speech-Language-Hearing Association
10801 Rockville Pike
Rockville, MD 20852
Frederick T. Spahr, Executive Director

National Association of the Deaf
814 Thayer Avenue
Silver Spring, MD 20910

National Center on Employment of the Deaf
National Technical Institute for the Deaf
Rochester Institute of Technology
One Lomb Memorial Drive
Rochester, NY 14623

National Information Center on Deafness
Gallaudet University
800 Florida Avenue, N.E.
Washington, DC 20002

Rehabilitation Services Administration
Department of Education
Mary E. Switzer Building
330 C Street, S.W., Room 3315
Mail Stop 2312
Washington, DC 20202

Rehabilitation Services Administration can refer to state-agency specialists in deafness (SCD) or rehabilitation counselors specializing in deafness (RCDs).

REFERENCES

Baker, C., & Cokely, D. (1980). *American sign language: A teacher's resource text on grammar and culture*. Silver Springs, MD: T. J. Publishers.

Balow, I. H., & Brill, R. G. (1975). An evaluation of reading and academic achievement levels of 16 graduating classes of the California School for the Deaf, Riverside. *The Volta Review, 77*, 266–276

Becker, S. (1981). Counseling the families of deaf children: A mental health worker speaks out. *Journal of Rehabilitation of the Deaf, 15*(1), 10–15.

Bodner-Johnson, B. (1982). Describing the home as a learning environment for hearing-impaired children. *Volta Review, 84*(7), 329–337.

Bodner-Johnson, B. (1985). Families that work for the hearing-impaired child. *The Volta Review, 87*(3), 131–137.

Danek, M. (1983). Rehabilitation counseling with deaf clients. *Journal of Applied Rehabilitation Counseling, 14*(3), 20–25.

Education for all handicapped children act of 1975. Public Law 94–142. 20 *U.S.C.A.* Section 1232, 1978.

Epstein, N., Bishop, D., & Baldwin, L. M. (1982). McMaster model of family functioning: A view of the normal family. In F. Walsh (Ed.), *Normal family processes*. New York: Guilford.

Greenberg, M. T. (1980). Hearing families with deaf children: Stress and functioning as related to communication method. *American Annals of the Deaf, 125*, 1063–1071.

Gregory, S. (1976). *The deaf child and his family*. London: George Allan & Unwin.

Guterman, S. S. (1983). The family environment and the self-esteem of the deaf child. *Directions, 3*(3), 75–80.

Higgins, P. C. (1980). *Outsiders in a hearing world: A sociology of deafness.* Beverly Hills, CA: Saga.

Kannapell, B. (1985). *Language choice reflects identity choice: A socio-linguistic study of deaf college students.* Unpublished doctoral dissertation, Georgetown University, Washington, DC.

Kubler-Ross, E. (1969). *On death and dying.* New York: Macmillan.

Luterman, D. (1969). *Counseling parents of hearing-impaired children.* Boston: Little, Brown.

Matheny, K. B., Aycock, D. W., Pugh, J. L., Curlett, W. L., & Cannella, K. A. (1986). Stress coping: A qualitative and quantitative synthesis with implications for treatment. *The Counseling Psychologist, 14*(4), 499–549.

Meadow, K. P. (1967). *The effect of early manual communication and family climate on the deaf child's development.* Unpublished doctoral dissertation, University of California, Berkeley.

Meadow, K. P. (1968). Early manual communication in relation to the deaf child's intellectual, social and communicative functioning. *American Annals of the Deaf, 113*, 29–41.

Meadow, K. P. (1969). Self-image, family climate and deafness. *Social Forces, 47*, 428–438.

Meadow-Orlans, K. P. (1985, April). *Impact of a child's hearing loss on the family.* Paper presented at the Biennial Meeting of the Society for Research in Child Development, Toronto, Ontario, Canada.

Mendolsohn, B., & Mendolsohn, B. (1986). Families in the transition process: Important partners. In L. Perlman & G. Austin (Eds.), *The transition to work and independence for youth with disabilities* (Report of the Tenth Mary E. Switzer Memorial Seminar, May, 1986). Alexandria, VA: National Rehabilitation Association.

Mindel, E. D., & Vernon, M. (1971). *They grow in silence: The deaf child and his family.* Silver Spring, MD: National Association of the Deaf.

Moores, D. F. (1976). *Educating the deaf: Psychology, principles, and practices.* Boston: Houghton Mifflin.

Murphy, A. T. (1979). The families of handicapped children: Context for disability. *Volta Review, 81*(5), 265–279.

Rawlings, B. W., & Jensema, C. J. (1977). *Two studies of the families of hearing impaired children.* Washington, DC: Gallaudet College, Office of Demographic Studies.

Schein, J. D., & Delk, M. T. (1974). *The deaf population of the United States.* Silver Spring, MD: National Association of the Deaf.

Schlesinger, H. S. (1978). The effects of deafness and childhood development: An Eriksonian perspective. In L. S. Liben (Ed.), *Deaf children: Developmental perspectives.* New York: Academic Press.

Schlesinger, H. S., & Meadow, K. P. (1972). *Sound and sign: Childhood deafness and mental health.* Berkeley, University of California Press.

Schwirian, P. (1976). Effects of the presence of a hearing-impaired preschool child in the family in behavior patterns of older "normal" siblings. *American Annals of the Deaf, 121*, 373–380.

Seligman, M. (1983). Sources of psychological disturbance among siblings of handicapped children. *The Personnel and Guidance Journal, 61*(9), 529–531.

Shontz, F. C. (1965). Reactions to crisis. *The Volta Review, 67,* 364–370.

Stuckless, E. R., & Birch, J. W. (1966). The influence of the early manual communication on the linguistic development of deaf children. *American Annals of the Deaf, 3,* 452–462.

Wallace, G. (1973). *Canadian study of hard of hearing and deaf.* Unpublished manuscript.

Wentworth, E. H. (1974). *Listen to your heart: A message to parents of handicapped children.* Boston: Houghton Mifflin.

Williams, D. M. L., & Darbyshire, J. O. (1982). Diagnosis of deafness: A study of family responses and needs. *The Volta Review, 84*(1), 24–30.

Personal Statement: Mechanisms for Coping with the Disability of a Child— A Mother's Perspective

Janet Miller

PRETRAUMA

Both my husband, Kurt, and I have come from upper-middle-class families of four children; he is the youngest of four boys, and I am the oldest child of my family, with a sister next and then two brothers. Neither of us had anything much more serious to deal with than the deaths of pets and grandparents before our marriage almost 13 years ago. As typical New England Yankees, we were taught stoicism and intellectualization for dealing with emotions undemonstrably. There was a high value on the Protestant work ethic, with work the means of coping with any difficulty; in each household and throughout the environment in which we grew up there has been heavy emphasis on the notion that "you can succeed at anything you want if you work hard enough at it." Emotions that could not be expressed through quiet strength of character were, in general, denied and intellectualized away.

Each of us has also totally compensated for a mild form of disability. Although I remember almost no direct conversations regarding my congenital hearing loss, I was taken regularly to Boston for tests and treatments. Probably before my school years I had taught myself to read lips and stay close to people whose words I wanted to hear. In school I always sat near the front of the class, managing well without undue difficulty. Reading difficulties plagued Kurt during his school years, and he received extensive tutoring and summer help. He, too, was able to succeed in school, intellectually able to fine tune his auditory learning abilities. Although not totally ignoring these problems, we each made a practice of "passing" as normal, choosing instead to work around the difficulties.

At the time of our marriage I was 21.5 years old and Kurt was 29. Our courtship had been a relatively short 10 months. Although we attempted to expand our family shortly after marriage, there were problems. The pregnancy difficulties were the first problems that either of us had really come across that could not be resolved by working harder. Action oriented, we tried all medical possibilities from tests to surgeries, capitalizing on the hope of each. We became closer than most couples, I think, but the closeness was largely nonverbal, in as much as we rarely discussed our disappointments but could see it in each others' faces, especially during the many times in the hospital, sitting quietly, sometimes holding hands. We considered it a sign of strength that we could maintain our optimistic facade, especially with others, even members of our families of origin who visited but were not overly attentive.

The most difficult trial during our early marriage came in January 1973, when I had to have emergency surgery for a ruptured ectopic pregnancy, surgery that ended not only the pregnancy but also our chances for having children at all. Undoubtedly I denied the possibility that I could have lost my own life. No amount of hard work could change our inability to have children, although becoming involved with some part-time tutoring and volunteer projects helped ease the depression I was under for over 2 months. Aware only of a sense of defeat and questions about what to do with my life, I sought no further than Kurt and the doctor for support for my bruised self-esteem. Initiating an adoption did introduce some hope into our lives, but the adoption was delayed for several months during which time we pondered this turn that symbolized the finality of our major defeat. Again we worked at staying busy during the interim of waiting for a child—for who knew how long?

The following fall another pregnancy began against all medical odds. This pregnancy, like the other, got off to a troublesome start, and we didn't dare hope it would continue. The pregnancy did continue, however, without any medical intervention, for which we would later be glad. As each month passed, and we could feel the baby moving, we became more and more sure that our troubles were over. By 7 months we felt as if we were home free, because even babies born that early often survived unscathed, and we went through Lamaze classes together. Those months in the last half of the pregnancy will probably always be remembered as our happiest, closest, and most deliciously carefree—with both of us wrapped up in the event to come.

Beth's delivery was medically unremarkable. For us it was a most remarkable achievement, all the more worthy because we had warded off all anesthesia and even the threatened forceps. Yet even as we congratulated each other and snapped a photo or two in the delivery room, we registered the silence of the staff that came only moments before the doctor told us what he had just discovered: Beth had been born with a meningomyelocele (open spine).

POSTTRAUMA: EARLY COPING MECHANISMS

The obstetrician was kind and gentle, putting his hand on my arm as he told us of the meningomyelocele. He told us nothing more, and my strong biology background registered a thud in the back of my mind but did not connect. All I could ask was whether Beth would be all right, whether she would live, to which I received affirmative answers. On a maternal high, I found the nurses to be annoyingly businesslike and was glad to finally return to my room to make phone calls. Kurt was back with me when we were told the baby would be sent by ambulance to Boston, and even then we assumed that Beth would be hospitalized for whatever was necessary and would come home later fine. The pediatrician arrived and began the jumble of what was to be our initiation into spina bifida. Although I recall that he gave a long description of the many organs and functions affected by the condition, I remember little else except his kindness and brutal honesty. A voice in my head kept repeating, "My baby won't be like that," and I was worrying about Kurt, who had been up all night and was expected to accompany the baby to Boston.

Kurt will never forget that trip to Boston, being asked whether to treat the baby—a decision, really, whether to let her live. He was told she was paralyzed from the waist down, would never walk, and would be retarded if she lived at all—and then he had to return to me to go through it all again. With essentially no guidance from anyone, we were asked to make a decision regarding a child for whom we had waited for 6 years and about a condition we had never heard of until just hours earlier. Neither of us had slept in 36 hours, and we had to decide within another 12. Coming to an agreement was only the first of many extreme difficulties, as we juggled our high value on this child against a future we could not begin to imagine. Beth's back was closed at the age of 24 hours. With this commitment I resolved that if she was to be disabled, at least I would see to it that she maximized every potential.

In those early days we did not cope: We existed. Minute followed minute and crisis followed crisis. We kept up our social life in an effort to maintain some semblance of an old reality, but I found those times dreamlike and irrelevant, because I was unable to think of anything but Beth and us. Kurt appeared to me to be intensely emotional, but he kept it in tight control; it was too big for us to discuss in anything but small snatches. A few times we cried together. I don't remember feeling anything at all, but I once considered writing a poem about a wood chip carried from the mountains to the ocean in a stream, sometimes whirled along, at other times submerged in white water, or circling in an endless eddy.

Our families were in their own shock and did not know how to help. Nor did we know how to ask for help. Our mothers visited Beth and me in the hospital, and I was grateful, especially sensing that they were ill-equipped to deal with the horror stories of others packed in around us at the nursery. I at least had had a medical background and could better understand both the hope and the limits of care given in answer to the insistent beeping of monitors. Meanwhile, our siblings received contradictory misinformation and tended either to minimize or exaggerate the facts of Beth's condition. Many people, family included, came to us with success stories about other children with spina bifida. Although I acknowledged the intent to help with hope, I also made a very conscious effort to put out of my mind these other stories, knowing that Beth was an individual and would be in her own way different from the others. The prognosis for Beth can never by anything more accurate than generally realistic. Somehow I knew this and felt compelled to find our own reality in her individual condition.

Within days of Beth's birth, our entire values system changed abruptly. All issues, problems, questions were related to matters of life and death. Nothing seemed more important than survival. Concurrently, the value we placed on friendship skyrocketed, for there seemed so few people who could even begin to understand what we were going through. We seemed to live at a layer many levels deeper and more vulnerable than ever before and became acutely sensitive, while at the same time attempting an incongruous facade of strength. We learned quickly that others needed to be put at ease with us, because they felt inadequate to help. Most did not know whether to send us a baby gift or flowers for condolence, whereas what was really important to us was that they cared enough to send anything. As time went on, we found, and still find, more and more people with problems of many kinds turning to us for solace, because they now somehow that we have grown sensitive ears.

In her first 18 months Beth had nine operations, including a shunt (and two revisions) for the hydrocephalus that developed at 3 weeks. She was hospitalized once with a severe urinary tract infection, and two or three other times I opted to keep her home and give her injections around the clock to avoid hospitalization. Every 2 weeks she had a different urinary tract infection necessitating a change in medication. We mastered Frejka pillows, splints, ROM (Range-of-Motion) exercises, shunts and their malfunctions, skin care, Crede's ophthalmic method, and later, night casts, a spica cast, glasses, patches, eye drops, suppositories, disimpaction, and intermittent catheterization four to five times daily. I have never ceased to be amazed at what one can learn to consider an ordinary part of life. Part of what was most difficult was keeping track of all the changes. When she first came home at the age of six weeks,

I initially had had little confidence in caring for this small girl. I felt as if she belonged more to the hospital than to us. The staff had been very supportive in teaching me, though, and by the end of the first year I had become quite an expert. My life was lived more moment to moment than day to day, with a motto of, "Tomorrow may not be any better, but at least it'll be different," or, "At least I'll never be bored." Planning even a day in advance was difficult because there were often many changes. But by the end of the first year I had developed a technique I called "putting my worries on hold." I was able to make an observation of impending crisis, set a reasonable time for a new evaluation of the problem, and literally put aside anxiety on the issue until the appointed time and the new information. I would then (1) act, (2) decide it was a false alarm, or (3) go back on hold until the next assessment.

Beth herself was a source of support in that she seemed rarely to actually suffer from any of this. She was a cheery and undemanding baby, very easy to be with except for the demands of her condition. I was determined to "accept" her condition and to avoid foisting my hang-ups on her, and to the extent that even at my worst I have managed to keep her independence in sight as my first priority for her, I have been quite successful in maintaining an attitude of optimism and open honesty.

Kurt, meanwhile, pulled together after the initial weeks into a stable strength. His attitude is generally more pessimistic and fatalistic than my complementary optimist activism. To this day, he starts with the worst possibilities and works toward reality, whereas I look to the most hopeful, backtracking toward reality where we meet minds. Although I do not entirely understand his ability to mentally analyze a problem and work toward a solution alone, I do see that this methods works for him. Says he about problems, "I think about them alone, in the car, uninterrupted, and I break the cycle" of going round and round on the same issue. He, meanwhile, does not entirely understand my need to, as he puts it, "sit around and talk about the same things."

Emotionally speaking the first year was relatively easy, with numbness and denial carrying me along. Little old ladies in stores bolstered me with comments about how cute she was; they could not see the scars and shaved head under the bonnet. There had been a turning point at age 6 months when I had become convinced that Beth would die during a shunt revision. I realized then that nothing, not even her death, could ever erase that she had ever existed—and that if she did die, I would have nothing left but memories of worries and crises. After the operation I was much more able to enjoy her charming personality, which was just beginning to emerge. At 1 year, however, I became increasingly aware of the many differences between her and her peers. Formerly quite competitive, I dropped out of the running altogether, so to speak, in the inevitable mothers' comparisons of height, weight, and developmental milestones. At about 1 year Beth decided to stop eating, something I am told has more to do with a desire to control some part of her life than it has to do with her medical condition. Nevertheless, it has been continually distressing to me to be unable to keep her size above the lines on the charts; even now she barely reaches the third percentile mark. I also began to become more and more resentful of people I considered to be friends who insisted on bragging to me about their seemingly perfect children. My reaction was to cut the conversation short and avoid the subject as much as possible. Still decidedly a people-pleaser, however, I was loath to withdraw from these friends altogether or to confront them.

When Beth was 18 months old she had to have double hip surgery, necessitating use of a spica cast and a Bradford frame for 2 months. Concurrently, Kurt was laid up with what was later diagnosed as a broken back, which could have left him a paraplegic as well. Both were in body casts at the same time. It was then that I began to seriously doubt my ability to continue. We had also just begun Beth's program of intermittent catheterization primarily to avoid what we considered to be destructive surgery on her bladder; even the urologist was skeptical; but although I became tied to the schedule Beth had far fewer infections. More tired than I ever knew was possible, I also felt especially lonely with Kurt's seemingly being someone else when he was on high doses of pain killers. My life seemed to consist of nothing besides nursing duties, and I knew that I was not functioning at all well.

Until this time I had had very little in the way of external support besides medical expertise and some baby-sitters on whom I depended heavily for some time out. Kurt's mother felt that she was too old to take on the responsibilities of Beth's care for any length of time, but offered to pay the $67.50 per day for nursing care if we would take a vacation. We didn't feel we could accept this generous offer and instead went off for 5 days once while Beth was in the hospital. My mother, enjoying the freedom of her new empty nest, said she wanted to help and once took Beth for 4 days during infancy. Mom's reaction has each time been hesitant, but she has looked after Beth for short trips to the store. She has also been quite helpful in accompanying Beth and me to clinics and appointments, which inevitably seem to necessitate carrying large quantities of heavy equipment, food, and baby trappings. Once there, Mom has been especially good at quietly entertaining Beth, enabling me to have less interrupted discussions with the doctors.

When Beth was about 7 months, I had started taking her to an infant-stimulation program run by the state's Department of Mental Hygiene (DMH), which helped me learn constructive ways to play with her. They had a nurse and social worker, but I was never sure of their functions and never capitalized on their resources. Because they felt Beth functioned at a relatively high level, they discouraged me from pursuing respite care through their residential center. Later, when Beth was considered more developmentally delayed than actually retarded, she was not eligible for respite care under DMH. Questions to the state bureaucracy about my own mental health went unanswered. I turned to the Visiting Nurses Association (VNA) but learned that nurses did not baby-sit and homemakers did not catheterize. Even now, 6 and a half years later, we have not found a source of respite care, the service I still consider the most essential.

For the most part we have relied on sitters and continue to do so. Kurt and I have insisted on maintaining our social life, with some time set aside for just the two of us. We have both found it essential to our sanity and to our marriage in spite of financial pressures and hassles in getting sitters. We have had extraordinarily good luck with students in high school or college. I hide nothing from them and describe what is involved to check their reactions before actually training them and putting them to work. For privacy's sake we have insisted on having only girls involved with the catheterization and find that once they have matured a bit beyond their own self-consciousness over puberty, they accept our medical regime easily. Older women, including our mothers, have had a more difficult time accepting the process, and nurses especially (e.g., at school) have had difficulty with the fact that a sterile technique is not necessary. Often the sitters are headed for a career in medicine or education, and their company is especially stimulating, which in turn helps me feel good about leaving.

Through our Lamaze teacher I became involved with an organization of parents of special-needs children. I had, of course, met many other parents of disabled children and had had meaningful conversations at clinics, in hospital corridors, and occasionally on the phone, but there was no sense of continuity with these people who were not otherwise parts of our lives. After a lecture sponsored by Parent to Parent on the subject of birth defects, I discovered a sense of warm, interested, understanding community spirit among the local parents in over an hour of conversation. The parents were as varied as the special needs their children represented. It was exhilarating to be face-to-face with a group of sane people who could cope (something I very much needed to know how to do), people who were just as much in awe of my situation as I was of theirs. It was like a club with horrible dues for membership in exchange for an almost instant bond of intimacy and shared concern for our children. That night friendships started that continue to this day. I would talk to my new friends for hours on the phone, as we shared our most private thoughts, often subjects too touchy even for our spouses, mothers, and closest friends.

Parent to Parent also helped open many doors to worlds of assorted resources. Even though I had since the beginning specialized in becoming an expert on the subjects of spina bifida and hydrocephalus from a medical standpoint, through the parent group I began to learn of consumer services, sources of adaptive equipment and clothing, and helpful hints to facilitate the translation of medical treatment into individual family living. It also felt good to be able to help others in small ways.

Shortly after the body cast episodes, a woman from the church sensed my feelings of being trapped and offered to take care of Beth one full day a week. She convinced me that she really wanted to do this, and she helped me learn to be helped by "allowing" me to pay her. I knew that the small fee I gave her went to the church, but she may never know how many millions it was worth to me to have that one day off a week for the better part of a year. Not only did she take on most of the dreary morning routine, but she also took Beth off on junkets and to play with her older children. For the first time in close to 2 years I had some real time alone in my own house, and it was rejuvenating.

By the time Beth was 2-and-a-half, our lives had stabilized some—with Kurt back on his feet and Beth home for a whole year without hospitalization. We had hired a cleaning woman, I went to an exercise class, and became satisfyingly involved with Parent to Parent, matching clients for phone support. Beth had begun to walk with braces to the waist, and her developmental age was gaining on her chronological age. She and I went weekly to an excellent infant-stimulation program provided through the United Cerebral Palsy Association, and I looked forward to having her in school the next year at a fine, integrated facility whose only drawback was the hour's drive each way. We were ready to expand and got a 6-week-old puppy at least partly to help Beth over her fear of dogs.

Two weeks after getting the puppy, we got a call from the adoption agency telling us that they had a 3-week-old baby girl for us to pick up in 4 days. She was adorable and very much wanted, even so suddenly, but those first months were awfully hectic for me, because Lindsey had her own set of problems: colic from the start, pneumonia requiring hospitalization at the age of 10 weeks, 4 months of incessant crying, and finally a discovery of an allergy to milk that lasted until she was over 2 years old. Actually, now I am glad for these problems because they established immediately a place for Lindsey in our family, which might otherwise have tended to put aside her needs for Beth's, which still seemed so urgent. Always, even during the hardest times, I knew that Lindsey's assertive presence was beneficial to all of us, although I worried about whether she got enough attention. I felt somewhat saddened and slightly cheated that Lindsey and I would never be as intimately involved as Beth and I had been. It was Kurt who helped me see that I was overinvolved with Beth, not that Lindsey was lacking my attention. Both girls were thriving, Beth as the oldest, Lindsey with the attentions of a big sister.

Once I gained some time and the distance that Beth's schooling provided at age 3-and-a-half, I was able to see the enmeshment more clearly. The diluting effect of Lindsey's arrival had been very healthy. I had not been prepared for the sense of responsibility I would feel toward a child, perhaps even an able-bodied one. The enmeshment had been understandably born out of our desires for a child and the realistic needs of this particular one, Beth. Enmeshment was also fostered by the system that taught me the care and treatments. I once realized that I was expected to carry out 9 hours work of assorted treatments per day, while meals, baths, groceries, social life, laundry, and recreation were to come out of the little remaining time. Kurt's role and mine did not change a great deal, but they expanded instead to include more tasks, some of which were traded or shared. Kurt spent many hours each week on the paper work and financial mix-ups of insurance, Handicapped Person plates, taxes, and the like. He could see my enmeshment but was unable to get through to my martyred state. His reasoning, cajoling, and insisting only made me cling the harder to what I considered virtuous conscientiousness.

INTERVENTION: COUNSELING

In spite of the many gains we had made toward the independence of both the girls, I continued to play the role of Wonder Woman. In the inevitable exhaustion my emotions eventually caught up with me, and I was unable to manage them. Angry explosions out of proportion to the situation would surprise me and shock Kurt, Beth, and Lindsey. At other times I was too depressed to remember what medications I had given and too tired to decide what to wear or what to serve for meals. I napped almost every afternoon but still felt too tired to complete the bedtime routine without lying down several times.

I had sought counseling twice before. Both times had been short term and neither had been terribly beneficial, I thought. The first time had been individual counseling back in the days of the body casts. The psychiatrist pursued my unidentified feelings, apparently appalled that I registered no real feelings around such issues as catheterization. In my mind it was something that simply had to be done, something in which feelings were irrelevant. He did, however, succeed in opening the door a crack before we terminated, and I suspected later that my growing awareness of intense feelings was due at least in part to the crack in the floodgates. The second experience with counseling was ostensibly marriage counseling, shortly after Lindsey's arrival, but the majority of the time was spent in discussion of my high expectations of myself and those around me. This woman, a clinical psychologist, helped me to better utilize the services around me, such as asking Kurt to do more child care, hiring more sitters, expecting physical therapy, occupational therapy, and teaching to be taken care of exclusively at school.

By the time Beth was 5 and Lindsey 2-and-a-half, I was mired in depression. My previously optimistic ability to make the most of a hard situation had burned out in negative musings on how badly we would lose this game of life with a disabled child—in spite of all the hard work. To my credit, I knew even then that Beth's disability was far from the whole problem (scapegoating), but I also knew that I needed professional help.

The most significant help came to me through a fine clinical psychologist who worked individually with me, primarily on the issue of self-esteem, helping me to better integrate my thinking with my feelings. From the start he offered me respect, as if I had as much to teach him as he had to teach me, and he responded with compassion and human reactions, from time to time with tears in his eyes. His positive regard for me supported his assumption that I could grow through this, and that, indeed, I already had. I was certain that I had crossed the line into insanity, wishing I could quietly evaporate. He got me an antidepressant, which helped me to go on and see that all of the overwhelming things I was feeling were, even in all their intensity, normal reactions to abnormal circumstances.

I had read many times about grief surrounding the birth of a child with defects, but the literature had not seemed to apply to me. My life certainly included denial, anger, bargaining, depression, and acceptance. But for me these were not milestones on a timeline, but were aspects of every day, sometimes every hour. Furthermore, there was little grief attached to the "expected baby." The grief was tied up in the whole mental picture I had for myself, my family, and our future. Feeling I had failed myself, Kurt, Beth, the family, and even society itself, what I really had lost was my whole sense of self-esteem, which I defined in terms of what I could do. The counselor taught me a whole new perspective on worth and value, one that rested on who I am, not on what I do. From this viewpoint, therefore, failures or disapproval could not change my value as a person.

Crucial to the counseling was my somewhat private but strong faith in God, a faith shared by the counselor but not by Kurt. Rigidly clinging to various misconceptions, I was less able to utilize effectively the resources of my faith. For instance, guilt was not an issue for me intellectually or even spiritually, because I believe in forgiveness. But emotionally I felt I deserved this disaster, not realizing I also had to forgive myself. I learned about peace and pacing as well as about my own human limitations, and I relearned a sense I had had long ago, that there is something to be learned in every situation. Knowing I was doing the best I could under the circumstances, I could let God take over the responsibility for the end results and put aside long-term worries. The counselor helped me gain a perspective, a sense of time with balance and meaning for my life. Contemplating the biblical concept of unconditional love also helped bolster my sense of self-esteem. By the time we terminated, I was able to see myself as a special and unique individual, equipped with my own set of strengths and weaknesses, grown and growing. These gifts could actually be used for the benefit of others, and a future began to form for the first time in 5 years. I had never before seen myself in this light, and it was a monumental turning point for me.

The counseling would undoubtedly have been more beneficial if it had been family counseling, but Kurt saw no need for that, and the girls were too young. Nevertheless, I have come away with a great deal which can almost be translated into skills. I feel now that it is my job as the "family communicator" to teach what I have learned to the rest of the family, big as the job may be. I hope to see each of us gain and maintain a sense of individuality and self-esteem based on who each of us is.

NOW AND LATER

The interaction between the girls has been decidedly normal, although frequently they seem closer than do many sisters, sharing well and being at times surprisingly considerate of each other. Beth's time in school has given me a chance to be with just Lindsey and to delight in her development, which, although less studied than Beth's, has been remarkable in its own right. The two of them fight and squabble like any other siblings and also gang up against us parents as well. If is a loud, irritating nuisance, but I realize a sense of gratefulness that they can be so normal. That each has an effect on the other is clear. In a burst of independence and perhaps competition with her sister, Beth learned to catheterize herself last fall, but tries on occasion to go "like Lindsey" without a catheter. Lindsey in the meantime was very slow in toilet training, and I wondered if she craved the attention Beth got at the toilet. Although I have made a concerted effort to help each view herself as an individual, I am seldom sure of how life looks from their angle. When Lindsey was over 4 and still needing a diaper at night, I took a calculated risk after she asked if Daddy and I were dry at night. I told her that everyone was dry at night unless there was something wrong with them. (Beth was not at home at the time.) She later asked to go through the same conversation again, and she has been dry with few mistakes since.

Beth is currently in her second year of kindergarten at the local elementary school, receiving help in physical therapy, occupational therapy, and learning disabilities outside the classroom. Most of her academics next year in first grade will take place in the resource room. Difficulty with eye-hand coordination makes most self-help skills laborious. Yet she can dress very quickly if she thinks she can get away without braces! The past year she has begun to abstract her self-image and has expressed marked anger at the equipment that still seems to dominate our lives. She has begun to learn to use words instead of shrieks to express frustration. My own role in this area has been difficult because it is so easy to put thoughts in her mind that were not necessarily already there. I have also been careful to direct disability-related anger at the equipment or the spina bifida itself, as opposed to Beth herself. I don't know yet whether she can herself make the distinction. Typically, she said several months ago, "I hate meatballs, applesauce, and myself," paused while my ears pricked up, "I don't know why I said that, Mummy." As casually as I could, I asked her what she didn't like about herself. "Oh," she thought, "casts and braces and catheters and stuff." We talked it out, cried it out, as I tried to help her separate these things from who she is. A few weeks later she asked, "Mummy, how come you always like to talk to me about braces and crutches and spina bifida?" Perception is perhaps Beth's greatest strength, and I knew as I chuckled that I'd been had. Yet it wasn't much later that she said, "You know, Mum, there are some good things about spina bifida. I get lots and lots of extra attention."

Lindsey is in the meantime becoming quite the athlete, and I have wondered how Beth would take to her sister's prowess on bikes, skis and roller skates. Beth has opted to try each to the best of her ability with our help, and since Lindsey's first steps "without anything," Beth has so far been quite proud of her sister. In a thousand little ways, such as grocery shopping (Who rides in the cart? Who walks?), Kurt and I have also had to face Lindsey's passing Beth in abilities, and we are reminded that it is personhood that is important, not ability. With this in mind, I can freely encourage Lindsey's weekly swimming with more enthusiasm than I might otherwise have.

Kurt and I, like Beth and Lindsey, lead parts of our lives together and other parts more separately. We have mustered a united front in house rules and discipline. Now that I have started back to school with the goal of eventually joining the work force, we are more likely to share child care and household chores. Because I spend more time outside the house, Kurt has to do more of these chores. Conversely, I hope in time to provide some income to offset the pressures on Kurt. Although it is still difficult to predict the future for either of our children, we have a hopeful coinciding picture of independence for each. We may be wrong, but we have probably considered most possible outcomes—although we generally put off till later the specifics of our picture. The more I study, the more I come to the comforting conviction that, despite some asynchrony, our family is indeed functional. It is far from perfect, and nothing is ever that simple. However, the strong alliance between Kurt and me, the clear but flexible boundaries, and the healthy dyads in each direction can all help build our coping strength.

These years, although they have frequently been overwhelming, have been a challenge to growth for each of us. Frankly, I am proud of the maturity we have each gained. I become more and more convinced that the lessons most worth learning are also the most painful ones. The pain will undoubtedly continue, but so, too, I think, will the growth.

PART II: Study Questions and Suggested Activities

1. After reading Linda Pelletier's statement, what were the characteristics of Linda's family that both hindered and facilitated her eventual adjustment to her disability?
2. If you have cerebral palsy, how would you want your family involved in your treatment and then your possible rehabilitation?
3. What would be the impact of a child challenged by a disability on your life at this time?
4. Discuss the issues related to the following statement: "A family is better able to cope with a seriously ill child during the early years of marriage."
5. Does the gender of a disabled child make a difference in the response of the family?
6. What are the issues faced by a family that has a child with a congenital anomaly as compared with the issues raised by a disability of sudden onset?
7. An emergency call has been received from a mother with a child being monitored for apnea in the hospital where you work. The clinic nurse who usually takes these calls is not available. The phone is handed to you. What questions do you need to ask in your assessment of the situation?
8. What skills do parents need to live with a child who is on a monitor?
9. What are the issues that distinguish childhood cancer from adult cancer?
10. In what ways may parents support and, conversely, interfere with, a child's efforts to cope with cancer?
11. Explain how the developmental stage of adolescence influences how a teenager with cancer views his or her disease process.
12. What are the factors that place families at *risk* when coping with childhood cancer?
13. Discuss factors that isolate families of children diagnosed with Human Immunodeficiency Virus. How can health care professionals work to overcome the obstacles these families encounter?

14. If your child had HIV infection, would you want the child to attend school in a regular classroom? Why? Why not? Who would you tell?

15. Identify the respite care needs of parents caring for an HIV-infected child. Would they be different if or when the child developed AIDS?

16. List the three primary routes of transmission of HIV, and appropriate at-home steps to reduce the risk of transmission.

17. Why would the diagnosis of deafness in a child bring relief to some parents? Would this relief facilitate parental acceptance of the deaf child? When and how might a feeling of relief interfere with the deaf child's development?

18. Why is it that professionals in the field of deafness have such divergent views on the best way to raise and educate a deaf child? Can these views be reconciled?

19. After reading the personal statement by Janet Miller, what could have been done to assist Janet in meeting the needs of her child, herself, and her family?

III

Emerging Family Issues During Adolescence and Adulthood

Introduction

Adolescence and adulthood are times of change, choice, consequence, as well as transition. As major stages in the normal developmental process, stress, strain, and uncertainty can tax both the emerging person as well as the family system. During this period, children make a major transition from the traditions, security, and structure of the home, and initiate a major interface with a variety of social systems. The success of this interface will prepare young persons to continue on their journeys to adulthood. However, conceptualization of the adolescent experience must attend to the earlier experiences of the child and the impact of the family on the formulation of values, resources, and goals. These earlier experiences are important because they determine how a child sees herself or himself within and outside of the family system. Understanding these earlier experiences are critical when the adolescent is experiencing disability. The goal of this section is to put into context examples of developmental needs, issues, and challenges faced by the adolescent and adult in the family system that has been challenged by illness and disability. In a personal and poignant statement, Robert Neumann, Ph.D., discusses sexuality from the frame of reference of an adolescent coping with not only adolescence and its complexities but also with the stress and uncertainty related to an emergency diagnosis of rheumatoid arthritis. Identified are many important issues concerning sexuality and the disabled adolescent, as well as the process of attempting to resolve some of them.

This personal statement is followed by Chapter 7, "Challenged Adolescents with Spina Bifida," which presents a comprehensive overview of the developmental needs of adolescents and their families when faced with the demands of a congenital anomaly. Written by Allen Johnson, who has personally experienced the process of living with spina bifida, as well as provided professional services to challenged adolescents and their families, this chapter puts into perspective the ongoing process of living with a disability, as well as its consequences and opportunities. Guided by the principle that all family members have a constructive role to play in the family's development, the author details concepts and approaches that can prevent families with a disabled child or adolescent from becoming disabled family systems. The chapter also provides an intervention framework for when helping professionals want to assist families with a disabled adolescent.

One of the most challenging aspects of living with the adolescents is the recognition of their sexual needs, issues, and concerns. This is difficult in the best of circumstances, but there are unique issues that must be attended to when the sexuality of an adolescent is complicated by a disability. In Chapter 8, "Insights and Intervention into the Sexual Needs of the Disabled Adolescent," Sue Bregman and Elaine E. Castles address the special needs of the disabled adolescent, as well as the specific skills needed by parents and helping professionals when working with this population. From their perspectives as a rehabilitation psychologist, a family therapist, and a nurse, the authors discuss many practical approaches, programmatic models, and needed resources.

An ever-present, but often subtle family dynamic is the impact of a handicapped child on adolescent siblings. Until recently, this subject has received little attention. Chapter 9, "The Impact of a Handicapped Child on Adolescent Siblings: Implications for Professional Intervention," by Carol Keydel, highlights the importance of understanding these influences and suggests intervention to create a healthy sibling interaction. The author has had extensive experience in her family practice with this special situation; she stresses those helping approaches that eventually create a family environment conducive for the growth of all its members.

Another major concern of the adolescent or young adult and their family faced with the demands of a disability is the development of delivery systems that facilitate the transition from school to work while creating the opportunity for mutual independence. Because of increased available funding from government and from private sectors, many intervention strategies are being developed to serve this population. But an integral factor in this transition process is the family of the adolescent. This resource, however, has received little attention in both the literature and the delivery of services. In Chapter 10, "Enabling the Family in Supporting Transition from School to Work," Edna Szymanski, David Hershenson, and Paul W. Power explain a model that incorporates the family as an indispensable resource for the process of transition from school to work. Family issues and needs are also identified and many intervention strategies are suggested. The chapter presents an important contribution to the field of special education and vocational rehabilitation when it highlights how the family can be a needed partner in the transitioning process.

Chapter 11, "Family Involvement in Mental Health Interventions for Women with Physical Disabilities," by Kay Harris Kriegsman and Beverly Celotta, identifies the mental health needs of this population and suggests varied interventions to meet these needs. One of the authors of the chapter, Kay Kriegsman, is a rehabilitation psychologist who has a personal perspective on physical disability; she also has extensive experience in assisting women who have disabilities to a more optimal life adjustment. In this chapter, the preparation of families for a more active role in the woman's adjustment process is discussed. All of the information contained in the chapter accentuates one of the book's themes, namely that families have the responsibility to become integrally involved in assisting the disabled or ill person toward rehabilitation goals.

A personal statement by Tosca Appel illustrates the anguish of a teenager challenged by multiple sclerosis. She explains how family dynamics made a difference at critical times in her own adjustment and how changes in family system caused by the aging illness of her parents necessitated her pursuit of an independent living arrangement. As an adolescent, young adult, and as an adult woman, Tosca was not only challenged by multiple sclerosis, but also by the variety of other life experiences that were part of her developmental process.

Part III concludes with discussion questions designed to facilitate further dialogue, thought, and insight into the emerging issues of the challenged adolescent, young adult, adult, and their families.

Personal Statement: Experiencing Sexuality as an Adolescent with Rheumatoid Arthritis

Robert J. Neumann

It was a walk I'd taken many times before, down to the train station of our town in suburban Chicago to watch the sleek yellow Milwaukee Road streamliners pass through. Usually it was nothing for the healthy 12-year-old kid that I was. Just seven or eight shady, tree-lined blocks—but today it felt like miles. With every step my right knee was aching more, feeling more stiff.

My friend Terry was walking along with me. I gritted my teeth against the rising pain and struggled to maintain a steady gait. I didn't want Terry to know. I sensed that this was no ordinary ache, and I feared he would not understand. I was right on both counts.

Finally, I could stand it no longer. "You know, Terry, my right knee's feeling awfully stiff and sore," I said.

Without missing a beat, my horror-film-aficionado friend shot back, "Must be rigor mortis!"

Happily, rigor mortis it wasn't, just rheumatoid arthritis. Yet it would be 5 painful months before I and my family had even the small comfort of that diagnosis. But, in a way, Terry was right: It was the demise of the lifestyle I had known for my entire previous 12 years.

By my 12th birthday, I was just beginning to feel that things were going really well. I enjoyed getting out of the house by taking long rides on my bicycle; the guys were actually beginning to seek me out to play baseball with them; and I was positively ecstatic when my parents allowed me to take my first long-distance train trip all alone to visit an aunt in Pittsburgh.

The arthritis changed all that. Literally within days my right knee became so stiff, swollen, and sore that it was all I could do to hobble from bedroom to bathroom to kitchen. I began seeing a bewildering succession of doctors who could not even arrive at a diagnosis, much less an effective treatment. They hypothesized tuberculosis or cancer of the bone. Their treatments were progressively more drastic—aspiration of the knee, a leg brace, exploratory surgery. None accomplished much more than aggravating the condition physically, and sending me emotionally even deeper into fear and depression. This was the late 1950s, and apparently in those days even the medical profession was less aware that rheumatoid arthritis can and does affect people of all ages, young as well as old.

Early in 1960 I went to the Mayo Clinic, where my arthritis was diagnosed at last, and where more appropriate treatment was prescribed. Nonetheless, even this was not able to halt the progression of the disease to my other joints. First it was my other knee, then my ankles, then my fingers, then my elbows, then my neck, then my hips, then . . . . With a sort of gallows humor, I'd say I had joined the Joint-of-the-Month Club. But behind this facade, I was terrified at how my body was progressively deteriorating before my eyes. Actually, I would avoid seeing it—or letting others see me—as much as possible. I would refuse all invitations to go to the beach or park for fear I would have to wear shorts that would expose my spindly, scarred legs. I would wear hot, long-sleeved shirts on even the most blistering summer days to avoid anyone's seeing my puny arms.

One day, almost by chance, I could avoid it no longer. I caught a good look at myself in a full-length mirror and was appalled at what I saw. I had remembered myself as having an able body. The person I saw looking back at me had a face swollen from high doses of cortisone, hands with unnaturally bent fingers, and legs that could barely support his weight.

I felt devastated. But as I look back on it now, I believe that experience of seeing myself as I really was, was the first step in becoming comfortable with the person I am. Of course, what I did not realize then was that I was a victim, not just of a disease, but of that even more insidious social phenomenon that Beatrice Wright (1983) has identified as the idolization of the normal physique. As a society, we celebrate the body beautiful, the body whole. As Dion, Berscheid, and Walster's (1972) research has demonstrated, we believe that what is beautiful in conventional terms is good, and we equate physical attractiveness with greater intelligence, financial success, and romantic opportunities. Media images of all types reinforce the notion that being young, active, and attractive is the ticket to the good life. Lose that attractiveness, lose that physical perfection, the images imply, and gone as well are the chances for success in love and life. This is definitely not the type of foundation upon which an adolescent's fragile self-concept is likely to develop a solid, confident base.

But, painful as it was, looking at myself in the mirror and seeing myself as I really was, was the prerequisite for self-acceptance. It was acknowledging the physical facts, if not liking them. It was not until years later when I was in graduate school that I attended a seminar given by a marvelous person named Jesse Potter, and came to understand our culture's body-beautiful emphasis is only one way—one narrow, constricting way—of viewing reality. She helped me redefine my experience and understand that a person's attractiveness, a person's value, depends on who one is, not how one appears. Simple as it sounds, for me that was a revelation and a liberation, to realize that in the words of the Velveteen Rabbit (Williams, 1975), "once you are real, you can't be ugly—except to those who don't understand."

If my rheumatoid arthritis was a trauma for me, its effects also extended to stress other members of the family. My mother was a quiet source of support, and preferred to keep her feelings about the disease to herself. Often she would cry alone in her room; she told me this only years later. But nowhere were the effects of the disease more evident than on my father. A traveling salesman with stubborn ways and volatile temperament, my father would frequently return from business trips edgy, angry, and generally out of sorts. This in turn caused me to dread these homecomings, because as an adolescent I had no way of predicting what mood he might be in or what might set him off. It was only after I had moved from home and was employed as a hospital-based psychologist that he felt free enough to tell me how he could do nothing but think of me at home while he was spending those long hours driving the expressways and lonely country roads, worried by how sick I was and frustrated by his own powerlessness to do anything about it. If only he had been able to express those feelings openly and directly 20 years earlier.

One subject my father *was* able to express himself directly on was the topic of education and my future. He put it in his customary unvarnished manner: "Bob, you don't have much of a body. But you got a good mind. If you're going to succeed, you've got to use it." And, as I was growing up, there never was any question I would succeed. It was simply assumed I would do well in school, go on to college, and get well-paid employment. Clearly I internalized these expectations for academic success even more than my father intended. But there is no doubt his high expectations functioned as a self-fulfilling prophecy. In large measure, I owe the Ph.D. behind my name, the jobs I have had, and many of the wonderful people I have met to my father's simple belief that I could and would. And today, when I work with clients, it is a particular frustration to see how many parents needlessly limit their disabled children's life possibilities through well-intentioned but misguided protectionism or realism that lowers expectations for success by focusing on all the problems rather than on the potentials.

During my high school days, my social life was virtually nonexistent. Because I received physical therapy at home in the afternoon and because my stamina was poor in any event, I only attended school until about 1 p.m. This eliminated any possibility of interacting with peers in extracurricular activities. To complicate the situation further, because my life revolved around classes and studying, I routinely received unusually good grades and routinely broke the class curve—much to the animosity of those peers I did interact with. But perhaps most significantly, the school I attended was a Catholic, all-boy high school. This removed me from any contact whatsoever with the female part of the population at a time when my interest was anything but dormant. I literally had only one date, with the daughter of family friends, during my entire four years of high school. This situation bothered me enough that I eventually discussed it with my biology teacher. A layman, he suggested that things would be better when I got to college, a response that was only partially more reassuring and accurate than that of the priests who counseled cold showers when issues like these arose.

These less than satisfying experiences have led me to be a strong advocate of mainstreaming. From one perspective I was fortunate to have experienced a limited form of mainstreaming in an era before the advent of Public Law 94-142. At least the interactions I had with male peers gave me a basic idea of how able-bodied adolescent males view the world. Unfortunately, neither the school authorities nor my parents understood how important it was to ensure that deficits in social skills would not develop through lack of informal, out-of-classroom socialization with male peers and the total lack of contact with any female ones. Meanwhile, I unsuspectingly continued to study and dream of the day I would start college and the active love life I had fantasized about for so long.

Finally, the big day arrived. Armed with a body of knowledge about women derived solely from TV, James Bond movies, and the *Playboy* magazines my younger brother smuggled in, I arrived at a small Midwestern college never dreaming I was, in reality, as green as the lovely pines that graced the campus.

It took only a short while before I noticed my actual accomplishments with women were falling far short, not only of my expectations, but also of the experiences of my friends and acquaintances. Within a few months most of the people I knew—both men and women—had developed ongoing intimate relationships. Everywhere the couples were obvious: sitting together in classes, dining together in the cafeteria, partying together at dances, studying together, walking together, sleeping together. I, on the other hand, became frustratingly adept at performing all these activities alone.

Actually, I was quite good at developing nonsexual friendships with women, especially those who had other boyfriends. I could relate well to them because there was no need for me to do the mating dance, no need for me to call on sociosexual skills I had never learned. These friendships were a mixed blessing. They provided emotional support and the beginning of much-needed learning about the opposite sex. But inevitably there were many poignant moments when my friend would go off to her lover, and I would go off alone.

As unpracticed as I was in picking up social cues, I continually confused friendship and romantic messages when meeting apparently available new women. A poem I wrote at that time unintentionally reflected the confusion:

LOST

I like you
   when we joked and laughed
   'bout people that we knew.

I wanted you
   when you softly said
   that you must have love too.

I love you—
   then you took his hand,
   and oh, I knew, I knew.

It was a depressing pattern. A woman would express an incipient interest; I would misread the cues and respond inappropriately, then feel crushed when the relationship died. Rejection and depression became themes that were only too familiar. I became convinced I was unloveable.

Finally, my roommate Michael decided to do something about the situation. A self-styled ladies' man with the body and bravado of a Greek god, Michael appointed himself my teacher. My first assignment was to read a book he provided me with called *Scoremanship*. Once I had finished the book, Michael proclaimed me ready for field experience. It was late on Friday afternoon, and Michael and I were having an early supper in the cafeteria.

"Bob," he nudged me. "Isn't that that Jane over there you've been wanting to go out with?"

"Yeah," I responded dubiously, looking at a woman several tables from us.

"Well, remember the book. Just go up and ask her to go to a movie tonight."

"Tonight?" I nearly choked. "But it's too late. She's probably got ten dozen things to do."

"Self-defeating talk is unknown to the Scoreman," Michael smiled serenely. "Just go and *do* it!"

Michael would not let me back out, so I figured I had no alternative but go forward and experience my next rejection. Slowly I walked over to her table.

"Oh, hi, Jane!" I said, as if I'd just noticed her. "You know, uh, seeing you here reminds me. I was thinking of going to a movie tonight. Would you like to come?" Listening to myself, I was sure she'd never buy this one.

"Why I'd *love* to!" she enthused. "Pick me up at my dorm in a half hour!"

I could hardly believe it. I rushed back to our table. "My God! She actually said yes. She actually said yes! What do I do now?"

Michael gazed at me with a smile of patient superiority. "You take her to the movie. Then you bring her back to our room. I'll fix everything up. Don't you worry about a thing."

The date itself was fine. The movie was enjoyable, the conversation relaxed and friendly. She even agreed to come back to the room for a drink.

I put the key in the door. As I opened it, I discovered just how much fixing Michael had done. Out billowed clouds of incense. Inside the room, candles everywhere cast their flickering light on *Playboy* magazines that had been artfully strewn about and opened to the most suggestive pages. Clothes and books were piled high on all the furniture except my bed. (So she would have to sit right beside me, Michael later explained.) But the crowning touch came when I noticed that on the night table beside my bed, Michael had arranged a little altar, complete with candles, a small *Playboy* calendar, and an opened package of condoms. I could have died.

Needless to say, seeing all this, Jane instantly developed a headache that required her immediate return to her dorm. After she had set out for her dorm, and though Michael had been trying to be a friend, I was embarrassed and set out to find him and relate my feelings.

Obviously, my role models were not always the most appropriate. And being the only disabled person on that small campus meant I did not have the benefit of interacting with and learning from other disabled peers. Nonetheless, I *was* learning, observing which things I did worked and which did not. Over time, even I could see that I was gradually improving my relationships.

My senior year eventually arrived, and I celebrated my 21st birthday—still without ever having experienced a physical relationship. Chronologically, I had come of age, but emotionally I still felt insecure, lacking the physical experience that symbolized manhood. I assumed my disability was largely to blame, since by then I knew I could develop nonsexual friendships with ease. Increasingly I came to view my virginity as a barrier in need of being surmounted. But this was not just a matter of desire, a stirring of hormones. To me it was also a matter of self-worth and self-esteem. For as long as I was valued by others *only* for my companionship and intelligence, I still was not being related to as a whole person, a person with sexual dimensions as well as emotional, intellectual, and spiritual ones—and I feared for whether I ever would be a whole person.

As it happened, that doubt was soon to be laid to rest in a manner I could never have foreseen. It was a Saturday night and my friend Justin and I had just finished viewing an on-campus theatrical production by the Garrick Players when we encountered Sarah in the foyer. Justin had been friends with her for some time, but I knew her only peripherally from having shared a class or two and an occasional meal in the cafeteria. Generally, Sarah traveled in a different circle than mine. But tonight she was alone, so after some discussion we three agreed it would be fun to drive to town to get a drink.

We stopped at the Nite-N-Gale, a popular campus hangout, and had a couple of glasses of wine. But mostly we just talked. The conversation was good: comfortable and convivial, a pleasant mix of the lighthearted and the more serious. After a while, we headed back to Sarah's room on campus and continued in the same vein. Midnight arrived, and Justin declared himself tired and left for his room, leaving Sarah and me alone.

The conversation turned more serious. She asked me what it was like to live with arthritis. I told her about the Joint-of-the-Month Club and looking in the mirror. She in turn shared some of the hurts she felt in growing up in poverty with parents in ill health. Finally, I noticed it was approaching 2 a.m. "Well, I guess it's time to go," I said.

"You don't sound too wild about it, Bob."

I was surprised she had picked up on a reluctance I thought I was not showing. "Yeah, you're right," I sighed. "It's just that when I get back to the room I'll find Michael there with his girlfriend. It's damn depressing. Hell, I met her before he did! I liked her too!"

For a long second, Sarah just stared at me. Then a smile, warm and tender like I had never before seen, began to cross her face. "Bob, you know you don't *have* to," she said.

I will never forget Sarah, perhaps more than most people will never forget their first. What we shared was physical, but also far more. With her, I did not have to worry about how to handle the issue of my disability because to my astonishment, she did not view my disability as an issue. The mere fact that our relationship was physical confirmed as nothing else could that this, too, was possible. The effect on my self-esteem was tremendous. As a disabled colleague once remarked, "When most of your problems have been on a physical level, it's on the physical level that you're most strongly reassured." That statement has always stayed with me, even though I would amend the thought somewhat. Self-esteem is most enhanced when one's positive expectations converge with the reality of one's experience. Lack one or the other, and the individual suffers. At any rate, I still recall how brilliantly the sun was shining the next day as Sarah and I walked across the campus.

RESOURCES

American Juvenile Arthritis Organization
Arthritis Foundation
1314 Spring Street, NW
Atlanta, GA 30309
(404) 872-7100

REFERENCES

Dion, K., Berscheid, E., & Walster, E. (1972). What is beautiful is good. *Journal of Personality and Social Psychology, 24*, 285–290.

Williams, M. (1975). *The velveteen rabbit.* New York: Avon.

Wright, B. (1983). *Physical disability: A psychosocial approach* (2nd ed). New York: Harper & Row.

7 Challenged Adolescents with Spina Bifida

Allen F. Johnson

In the United States spina bifida cystica is one of the most common and one of the most serious birth defects. It is the major cause of paraplegia in the young child and now surpasses cerebral palsy in incidence rate. The incidence of spina bifida among live births is approximately 2.5 to 2.7 per thousand, or a total of 11,000 births per year. Before 1985, most infants with this condition died in the first weeks of life because no treatment was available (Guiney, Fitzgerald, Blake, & Goldberg, 1986).

Spina bifida denotes a variety of congenital abnormalities. The common denominator is a failure of complete fusion of the spine's vertebral arches. The condition may entail the following: (1) partial or total paralysis of the legs, necessitating surgery and orthopedic appliances; (2) hydrocephalus or retention of fluid in the skull cavity, which may cause retardation; and (3) numerous related congenital abnormalities, such as orthopedic malformations, strabismus and poor eyesight, intestinal abnormalities, partial or total incontinence of bowel and bladder functioning, genitourinary dysfunctions, and other conditions (Clopton, 1981; Matson, 1969).

Today there are some infants with spina bifida who are so severely disabled at birth that even the most heroic surgical interventions cannot ensure their survival. However, a large proportion of children with this condition now have a good chance of survival, and their disabilities can be minimized by surgical intervention, medical management, and a supportive social network. When treated properly most of these children will have normal intelligence and can benefit from a standard education. However, the anomaly can impede the biopsychosocial development of these children (Allum, 1975; Anderson & Spain, 1977; Lorber, 1972; Williamson, 1987).

In the process of conducting research with children and adolescents who have severe physical disabilities as a consequence of being born with the challenge of spina bifida, I began to describe social, psychological, and spiritual aspects of chronic disability in childhood and adolescence (Johnson, 1979a,

1979b, 1980a, 1980b, 1984). I have also explored many routes to adaptation that these young people and their families have found. I have learned that adaptive, developmental routes do exist for severely challenged youngsters, and that the epigenetic development of these persons would be influenced by the adequacy of the parental support provided them. The adequacy of that support appears to be related to many factors, but mainly to the parents' and families' abilities to accept the condition and its manifestations, their psychological health, the special meaning the handicap has for them, the child's constitutional fortitude, and other intrafamilial and socioeconomic influences (Bode, 1980; Myers, Cerone, & Olson, 1981; Nevin & McCubbin, 1981).

Now the literature establishes a framework for understanding what occurs in the interactive process between the parents, siblings, grandparents, and the challenged child (Nevin, 1983; Roberts, 1983; Scheers, Beeker, & Hertogh, 1984), and issues can be identified that have been found to be the most critical for the adolescent with this condition. These issues are: (1) the acceptance of their personhood by others; (2) the integration of their body image and self-concept; (3) their interdependence; (4) their sexual affirmation; and (5) their spiritual awareness. Throughout this chapter, I will refer to disabled individuals as the *challenged* ones to highlight their abilities rather than their disabilities.

I. ACCEPTANCE OF THEIR PERSONHOOD BY OTHERS

Adolescence is a period typified by the search for self-identity, one in which individuals are concerned with how others perceive and accept them. This perception and acceptance by others is complicated for the congenitally challenged adolescent by what I now refer to as *disaphobia*. Disaphobia is defined as that social anxiety, prejudice, and ignorance that able-bodied persons feel toward the challenged child, adolescent, the adult. In turn, this phobic reaction will be felt by the challenged person in one's interaction with the able-bodied majority. The literature highlights the negative impact of disaphobia for both the challenged as well as the able-bodied. Many researchers (Clive, 1982; Dembo, Leviton, & Wright, 1956; Epstein, 1983; Roth, 1982) have commented that society does not value physically challenged persons and their family members. A person whose body differs from the majority has a minority status and, as such, is subject to the social-psychological dynamics that hold for any minority member.

Although being a minority member has its stigmatizing effects, it also can be a positive experience. Because in the past decade the black minority has made positive strides toward equality, the disabled minority has benefited from their progress. Although there is much to be accomplished, because children with a disabling challenge can identify with other minority persons in their struggles and subsequent accomplishments, this identification can be positive for the adolescent's self-identity.

Nevertheless, there is a unique way in which the youngster with a disability is sadly set apart from other minority persons. In every other minority group there are other family members who are themselves minority members who live together within a subgroup of minority persons. For example, typically black children have mothers and fathers who are black as well. They attend a school where they come into daily contact with black classmates, as well as with black role models, such as teachers, cafeteria workers, or bus drivers. However, children with disabilities may not have family members, societal role models, or peers who are themselves disabled. Often children with a specific disability have not met another individual with the same disability while growing up. The resultant feelings of isolation and aloneness these children and their family members experience in this regard are understandable when viewed in this context.

Because of the disaphobic reaction, these challenged adolescents are rejected by peers more often than they are accepted by them. And the times that they do appear to be accepted by their peers, the challenged classmate is placed in the helper-helped position, and is typically the helped individual. Hence, the challenged adolescent is isolated from normal peer interactions because of the uncomfortable feelings that able-bodied peers experience in dealing directly and naturally with the disability itself. Too often the challenged adolescents' environment relates to *them as disability*, rather than to them as an adolescent who just happens to have a disability. Due to this isolation, they may lack the social skills to interact with others, which creates even further isolation. In turn, a lack of social acceptance leads to a lowered feeling of self-esteem.

II. INTEGRATION OF THEIR BODY IMAGE AND SELF-CONCEPT

Closely tied into the acceptance of challenged adolescents by society is their acceptance of themselves. The development of one's adaptive capacities, a realistic self-concept, and a reasonable evaluation of one's capabilities and limitations depends on the earliest formation of one's body image. The body image is that aspect of the self that pertains to the attitudes and experiences involving the body.

Campbell, Hayden, and Davenport (1977), in their study of self-esteem, tested 20 adolescents with spina bifida aged 10 to 18 years, with 20 able-bodied controls matched for age and sex. They found that the able-bodied youngsters had generally better self-concepts than the challenged youngsters. And even among the challenged youngsters, boys displayed more concern for their body image than the girls, but girls showed more emotional disturbance than the boys. Pearson, Carr, and Halliwell (1985), in their research on adolescents with this condition, found that the length of time the children spent in the hospital during their first 6 years of life was negatively associated with their self-concept in adolescence. They stated, "This finding is in accord with the conclusion that early experiences (including parental attitudes and behavior) are crucially related to self-concept" (p. 29). I conclude that the more severely involved adolescent, who must be hospitalized more frequently in those early years, has more difficulty forming a positive body image and, hence, self-concept.

Moreover, society's point of view becomes part of the parents' own attitudes. The power of stigmatization creates feelings of shame, lowered self-worth, and depression, and thus affects the parents' administration of care. This stigmatization is fostered by the taboo against discussing the disability or anyone's feelings about it. As a result, few parents discuss adolescents' inner concerns with them or their siblings. In turn, their feelings of emotional isolation and aloneness add to their feelings of unacceptability, and thus they internalize the social injunctions. This contributes to a downward spiral of low self-esteem, low performance, and poor adjustment to the challenges of the disability and life in general.

Thus, the challenged adolescent is a marginal person, one who may claim partial membership in two worlds but is not completely accepted by either. The adolescent with a moderate handicap, which spina bifida often creates, is marginal both to the nondisabled and to the world of the severely challenged. Their intermediate status creates ambiguity for them as well as their family members, who also are placed in this marginal position. Myerson (1963) stated that "the disabled person lives in two psychological worlds. Like everyone else he lives in the world of the non-disabled majority. He also lives in the special psychological world that his disability creates for him" (p. 42). Fewell and Gelb (1983) point out that the moderately challenged person cannot be sure whether he or she will be treated according to "normal" or "handicapped" expectations in many given situations. For example, adolescents with moderate spina bifida would be uncertain whether the school and classmates would accept them for their normal capabilities or would reject them as fit only for a segregated classroom. The reaction of society to the severely challenged adolescent is much more predictable, in that they will nearly always be rejected by the able-bodied majority (Cowen & Brobrove, 1966).

Parents often cannot assist the challenged adolescent to resolve these feelings of marginality because they too experience uneasiness with regard to the child's marginal status. Fewell and Gelb (1983) found that parents who know the severity of their child's condition cope with the challenges imposed more easily than those where the uncertainty of the condition, because of its moderateness, leaves much to the imagination.

I believe that the use of other body parts and appliances to compensate for lost body functions is an adaptive alternative for achieving the standard developmental goals. Adaptive adolescents learn to supplement leg muscles with braces and crutches, and learn to empty urine from their appliance or to catheterize themselves in place of learning to control internal sphincter muscles. Considering their extensive physical and emotional traumata, these compensations show resilience, determination, and the capacity to take full advantage of opportunities and developmental routes open to them. Thus, I have found that the difference between the able-bodied child and adolescent and the challenged is not one of kind, but one of degree. Spina bifida cystica puts no ceiling on the child's psychosocial development.

Parker (1971) reported a case study of a very adaptive 29-year-old female, Julie, who was born with spina bifida and was often depressed during adolescence. Her depression was tied into her negative body image and sense of self. Because Parker believed that maternal depression is "contagious" to an infant child, Parker concluded that Julie's depressive mood was established during infancy. Parker understood this mood to be somewhat adaptive. Often during adolescence, Julie considered suicide because of her lifelong depression about her physical challenges. Suicide wishes and fantasies served an important function. It gave her a feeling of control over the anticipation of her own passive victimization.

Parker (1971) found that an internalized, positive self-concept can be nurtured by parental love and consistency:

> A grossly distorted body-image cannot help but result in some degree of disturbed character formation and psychopathology. . . . When such internal stability has been created by the maintenance of firm limits in a framework of love and consistency towards the child on the part of both parents, severe ego defects can be greatly mitigated. (p. 320)

I believe that working through the grief process with regard to the disability is crucial for adolescents with spina bifida because it will determine whether they can integrate their negative body image into a more positive self-concept (Bristor, 1984; Bugen, 1980). The grieving process must deal with at least two critical issues: (1) a resolution of the depressive nucleus passed on to the adolescents by their maternal object during childhood, and (2) a resolution of their wish to be "normal" while accepting their differentness from their able-bodied family members and peers. Nevertheless, I believe that acceptance—the final phase of the grieving process—can never completely be attained by congenitally challenged persons nor by their families because each day they must reaccept the condition and its challenges as they occur on that very day.

Adolescence is a time of comparing one's self with one's peers and resolving the differences. Most beneficial in this process for challenged adolescents is to identify personal assets they possess, such as determination, resilience, or cheerfulness, in place of the comparative values, such as wearing the latest fashions. Whereas for the able-bodied this process of comparing themselves with others occurs during adolescence, for the congenitally challenged it begins during latency (Minde, Hachett, Killon, Silver, 1972).

III. THEIR INTERDEPENDENCE

In the literature (Bode, 1980; Dorner, 1976; Fallstrom, 1980; Gerber, 1973; McAnarney, 1984; Oakland & Sherman, 1969; Pearson, et al., 1985), adolescents with a physical disability, particularly those with spina bifida, are viewed as extremely dependent. Wright (1982), in her paper on the interdependence of the challenged individual, states:

> What I am proposing is that the concepts of overprotection, dependency, and interdependence need to be reexamined and that the concept of interdependence be included as an important part of the matrix of satisfying and constructive interpersonal relations. (p. 99)

Wright (1982) explains that, in our culture, dependence is devalued as a sign of immaturity whereas independence is valued as a sign of ability and accomplishment. She defines interdependence as "mutual dependency," and concludes that:

> Until the values of independence, dependence, and interdependence are seen in relationship to each other and as equally important, human relationships must remain distorted. . . . It is then that the balance needed in independent, dependent and interdependent relations can begin to be gauged and adjusted according to our best understanding of growth-promoting opportunities. (p. 103)

The challenged individual of whatever age, consequently, must be assessed in terms of this interdependence continuum, rather than the more standard dependence–independence scale. Many of the typical achievements in development are either delayed or not achievable by the challenged individual, and hence a different set of criteria must be used in this assessment process (Wright, 1982).

Moreover, clinicians may overlook that the prolonged dependence of these children and adolescents frustrates other modes of expressing autonomy. Parents and doctors expect and reward passivity and compliance to facilitate their numerous medical interventions, a process that can be referred to as the making of a patient patient. The limits imposed by their walking difficulties, incontinence, hospitalizations, separations from siblings and friends, and long recoveries do not provide these children with the experience to learn peer roles and behavior styles to replace the deference and dependency behaviors they learn in the role of the chronically challenged child and adolescent. And although adolescents may have some locomotor potential, they may feel the need to control this aggressive, mobile activity because they think the activity is too risky, suggestive of hostility and rebellion (Burlingham, 1961; Eckart, 1987; Johnson, 1980b).

It is to be noted that these adolescents' body images and self-concept are closely tied to the issue of interdependence. For example, they may need assistance with their personal hygiene because of their incontinence. Yet, sensitive parents can promote self-care skills early in their children's lives, so that by the time they reach adolescence they will not need to be assisted to any large extent in toileting. In addition, interdependence is displayed as challenged adolescents read more about their disability, take on responsibility for their medical management, and learn to drive a car (which is a mainstreaming experience).

IV. THEIR SEXUAL AFFIRMATION

Sex and disability are often taboo subjects. Spina bifida does impair the genitourinary system, but sexual functioning can still be present and the genital sensations—limited as they are—may be aroused. In adolescent boys with this condition, 75% can obtain a partial or full erection (Anderson & Newman, 1978; Kaplan, 1974). Yet the uncertainty about sexual functioning for both these male and female adolescents may contribute to even lowered feelings of self-worth. For these adolescents, the genitals are often fraught with a great deal of conflicted feelings, because from an early age the disability has focused negatively on both the genital and anal areas (Comfort, 1978; Johnson, 1980b). Moreover, because of the use of disposable diapers for excretory accidents, adolescents may still feel like a youngster rather than a sexual adolescent. The ideal loop appliance is often considered ugly by adolescents, creating further ambivalence toward the genitourinary area. Moreover, because parents, typically the mother, still may be assisting the adolescent with toileting by washing after excretory accidents or checking for bed sores, physical privacy is lacking. Because of developmental considerations, I recommend that, when the challenged child reaches age 4, the father assist the son with toileting problems and the mother assist the daughter, which can promote their child's feeling of interdependence, as well as gender identity with the parent of the same sex. This interaction with the parent of the same sex also can assist with the adolescent's age-appropriate need for physical privacy, which often is impeded by the disability.

Although parents of the able-bodied are conflicted about their adolescent's sexuality, even more so are parents of the challenged (DeLoach & Greer, 1981). Open communication between the parents and the challenged adolescent is crucial for positive sexual identity. Recognizing how difficult this task is, it is the parents' responsibility to take the initiative in a discussion of sexual issues. Most likely, however, such a discussion will be avoided by both the parents and the adolescents because challenged adolescents typically suppress their feelings about both the disability and their sexuality. Yet Fishman and Fishman (1971), in their study of children with spina bifida, found that open discussion of the abnormality and its manifestations is essential for self-acceptance and positive biopsychosocial development. An openness suggests to them that their anomaly is a legitimate topic of discussion, one not too shameful, not too frightening, not too ugly to talk about. They are permitted to express their fears and frustrations that, if left unexpressed, can grow to fantastic proportions. I have noted that to expect the child to lead in such a discussion is unrealistic (Johnson, 1980a, 1980b, 1984).

Friendship for adolescents of both sexes is a prerequisite for mature intimate relationships during adolescence and beyond. The formation of mature relationships between both sexes is a task of adolescence that is often made difficult because of both the social isolation and the subsequent social immaturity of the challenged adolescent, as well as the disaphobic reaction of the able-bodied. When challenged adolescents have not worked through their grief over the disability, they often attempt to form relationships with more attractive nondisabled peers. Typically, this attempt leaves the adolescent disappointed and with lowered feelings of self-worth.

I have found that challenged adolescents' peer relationships are enhanced when they relate both to challenged individuals like themselves and to able-bodied persons whom society also stigmatize, such as obese adolescents. Assuming that, when challenged adolescents become adults, they will have more egalitarian relationships with a wider range of friends, being friends with other peers challenged by disabling conditions can be beneficial if such peers are positive role models. In addition, relating to adults with a similar disability can be helpful because the challenged adult can be an adaptive role model for both these adolescents and their parents. For example, parents of children and adolescents with spina bifida whom I have seen clinically have expressed the feeling that they began to realize that their child or adolescent had more potential after meeting an adult challenged by spina bifida (Johnson, 1980a, 1980b).

V. THEIR SPIRITUAL AWARENESS

Parents of the challenged, as well as the challenged themselves, often perceive God as being a God of wrath. These individuals then look for reasons in their lives for which they feel they need to be punished by God. An example of such a situation was the case of Paul in my study of children with spina bifida (Johnson, 1980b). His parents blamed God for the defect. They questioned whether, because of a cousin's out-of-wedlock pregnancy, they were given two sons with spina bifida—due to God's anger toward their family. Often parents must live with this anger and the guilt that it entails indefinitely because others, including extended-family members, may frequently reinforce such an idea.

Contrary to this view, I and others (Long, 1986; McCubbin, 1979; Ross, 1984; Tada, 1986; Wheeler, 1980, 1983) have noted that spiritual faith in the present and hope for the future, maintained by these parents and conveyed to the challenged child and adolescent, can be of great value and can give each of them a sense of meaning and purpose to what, at times, appears to be a meaningless and purposeless existence. Because trustworthiness in society often is shaken, moreover, because of the reality of disaphobic reactions toward these challenged families, Erikson's (1959) understanding of the importance of religion and tradition is noteworthy:

> The psychological observer must ask whether or not in any area under observation religion and tradition are living psychological forces creating the kind of faith and conviction which permeates a parent's personality and thus reinforces the child's basic trust in the world's trustworthiness. (p. 64)

Such a psychological force, displayed by these challenged families, makes spirituality an adaptive coping skill rather than a defensive maneuver.

In addition to establishing more spiritual value in life, which can be in itself supportive for these challenged families, the social aspects of church life also can be valuable. Attendance at church functions can assist the challenged adolescent in developing socialization skills. By being involved in these activities, the adolescent forms a more egalitarian relationship with peers in which to practice social skills. Within such a small group setting, one can also begin to practice assertiveness skills, which may be beyond one's capacity in other situations, such as in the larger school system.

In summary, the difference between the emotionally well-adapted challenged adolescent and the one with serious limitations is that the former continues to find various adaptive solutions to the physical, emotional, familial, social, and spiritual crises one experiences; the latter reaches a developmental impasse. Consequently, the poorly adapted adolescent does not experience this sense of wholeness and empowerment within oneself or one's environment. Well-adapted adolescents, however, feel a sense of wholeness and empowerment within themselves, which they share with their parents, siblings, extended-family members, as well as with able-bodied peers and adults in their environment.

IMPLICATIONS FOR SUPPORT SERVICES

Voysey (1975) states that to adapt positively to a disabling condition, parents of the challenged must feel more control, not only over their own lives, but also over the disability itself. Hence, Voysey presents six values on an ideological framework, often experienced in a religious context, that provides this needed sense of control and order. Voysey regards these elements as adaptive because they provide meaning to the disabling condition, and she suggests that helpers convey their importance to these challenged individuals. These elements are (1) the "acceptance of the inevitable," or submission of an individual to the inscrutability of fate; (2) the "partial loss of the taken-for-granted," or the suspension of the belief that life is predictable; (3) the "redefinition of good and evil," or the recognition of other forms of suffering compared to which their own is said to be less; (4) the "discovery of true values," or maintaining a deeper awareness of the moral order in the nature of God, rather than as being in the hands of humankind; (5) the "positive value of suffering," or a means by which individuals earn rewards for the struggles in their lives; and (6) the "positive value of differentness," or an identity that transcends the negative societal norm conferred upon the challenged individual. These values can be shared by these parents with the adolescent, siblings and other family members and thereby bring sense to what appears to be at times a senseless situation.

As a framework for intervention approaches, Schild (1977) identifies five major psychosocial tasks in dealing with the crises that the challenging condition imposes within the family system on the adolescent. These are:

1. Reaffirming the parents' individual self-worth.
2. Promoting the family members' acceptance of the limitations of the disability, which, in turn, involves grieving the loss.
3. Helping adolescents to organize their self-concept by accepting a different, more positive body image.
4. Assisting the family to adjust to the aspects of differentness, including positively coping with social stigma and disaphobia, and
5. Supporting the parents in mastering their parental roles in a way that

does not interfere with the challenged adolescent's normal growth and development or inhibit one's identity as a challenged individual.

Schild (1977) also explains five situational tasks that face these challenged parents. They are (1) obtaining and carrying out treatment; (2) handling medical, financial, and concrete needs, such as transportation; (3) coping with reactions and attitudes of significant others; (4) changing the family lifestyle to accommodate the challenge of the disability and its manifestations; and (5) ensuring access to medical, psychological, and community resources, such as respite care.

An additional step toward the parents' and sibling's adaptive coping is the development of family competence. This can be facilitated by a professional who instills trust in what the parents are attempting to do for the child, who relates to their natural ambivalence about the disability and its manifestations, who is knowledgeable about appropriate developmental tasks unique to the challenged adolescent, and who is aware of each family member's need for information and support. Through nonjudgmental, dynamic listening, the helper should be able to share all types of concerns, thoughts, and feelings that are often unacceptable to either extended-family members or to the public at large. In this atmosphere of acquired confidence, parents can then take risks and perhaps raise their expectations for the challenged member, expectations that are often shattered by the diagnosis and prognosis. Older siblings need also to be included in this development of competence because they are often able to provide acceptance and support, which in turn might promote a higher level of adaptation than was anticipated for their challenged sibling (Kolin, 1971). Such a development of competence will be contagious and, thereby, assist the challenged one to mature while feeling more competent.

Travis (1976), in discussing the psychosocial implications of spina bifida and the clinical issues related to it, recognizes the problem of involving families in supportive casework services. She emphasizes forming a working alliance with parents by providing them with concrete services, such as financial assistance, the acquisition of appliances, and knowledge about the condition. This supportive work, in turn, builds an empathic relationship in which parents can express their doubts, fears, and resentments, and thereby come to a better resolution of these thoughts and feelings.

The good intentions of the helping professional to provide treatment, however, may not be accepted so readily by parents traumatized by the physical, medical, psychosocial, and economic crises involved with a challenged individual. Koop (1983) states, "Even if they have made a commitment to care for their child and give it all the love it needs, they may be overwhelmed by the complexity of our social service delivery system. Society, in a sense, may actually conspire against their humanity" (p. 71). In my clinical work with this population, I have found that it is often the sensitivity of the allied health professional, such as the occupational or physical therapist, and their supportive encouragement that help these overwhelmed parents to seek needed counseling services for themselves and their family (Johnson, 1980a, 1980b).

Frequently, groups that are developed for challenged parents can be of invaluable assistance in relieving their concerns (Dell Orto & Power, 1980; Lasky & Dell Orto, 1979; Meyer, Vadasy, & Fewell, 1985). Clinicians who work with this population underscore the growing need not only for parent groups, but also for groups for the challenged children and adolescents themselves (Lasky & Dell Orto, 1979; Roback, 1984; Schreiber & Feeley, 1965; Wright, 1983), their siblings (Meyer, Vadasy, & Fewell, 1985; Powell, 1986), as well as their extended-family members (Meyer, & Vadasy, 1986; Vadasy, Fewell, & Meyer, 1986). Sweeney (1986), a challenged father, describes his experience in a group by saying, "For me, the . . . group enhances that strength by offering us time to share. My experience, much to my surprise, has provided the support to be braver, stronger, and ultimately a better father. . . . I am talking about a gradual process of healing" (p. 5).

Such a positive outcome in self-help groups for family members who are similarly challenged has been demonstrated as well (Schleifer & Klein, 1986; Sterzin, Woodruff, Carey-Neville, Young, Clabeaux, 1980). Referring the parents to such a group should be made early in the intervention process. I have found that a shared concern provides both strength and insight for the many tasks that must be accomplished if challenged family members are to reach their full potential (Des Jardins, 1980).

A further step toward adaptive coping is identified by Friedman, Chodoff, Mason, and Hamburg (1971) as "shared family mourning," namely, a healthy, adaptive, and mature response to the initial news of chronic illness and disability. Mutual support from family members during the grieving process has been found to be beneficial for the parents, siblings, and extended-family members. When chronic sorrow and mourning are not shared and resolved, they may lead to complications in the family members' ways of relating to the challenged individual (Panides, 1983).

Travis (1976) suggests that, although challenged family members need to express to the helping professional their ambivalent feelings about the condition and the many crises it creates, it should be done at a time when they can understand and accept such emotions without being overwhelmed. Furthermore, parents who receive early supportive services are assisted in burying their feelings to some extent, and hence postpone confronting them and the reality of the child's condition.

When working with challenged families, I have found that the use of the defenses of denial, avoidance, overcompensation, and reaction formation to suppress conflicted feelings about the disability may be adaptive until the shock of the child's, or adolescent's condition and its manifestations can be incorporated into each family member's self-concept. The well-adapted challenged ones may deny their abnormality, their fantasy world may often exclude the defect, and they may use reaction formation against feelings of insecurity and inferiority (Lussier, 1977). Parents and helpers alike can be beneficial in this growth-promoting process by identifying the compensatory skills that the challenged can realistically pursue, such as handicrafts, creative writing, or an interest in raising animals. Moreover, it is important that the helper never confront defenses unless clients—whether they be the parents, child, siblings, or extended-family members—have a more adaptive coping skill with which to replace the defensive maneuver.

The helping professional, therefore, attempts to synthesize for the parents the many divergent biopsychosocial perspectives, recommendations, and procedures necessary for the treatment of the multiply challenged child and adolescent (Panides, 1980; Ratliff, Timberlake, & Jentsch, 1982). Fraiberg (1971) identifies the helper's role as that of an advocate and an interpreter of the experiences, thoughts, feelings, and behaviors. In addressing intervention issues with the challenged child and adolescent, Woods (1975) adds that:

> Assimilation of the defect . . . is a major task in the adjustment process. . . . The child . . . needs to be made aware that while part of his body is different, other parts are available for mastery and he can have emotional experiences common to other individuals. (p. 19)

I believe that the clinician can thereby promote a positive body-self concept within the challenged individual, as well as within the parents and siblings.

Importantly, when intervening with the challenged family and adolescent, Travis (1976) cautions the helper to be realistic about the adolescent's abilities to be autonomous. The young person's wish for independence may be great, but there also may be limitations that should not be underemphasized. Travis notes that emotional immaturity is often associated with inadequate socialization. Therefore, the helper should assist the challenged and their parents to find appropriate avenues for socialization with peers in an attempt to spur further autonomy.

The clinician, moreover, must communicate to the family concrete information not only about the terminology associated with the disability, but also about the child's developmental issues and the sibling's concerns about the condition, as well as about maturational needs. The helper also should be aware of the varied tasks that all children and adolescents must negotiate as they mature, as well as be cognizant of the additional tasks the challenged one must work through as related to the condition itself (Goldberg, 1981).

For example, I believe that a crucial area to focus on is the adolescent's sexuality. Sexologist Ruth Westheimer (1984) says about the professional's discussion of sex with the disabled—whom she refers to as patients—that:

> Human beings are born with a libido and they die with a libido. When health professionals understand this concept and incorporate it into their dealings with patients, they will have made significant progress toward achieving a healthy attitude about sexuality for all people. (p. 530)

In any discussion of sex with the challenged person, the parents, seated together with the adolescent, must differentiate between the sex drive, the sex act, and sexuality. In fact, the sex act may be the only area that is affected by the condition. The drive and the adolescent's sexuality may not be affected at all (Heslinga, 1974; Kaplan, 1974).

It is important to inform these adolescents that one's sexuality must be viewed in the context of an intimate relationship. The parents need to remind the adolescent that romantic sex and sexuality, so prevalent in the mass media, usually last for a relatively short period of time in a relationship between two people, no matter how attractive they are. Concerning the sex drive, self-pleasuring and masturbatory activities are natural for all adolescents. Heslinga (1974) and Westheimer (1983) indicate the importance of self-pleasuring for challenged individuals as a means by which they can achieve sexual fulfillment. Frequently this type of sexual fulfillment may of necessity last an entire lifetime or until they are ready and able to relate to another person on a sexual level rather than on a purely relational level.

What is most critical for these parents to discuss with the adolescent is whether these individuals can be companions. When sex wanes, companionship must remain. A relationship between two people will only survive when there are other things between them that form the basis of their friendship and make each a companion to the partner. That is not to say that sex is not important, but it is to emphasize that the companionship aspect of the relationship must last longer than the hormonal one.

CONCLUSION

U.S. Surgeon General C. Everett Koop (1983) ties together the many complex issues discussed in this chapter when he states, "It is profoundly important for our society that we tend to these issues, and that these children not be forgotten and not pushed aside and that we retain our belief in the strength of the family to absorb whatever life has to offer" (p. 73).

The parents, adolescents, siblings, and extended-family members who have been examined in this chapter are challenged people. With effective interventions, these individuals can adapt well to their many biopsychosocial challenges. In turn, they challenge the able-bodied majority to accept differentness, and thereby to value those that until now have been devalued by society. When will society accept this challenge?

RESOURCES

American Coalition of Citizens
with Disabilities
1345 Connecticut Ave., N.W.
Washington, DC 20036

Association of Mental Health
Practitioners with Disabilities
c/o Adrienne Asch
316 W. 104 St.
New York, NY 10025

The Coalition on Sexuality and
Disability, Inc.
841 Broadway, Suite 205
New York, NY 10003
(212) 242-3900

Division on Physically Handicapped
c/o the Council for Exceptional
Children
1920 Association Drive
Reston, VA 22091

Healing Community
30 E. 29 St., Rm. 200
New York, NY 10016

Information Center for Individuals
with Disabilities
20 Providence St., Rm. 329
Boston, MA 02116
1-800-462-5015

International Association for Pediatric
Social Services, Inc.
6 South Terrace
Auburn, MA 01501
(508) 832-4297

Joni and Friends
P.O. Box 3225
Woodland Hills, CA 91365

National Council on the Handicapped
800 Independence Ave., S.W., Suite 814
Washington, DC 20591

National Information Center
for Handicapped Children and Youth
P.O. Box 1492
Washington, DC 20013

Parentele, Network of Parents &
Friends of Those with Special Needs
5538 No. Pennsylvania St.
Indianapolis, IN 46220

A Positive Approach (magazine serving
the challenged)
CTEC
1600 Malone St., Municipal Airport
Millville, NJ 08332
(609) 327-4040

Rehab Brief
National Institute
of Handicapped Research
Office of Special Education
& Rehabilitative Services
Department of Education
Washington, DC 20202

REFERENCES

Allum, N. (1975). *Spina bifida: The treatment and care of spina bifida children.* London: George Allen & Unwin.

Anderson, E. M., & Newman, B. (1978). *Sex and spina bifida.* London: Association for Spina Bifida & Hydrocephalus.

Anderson, E. M., & Spain, B. (1977). *The child with spina bifida.* London: Methuen.

Bode, B. (1980). Identity crisis in disabled adolescents. *Pediatric Social Work, 1*(2), 47–5.

Bristor, M. W. (1984). The birth of a handicapped child—A holistic model for grieving. *Family Relations, 33,* 24–32.

Bugen, L. A. (1980). Human grief: A model for prediction & intervention. In P. W. Power & A. E. Dell Orto (Eds.), *Role of the family in the rehabilitation of the physically disabled* (pp. 489–501). Baltimore: University Park Press.

Burlingham, D. (1961). Some notes on the development of the blind. In R. Eissler, A. Freud, H. Hartmann, & E. Kris (Eds.), *The psychoanalytic study of the child, XVI,* New York: International Universities Press.

Campbell, M. M., Hayden, P. W., & Davenport, S. L. H. (1977). Psychological adjustment of adolescents with myelodysplasia. *Journal of Youth & Adolescence, 6*(4), 397–407.

Clive, A. (1982). A tale of two prospects for disabled Americans. *Pediatric Social Work, 2*(4), 133–136.

Clopton, N. (1981). *Caring for your child with spina bifida.* Oak Brook, IL: Eterna Press.

Comfort, A. (1978). *Sexual consequences of disability.* Philadelphia: George F. Stickley.

Cowen, E. L., & Brobrove, P. H. (1966). Marginality of disability and adjustment. *Perceptual & Motor Skills, 23,* 869–870.

DeLoach, C., & Greer, B. G. (1981). *Adjustment to severe disability: A metamorphosis.* New York: McGraw-Hill.

Dell Orto, A. E., & Power, P. W. (1980). Physical disabilities and group counseling: A proactive alternative for families of the disabled. In P. W. Power & A. E. Dell Orto (Eds.), *Role of the family in the rehabilitation of the physically disabled* (pp. 419–432). Austin, TX: Pro. Ed.

Dembo, T., Leviton, G. L., & Wright, B. A. (1956). Adjustment to misfortune—a problem of social-psychological rehabilitation. *Artificial Limbs, 3*(2), 4–62.

Des Jardins, C. (1980). *How to get services by being assertive.* Chicago: Coordinating Council for Handicapped Children.

Dorner, S. (1976). Adolescents with spina bifida—how they see their situation. *Archives of Diseases in Childhood, 51,* 439–444.

Eckart, M. L. (1987, February). Study of children with spina bifida. *MSBA News,* pp. 6–7.

Epstein, L. (1983). Short-term treatment in health settings: Issues, concepts, dilemmas. In G. Rosenberg & H. Rehr (Eds.), *Advancing social work practice in the health care field* (pp. 77–106). New York: Haworth Press.

Erikson, E. (1959). The problems of ego identity. *Psychological Issues, 1*(1).

Fallstrom, K. (1980). Psychological problems for children and parents. In A. Martinson (Ed.), *Spina bifida and hydrocephalus: Medical and social problems* (pp. 91–101). Stockholm: International Federation for Hydrocephalus & Spina Bifida.

Fewell, R., & Gelb, S. (1983). Parenting moderately handicapped persons. In M. Seligman (Ed.), *The family with a handicapped child: Understanding & treatment* (pp. 175–202). New York: Grune & Stratton.

Fishman, C., & Fishman, D. B. (1971). Maternal correlates of self-esteem and overall adjustment in children with birth defects. *Child Psychiatry & Human Development, 1*(4), 255–265.

Fraiberg, S., et al. (1971). Behavioral observations of parents anticipating the death of a child. In R. I. Noland (Ed.), *Counseling Parents of the Ill and Handicapped* (pp. 453–480). Springfield, IL: Charles C. Thomas.

Friedman, S. B., Chodoff, P., Mason, J. W., & Hamburg, D. A. (1971). Behavioral observations on parents anticipating the death of a child. In R. L. Noland (Ed.), *Counseling parents of the ill and the handicapped* (pp. 453–480). Springfield, IL: Charles C. Thomas.

Gerber, L. A. (1973). Issues in the psychotherapy of patients with previous successful spina bifida surgery. *Psychiatric Quarterly, 47*(1), 117–123.

Goldberg, R. T. (1981). Toward an understanding of the rehabilitation of the disabled adolescent. *Rehabilitation Literature, 42*(3–4), 66–74.

Guiney, E. J., Fitzgerald, R. J., Blake, N. S., & Goldberg, C. (1986). Status of a group of spina bifida children not managed by early surgery. *Surgery in Infancy & Childhood, 41*(Suppl. 1), 16–17.

Heslinga, K. (1974). *Not made of stone: The sexual problems of handicapped people.* Springfield, IL: Charles C. Thomas.

Johnson, A. F. (1979a). A case study of developmental achievement in latency-aged spina bifida children. *Spina Bifida Therapy, 2*(1), 19–26.

Johnson, A. F. (1979b). *Developmental achievement in latency-aged spina bifida children.* Unpublished doctoral dissertation, School for Social Work, Smith College.

Johnson, A. F. (1980a). Coping with chronic illness in the family: Implications for social work practice. *Pediatric Social Work, 1*(2), 41–46.

Johnson, A. F. (1980b). *Developmental achievement in the child with spina bifida: A spina bifida therapy monograph.* Oak Brook, IL: Eterna Press.

Johnson, A. F. (1984). Psycho-social achievement in the latency-aged child with spina bifida within the family structure. *Surgery in Infancy & Childhood, 39*(Suppl. 11), 138–140.

Kaplan, H. S. (1974). *The new sex therapy: Active treatment of sexual dysfunctions.* New York: Brunner/Mazel.

Kolin, I. S. (1971). Studies of the school-aged child with meningomyelocele: Social & emotional adaptation. *Pediatrics, 78*(6), 1013–1019.

Koop, C. E. (1983). Dealing with modern dilemmas in child health care. *Pediatric Social Work, 3*(3), 69–73.

Lasky, R. G., & Dell Orto, A. E. (1979). *Group counseling and physical disability: A rehabilitation and health care perspective.* North Scituate, MA: Duxbury Press.

Long, J. (1986). *How could God let this happen?* Wheaton, IL: Campus Life Books.

Lorber, J. (1972). *Your child with spina bifida: A practical guide to parents.* London: Association for Spina Bifida & Hydrocephalus.

Lussier, A. (1977). Analysis of a boy with a congenital deformity. In R. Eissler et al. (Eds.), *Physical illness & handicap in childhood* (pp. 195–218). New Haven: Yale University Press.

Matson, D. D. (1969). Spina bifida and myelomeningocele. *Neurosurgery of infancy and childhood* (2nd ed., pp. 5–60). Springfield, IL: Charles C. Thomas.

McAnarney, E. R. (1984). Social maturation: A challenge for handicapped and chronically ill adolescents. *Journal of Adolescent Care, 6*(2), 9–101.

McCubbin, H. (1979). Integrating coping behavior in family stress theory. *Journal on Marriage & Family Therapy*, May, 237–244.

Meyer, D. J., & Vadasy, P. F. (1986). *Grandparent workshops: How to organize workshops for grandparents of children with handicaps.* Seattle: University of Washington Press.

Meyer, D. J., Vadasy, P. F., & Fewell, P. R. (1985). *Living with a brother or sister with special needs: A book for siblings.* Seattle: University of Washington Press.

Minde, K. K., Hackett, J. D., Killon, D., & Silver, S. (1972). How they grow up: 41 physically handicapped children and their families. *American Journal of Psychiatry, 128*(12), 104–110.

Mullins, J. B. (1983). The uses of bibliotherapy in counseling families confronted with handicaps. In M. Seligman (Ed.), *The family with a handicapped child: Understanding and treatment* (pp. 235–260). New York: Grune & Stratton.

Myers, G. J., Cerone, S. B., & Olson, A. L. (1981). *A guide for helping the child with spina bifida.* Springfield, IL: Charles C. Thomas.

Myerson, L. (1963). Somatopsychology of physical disability. In W. Cruickshank (Ed.), *Psychology of exceptional children and youth*, Englewood Cliffs, NJ: Prentice-Hall.

Nevin, R. S. (1983). Assessment and promotion of family coping with stressors of disability. *Pediatric Social Work, 3*(1), 23–30.

Nevin, R. S., & McCubbin, H. I. (1980) Parental coping with physical handicaps: Social policy implications. *Pediatric Social Work, 1*(1), 17–25.

Nevin, R. S., & McCubbin, H. I. (1981) *Families coping with myelomeningocele.* St. Paul: School of Social Work, University of Minnesota.

Oakland, J. A., & Sherman, W. D. (1969, April). *An examination of Erikson's theory from the perspective of a study of congenitally paraplegic children.* Paper presented at the 46th Annual Meeting of the American Orthopsychiatric Association.

Panides, W. (1980). Chronic life-threatening illness in children: A model for pediatric social work practice. *Pediatric Social Work, 1*(3), 53–60.

Panides, W. (1983). Helping parents deal with loss: A psychoanalytic perspective. *Pediatric Social Work, 3*(2), 53–58.

Parker, B. (1971). A case of congenital spina bifida: Imprint of the defect on psychic development. *International Journal of Psychoanalysis, 52*, 307–320.

Pearson, A., Carr, J., & Halliwell, M. (1985). The self concept of adolescents with spina bifida. *Surgery in Infancy & Childhood, 40*(Suppl. 3–4), 27–30.

Powell, T. (1986). Specifically for sibs. *Sibling Information Network Newsletter, 5*(2), 7.

Ratcliff, B. W., Timberlake, E. M., & Jentsch, D. P. (1982). *Social work in hospitals.* Springfield, IL: Charles C. Thomas.

Roback, H. B. (1984). Critical issues in group approaches to disease management. In H. B. Roback (Ed.), *Helping patients and their families cope with medical problems.* San Francisco: Jossey-Bass.

Roberts, C. S. (1983). *Family functioning and the rehabilitation of the child with myelodysplasia.* Oak Brook, IL: Eterna Press.

Ross, B. M. (1984). *Our special child: A guide to successful parenting of handicapped children.* Old Tappan, NJ: Revell.

Roth, W. (1982). Almsgiving in the 1980's: Social, political and policy aspects of being disabled in an able-bodied world. *Pediatric Social Work, 2*(4), 105–110.

Scheers, M. M., Beeker, T. W., & Hertogh, C. M. (1984). Spina bifida: Feelings, opinions and expectations of parents. *Surgery in Infancy & Childhood, 39*(Suppl. 11), 120–121.

Schild, S. (1977). The family of the retarded child. In R. Koch & J. Dobson (Eds.), *The mentally retarded child & his family.* New York: Brunner/Mazel.

Schleifer, M., & Klein, S. (1986). *The disabled child and the family: An exceptional parent reader.* Boston: Exceptional Parent Press.

Schreiber, M., & Feeley, M. (1965). A guided group experience. *Children, 12*, 221–225.

Sterzin, D., et al. (1980). *Parent involvement manual.* Quincy, MA: Project Optimus.

Sweeney, M. (1986). Father concerns: The shared bravery of fathers. *Siblings Information Network Newsletter, 5*(2), 4–5.

Tada, J. E. (1986). *Choices . . . Changes.* Grand Rapids, MI: Zondervan Press.

Travis, G. (1976). *Chronic illness in children: Its impact on child and family.* Stanford, CA: Stanford University Press.

Vadasy, P. F. Fewell, R. R., & Meyer, D. J. (1986). Supporting extended family members' roles: Intergenerational supports provided by grandparents of handicapped children. *Journal of the Division of Early Childhood, 10*(1), 36–44.

Voysey, M. (1975). *A constant burden: The reconstitution of family life.* Boston: Routledge & Kegan Paul.

Westheimer, R. (1983). *Dr. Ruth's guide to good sex.* New York: Warner.

Westheimer, R. (1984). Sex. In A. P. Ruskin (Ed.), *Current therapy in physiatry: Physical medicine and rehabilitation* (pp. 530–535). Philadelphia: Saunders.

Wheeler, B. (1980). *Braces and blessings.* Chappaqua, NY: Christian Herald Books.

Wheeler, B. (1983). *Challenged parenting: A practical handbook for parents of children with handicaps.* Ventura, CA: Regal.

Williamson, G. G. (1987). *Children with spina bifida: Early intervention and preschool programming*. Baltimore: Brookes.

Wright, B. A. (1982). What is wrong with the concept of independence? What will make it right? *Pediatric Social Work, 2*(4), 99–104.

Wright, B. A. (1983). *Physical disability: A psychosocial approach* (2nd ed.). New York: Harper & Row.

Woods, T. L. (1975). Comments on the dynamics and treatment of disfigured children. *Clinical Social Work Journal, 31*(1), 16–23.

8 Insights and Intervention into the Sexual Needs of the Disabled Adolescent

Sue Bregman and Elaine E. Castles

One of the primary developmental tasks for all adolescents is to learn to deal appropriately with their emerging sexuality. These issues of sexuality can be very difficult for families to handle even when their teenager does not have a handicap. When the adolescent child is mentally or physically disabled, parental fears and concerns may be even more intense. Thus, helping handicapped adolescents and their families to deal appropriately with issues of sexual knowledge, behavior, and values can be one of the major tasks confronting an allied health professional who works with this population.

SOCIETAL RESPONSES TO THE SEXUALITY OF PERSONS WITH DISABILITIES

Historically, society has had a difficult time accepting that persons with disabilities are and have the right to be sexual beings. This has been particularly true for mentally retarded persons. In the early part of this century, retarded persons were commonly regarded as "moral morons" who lacked sexual inhibitions or the ability to control their impulses; it was feared that if they were left unsupervised they would commit sexual crimes and reproduce indiscriminately, producing large numbers of mentally retarded offspring. These widespread fears led to mass-institutionalization and passage of compulsory-sterilization laws in many states in the first part of the 20th century. A more recent (and diametrically opposite) theory holds that mentally retarded persons are "eternal children" for whom sexual expression is inappropriate and unnecessary. Because this theory views retarded persons as basically asexual, prohibitions on sexual activity are not seen as causing any real hardship for them.

A similar Peter Pan myth is frequently applied to youngsters who have severe physical disabilities that necessitate extended dependency. Parents often attempt to shield such children from the ordinary unpleasant, unhappy, or difficult events of life. This extended dependency may make it very difficult for society and the family to view physically disabled adolescents and adults as sexual beings who experience the same sexual needs and desires as able-bodied members of society.

Despite these myths, research has shown that, like most young adults, physically disabled and mentally retarded adolescents are concerned about sexual issues and want sexual contact (Heshusius, 1982; Johnson & Kempton, 1981). Furthermore, their attitudes about such topics as masturbation, homosexuality, pre-marital sex, and childbearing are very similar to those of other persons their age (Hall, Morris, & Barker, 1973; Johnson & Kempton, 1981). The great majority of mildly and moderately retarded persons, as well as people with physical disabilities, develop physically in the same way that other persons do and thus have a normal desire for sexual expression (Chipouras, Cornelius, Daniels, & Mahas, 1979; Hall, Morris, & Barker, 1973; Mosier, Grossman, & Dingman, 1962). Finally, many mentally retarded and physically disabled persons marry, and many of these eventually have children. Thus it is evident that to ignore the sexuality of adolescents with disabilities is to ignore a crucial aspect of their lives.

SEXUALITY AND THE MAINSTREAMING AND NORMALIZATION MOVEMENTS

In recent years, workers in the field of rehabilitation have come increasingly to accept the theories of *mainstreaming* and *normalization*. These concepts hold that, to the extent possible, persons with disabilities have the right to live and work in ways similar to those of nonhandicapped persons of the same age. According to this theory, disabled individuals should be able to live in the community, hold jobs, engage in age-appropriate leisure-time activities, and in general be encouraged to participate as fully as possible in normal life. Because the right to appropriate and responsible sexual expression is one of the most basic aspects of adult functioning, normalization theory holds that persons with disabilities have a fundamental right to responsible sexual gratification. It is difficult to find a current author in the field of rehabilitation who does not support sexuality as a basic right of all disabled persons who desire it (de la Cruz & LaVeck, 1973; Johnson & Kempton, 1981; Perske, 1973; Szymanski & Jansen, 1980).

In the area of sex, however, expressed values and actual practice frequently fail to coincide. This is particularly the case with mentally retarded persons.

Studies indicate that there are still a great many persons (parents, direct care workers, and institutional administrators) whose actual practice is to forbid any sort of sexual behavior by the retarded persons under their care (Mitchell, Doctor, & Butler, 1978; Mulhern, 1975; Smith, Valenti-Heim, & Heller, 1985). It appears that the general societal discomfort with sex asserts itself particularly strongly when applied to mentally retarded persons (or indeed, any other "different-from-ordinary" members of society).

SPECIAL PROBLEMS FOR DISABLED ADOLESCENTS IN THE AREA OF SEXUALITY

We strongly agree that people with disabilities have the same sexual needs, rights, and responsibilities as do nondisabled persons. However, it is also true that the nature of the disability creates some special problems that affect the sexual development and behavior of the handicapped teenager. These problems are often a major focus of concern among families who come to professionals for help in dealing with their physically or mentally disabled adolescent.

For example, it is well known that the level of sex education offered even to nondisabled adolescents is abysmal. Teenagers with disabilities have even fewer opportunities for obtaining reliable information about sexuality. Both mentally retarded adolescents and those with severe physical or sensory impairments tend to lack access to the many informal sources of information available to their able-bodied peers (e.g., older and more knowledgeable friends, or the print medium). Research has shown that persons with disabilities particularly lack knowledge about conception, birth control, and venereal disease, the very subjects about which they most need to be informed for their own protection (Edmondson, McCombs, & Wish, 1979; Edmondson & Wish, 1975; Hall, Morris, & Barker, 1973). This lack of appropriate sex education poses an especially difficult problem for retarded adolescents, whose cognitive limitations make direct and explicit instruction about sexuality even more essential than for intellectually normal persons.

Because of the limited lifestyle available to them as a result of emotional, social, and architectural barriers, teenagers with disabilities may have fewer opportunities than their normal age-mates to learn appropriate social behavior through interaction with their peers at discos, libraries, or sporting events. This lack of social experience may leave such youngsters emotionally unprepared for the intimacy and involvement of sexual relationships. Lack of appropriate sex education and social isolation may also lead some adolescents with disabilities to have difficulty in knowing which behaviors are appropriate and which are inappropriate, and in discriminating between public and private situations (Chipouras et al., 1979; Kempton, 1975; Smith,

Valenti-Heim, & Heller, 1985). Because of their cognitive limitations, such discriminations may be particularly difficult for mentally retarded youngsters. This problem is sometimes exacerbated by families who allow their retarded children to be affectionate in age-inappropriate ways (Smith et al., 1985) or by institutions that passively allow behavior (e.g., public masturbation) that is unacceptable in the larger society (Chipouras et al., 1979). Thus, out of ignorance and inappropriate training, persons with disabilities (particularly those who are mentally retarded) may engage in sexual behavior that society finds to be inappropriate, unacceptable, or even frightening.

All adolescents have a need to be liked and to feel that they are accepted by their peers. Because of the social rejection and stigmatization that accompanies disability, this tends to be an even greater problem for youngsters with disabilities than for their able-bodied peers (Abramson, Ash, & Nash, 1979; Chipouras et al., 1979; Greengross, 1976). Many physically disabled youngsters are convinced that their crutches, awkward speech, ostomy surgery, wheelchairs, appliances, and so forth, cause them to be unattractive to others. To compound the problem, individuals adjusting to a new disability (e.g., a traumatic spinal cord injury) might experience a mourning process that interferes with readjustment to the new body image (Chipouras et al., 1979). During the stages of anger and denial, the pain of rejection can be extremely distressing. Embarrassment and shyness may overwhelm newly disabled adolescents, leading them to believe that their able-bodied peers will not want to become friends or to date them. Their search for acceptance and affection, along with naivete and poor social judgment, may lead some persons with disabilities (especially those who are mentally retarded) into situations in which they are sexually exploited. In fact, one of the major concerns expressed by the parents of retarded young women is fear that their daughters will be taken advantage of sexually (Katz, 1968; Kempton, 1975).

Another problem commonly faced by persons with disabilities is that because of social isolation, parental overprotectiveness, and in some cases institutionalization, they frequently lack the opportunity to find appropriate sexual partners. A recent survey done by Castles and Glass (1986) has shown that retarded young persons consider difficulty in finding a girlfriend or boyfriend to be among their most significant social problems. Placement in an institution where residents are generally denied opportunities for sexual contact with members of the opposite sex frequently leads to homosexual behavior in persons whose inclinations might otherwise be heterosexual (Chipouras et al., 1979; Szymanski & Jansen, 1980). Lack of appropriate sexual partners may also occasionally lead a retarded adolescent to seek sex with a younger child (Zetlin & Turner, 1985). It is usually lack of opportunity for appropriate sexual expression, rather than any true sexual deviance, that leads retarded persons into socially unacceptable behaviors.

Finally, most nondisabled adolescents do not require the overt knowledge or consent of their parents in order to develop satisfying sexual lives. Children and parents frequently avoid open value conflicts about issues such as masturbation and premarital sex by means of a tacit agreement whereby parents will simply "not see" behaviors that may be upsetting to them. However, adolescents who have disabilities are frequently less independent, and their parents are much more likely to be aware of their sexual activities. Thus, parents of disabled teenagers may be unable to close their eyes to sexual behaviors about which their own feelings are confused or ambivalent. Furthermore, because marriage is not a realistic option for some very severely disabled persons, their sexual behavior may have to take nonmarital forms, which many persons in our society have difficulty accepting. Because the development of a satisfactory sexual life among persons with severe disabilities may require the active knowledge and consent of their parents or caregivers, the potential for value conflicts is very great.

THE ROLE OF THE ALLIED HEALTH PROFESSIONAL

Parents of adolescents with disabilities are likely to have many concerns about the sexuality of their sons or daughters, and they frequently seek the help of allied health professionals in dealing with these concerns. The assistance that can be offered by the professional falls into three major categories: (1) guidance in obtaining appropriate sex education for the child; (2) assistance in raising the disabled adolescent's self-esteem and increasing opportunities for social interaction; and (3) help for the family in clarifying their own values and in improving communication about sexual issues.

Sex Education

Contrary to popular belief, surveys show that parents of mentally retarded adolescents are almost unanimous in their desire for assistance with sex education (Alcorn, 1974; Hall, Morris, & Barker, 1973; Szymanski & Jansen, 1980). Although they are aware that their children need information about sexual issues, they do not feel competent to provide this instruction themselves; indeed, it appears that, despite their good intentions, parents of disabled children provide very little sex education in the home (Alcorn, 1974; Zetlin & Turner, 1985). In addition, like normal adolescents, because many teenagers with disabilities find it difficult to talk to their parents about sex in these cases, an outside person can be very helpful (Kempton, 1975; Buscaglia, 1975).

Virtually all parents agree that their disabled adolescents need information about the nuts and bolts of sex, including such issues as male and female physical differences, puberty, menstruation, conception, and birth. They must also learn about the responsibilities associated with their sexual activities (e.g., protection from unwanted pregnancy and from sexually transmitted diseases, and avoidance of exploitation). There are now curriculum guides covering these subjects, written specifically for use with mentally retarded persons (e.g., Kempton, 1975) or those with visual impairments (Library for the Blind and Physically Handicapped, 1980). The guides for mentally retarded persons emphasize a number of instructional principles, including the use of very direct language and concrete visual aids, the presentation of small amounts of material at one time, numerous repetitions, and an emphasis on presenting information that is appropriate to the developmental level of the students. The guides developed for visually impaired students make use of braille. In Holland, live models are brought to classrooms so that blind students can actually find out how the opposite sex "looks" in the nude (Dalton, 1977).

It is generally agreed that disabled adolescents need assistance in handling the interpersonal aspects of their sexuality, including skills in establishing appropriate relationships, learning the difference between public and private behavior, and avoiding sexual exploitation. Because of their social isolation and stigmatization, many teenagers with disabilities have not had an opportunity to learn the social conventions associated with sexual behavior in our society. Furthermore, handicapped teenagers may have difficulty in picking up cues from their peers; for example, blind adolescents cannot see the special glance, the sheer blouse, or other sexual symbols. Because of their perceptual difficulties, learning-disabled youngsters may often misinterpret such cues. A number of techniques have been developed to help persons with disabilities deal with these issues, including role playing (Castles & Glass, 1986), assertiveness training (Zisfein & Rosen, 1974), and board games (Foxx, McMorrow, Storey, & Rogers, 1984).

Building Self-Esteem and Social Interaction

Formal sex education is one essential component in helping adolescents with disabilities to deal with their emerging sexuality. However, parents and allied health professionals also need to assist these teenagers in coping with the emotional difficulties that can result from a handicapping condition. For example, hugging, kissing, and caressing are important in the normal development of an individual, both in attitudes toward the self and in attitudes toward others (Chipouras et al., 1979). However, because of their social isolation, many disabled individuals suffer from a deprivation of touching. The hormonal and anatomical changes that occur during puberty make sexual gratification a very salient issue for all teenagers. Mass media, such as films, television, magazines, and newspapers reinforce this need and its importance. Yet because of the stigma associated with their handicaps, disabled adolescents may have a fear of never achieving a satisfactory sexual relationship. "The sex problems that the handicapped face are only different in that for too long society has not credited them with the capacity for falling in and out of love, for feeling sexual urges, for wanting emotional satisfaction, marriage and even children" (Greengross, 1976, p. 4). Such concerns and societal attitudes lead almost inevitably to difficulties with self-esteem.

The media portray the *whole* as being beautiful, and anything less is considered unpleasant and distasteful. This belief system of beauty and perfection expressed by our society is often internalized by the disabled individual, resulting in guilt associated with normal sexual feelings (Buscaglia, 1975; Greengross, 1976). Disabled persons may thus be locked into an unreal image and feel shut off from others. Bowel and bladder dysfunction due to spinal cord injury, ostomy surgery, or related conditions increase self-esteem problems relating to developing bodies and self-image. "The disabled person's first hurdle in overcoming these obstacles is self-deprogramming—rejecting the idea that he or she is not a potentially sexual person and is not loveable by any person" (Mooney, Cole, & Chilgren, 1975, p. 26).

Counselors, allied health professionals and parents need to help adolescents to learn that, although they may be limited by their handicaps, they are still capable of achieving emotional and psychological independence, as well as a full sexual life. This message is conveyed on a day-to-day basis by the attitude the family expresses toward the youngster. This attitude says, "Yes, you have a disability, but you are not disabled. You are capable of doing many things with your life. I believe in your ability to be an independent person. I trust you and will support you." Such families help their youngsters to learn more about themselves, make independent decisions, and develop opportunities to establish satisfying interpersonal relationships.

According to several authors, healthy parental affection, attention, and love help develop in the young person the ability to form positive relationships, a high level of self-esteem, and a sense of confidence and identity (Pinkerton, 1971; Reuter, 1969). When family members are able to do things together and be available to each other, their youngsters will feel comfortable talking about whatever is on their minds. If the young person is able to accept the disability, her self-esteem will have an opportunity to continue to develop. Research findings support this relationship between acceptance of disability and self-esteem (Linkowski & Dunn, 1974), which relates to the young person's body image and sense of autonomy (Rosenberg, 1979).

Clarification of Family Values, Attitudes, and Concerns

Because it is the parent who is usually the primary adult figure to have regular contact with the youngster throughout her growing-up experience, sex education begins in the home. "Children begin learning about sexuality when they are born, from the way they are touched by others, the way their bodies feel to them, what is okay and not okay to do, the words different members use (and do not use) to refer to parts of the body, who hugs whom in what ways, who does what chores, and so on" (Keane, 1984). Parents play an extremely influential role in their child's sexual development and maintenance of self-image. However, the child's disability can inhibit parents from discussing sexual issues. Overprotectiveness, embarrassment, lack of information, and misconceptions all contribute to the avoidance of discussions of sexuality by the parent of a disabled child (Chipouras, Cornelius, Makas, & Daniels, 1982).

Parents are at times shocked when their disabled child displays adult activities such as smoking, having a drink, wanting to get an apartment alone (Chipouras et al., 1982). "Most parents of handicapped children can wish them an education, a job, and a home of their own, but not that their children should find a partner or live a sexual life. Some parents can accept their children having a sexual life, but not the power of reproduction" (Nordquist, 1972, p. 30). Some parents fear that their youngster will have a disabled child and the cycle will be repeated. However, genetic counseling can provide helpful information to assist prospective parents in their plans and, if need be, they can choose not to have children. The prospect of their disabled youngster's having children is a particular concern to parents of mentally retarded adolescents. Although only about 4% of mental retardation is due to genetic factors, the combined effects of heredity and environment lead to a much higher than average incidence of mental retardation among the offspring of retarded parents (Szymanski & Jansen, 1980). If a mentally retarded couple does choose to have children, they will most likely need extensive support from their parents and from community agencies.

With regard to sexuality, straightforward education and information are essential, but this can take the family only so far. At some point, all parents of disabled individuals must confront their attitudes about their own sons and daughters engaging in such behaviors as masturbation, petting, intercourse, and entering marriage. Many professionals in the field now endorse the approach of Gordon (1973), who feels that physically disabled adolescents (as well as those who are mentally retarded) should be given the following information:

1. Masturbation is normal.
2. Sexual behavior should take place in privacy.

3. Sexual activity risks pregnancy.
4. Use birth control unless you are ready to have a baby.
5. Society says you should not have intercourse before the age of 18.
6. Sexual exploitation is not acceptable.
7. Sexual behavior between consenting adults is no one else's business if birth control is used.

Although many parents would also agree with these statements, others may be extremely uncomfortable with this approach. It is not the job of the professional to tell families what their values should be. However, the professional can be helpful in providing parents with realistic information about the sexuality of their children, correcting misconceptions, providing an opportunity for open and honest communication, and assisting families in arriving at a position that is respectful of their own ethical values and of the rights of their adolescents.

COUNSELING TECHNIQUES AND RESOURCES

Counseling the Adolescent Who Has Disabilities

By introducing sexual issues and concerns in interactions with the disabled youngster, the allied health professional is able to provide an atmosphere of permission in which the exploration of these issues is greatly facilitated. When working with the teenager, the interrelationship between self-esteem and sexuality, as well as an appreciation for each individual's unique needs, must constantly be considered.

Youngsters will thrive in a permissive atmosphere where they can express concerns about both the positive and negative aspects of their lives openly, without fear of criticism. Adolescents with disabilities need assistance in sorting out issues relating to real and ideal self-concepts and how they compare themselves to able-bodied peers. Jack Annon (1976) has developed a model of treatment that is very helpful in terms of assisting people with sexual counseling. It is called the PLISSIT model. Annon provides for four levels of approach and each letter or pair of letters designates a suggested method for handling presenting sexual concerns. The four levels are (1) *P*ermission, (2) *L*imited *I*nformation, (3) *S*pecific *S*uggestions, and (4) *I*ntensive *T*herapy. This model may be applied in a variety of settings. A professional may encounter different presenting sexual concerns over a period of time. Depending upon one's setting, profession, and specialty, these problems may represent what one meets in one day, one month, one year, or even during one's professional career. It would be inappropriate to attempt to assess and treat each problem in exactly the same way. The first three levels (or phases) of this model—P, LI, and SS—can be viewed as brief therapy, as contrasted with the fourth level, IT, which is intensive therapy.

The first phase or level of the model is P, which stands for *permission*. During this phase, one informs the patient that sex is important, that it is all right to talk about sexual matters, and that you are available as a resource person. People want to know that what they are experiencing is normal. With permission, patients feel more secure about being able to share their concerns about what they are feeling, thinking, or fantasizing.

The LI stand for *limited information*. In providing limited information, it is important that one do just that—provide "limited" information that is *directly* relevant to the client's concern. There is evidence indicating that presenting a broad range of sexual information has little direct influence on changing a client's problem and can affect significant change in relevant attitudes and behavior (Annon, 1976). Common areas of concern where limited information can be helpful are issues regarding masturbation, sexual frequency and performance, and breast and genital size and shape. By providing limited information, myths about physically disabled people's abilities to have sex also can be dispelled.

The SS stands for *specific suggestions*. In this phase, specific suggestions are provided to the patient. Many times through understanding, reading, and talking, many issues can be resolved. However, if the problem is more complex, the individual may require *intensive therapy* (IT), which can be provided by a sex therapist. When asking questions, remember to ask the least threatening ones first and work your way up to the more threatening ones only if it is appropriate to do so. Do not impose your values regarding sex on people. You have to take the approach that they will respond to you if you go along with their way of thinking.

Often, youngsters want to be heard and understood (the P section of the PLISSIT model) more than anything else. The books mentioned in the Resources section at the end of this chapter should provide enough extra information to fill the LI and some of the SS material.

The allied health professional can help youngsters with physical disabilities to understand that their sex lives are not over, despite disability. Many individuals with a whole variety of disabilities have full and satisfying sexual relationships. There is a great deal of information available about different techniques and alternative positions that may make intercourse possible. Also, intercourse is only one facet of a sexual relationship. Many persons, whether they are disabled or able-bodied, find other forms of sexual expression to be enjoyable. Allied health professionals, as well as doctors, have to be aware of both the wide range of sexual options available to patients and the impact that a positive statement about these options can have on a patient's self-esteem. Adolescents may not be interested in sexual activity at this time in their lives, but it is important that they know that sexuality is a potential part of their life. This will assist them in making plans for the future and in knowing their possibilities. A statement made by one of 31 spinal cord injured persons in a survey on sexual ability conducted by Bregman (1975) summed it up. She said: "Your acrobatic days are over, but it is still fun."

In addition to individual counseling, peer counseling is another option that should be strongly considered because it offers varied opportunities for role modeling. A peer-counseling group can be developed by almost any allied health professional (e.g., social worker, nurse, or occupational therapist). The purpose of the group is to set a context where youngsters can make contact with each other and provide mutual help and understanding of their personal as well as their physical problems and adjustments. The professional serves as a facilitator in these groups—a person who encourages interaction among the group members.

The vocational-rehabilitation counselor or the occupational therapist, assigned to a caseload of 300 clients, will not find the time to serve adequately the sexuality concerns of those patients. But one can provide pamphlets and other publications about sexuality and disability. One can also help to organize a group of clients interested in discussing sexual concerns. A community referral list can be compiled that may be passed on to the clients as well.

Counseling with the Family

It is crucial as well to involve the family of the disabled adolescent in discussions of sexuality. The nurse, occupational therapist, physical therapist, social worker, or whoever is closest to the young person and feels the most comfortable interacting about personal and sexual issues should contact the family and arrange a meeting. This meeting can be in the form of an open forum where the members have an opportunity to talk about any concerns and problems that are on their mind. The health professional's role is that of facilitator and listener. Holding such a meeting one or several times can be extremely helpful. So often families of disabled adolescents feel isolated; they do not know where to turn, are afraid to bother the medical staff, and need advice, help, or sometimes just someone who is willing to listen to their concerns. Such meetings can open the door to a close relationship with the allied health professional and provide a permissive atmosphere in which the patient can feel more comfortable expressing all kinds of concerns, including those having to do with sexuality. Allied health professionals might not have the time to set up such meetings with all families. A way to deal with this is to have family group meetings, where three families meet together for part of the time and then at other times one family meets with the staff member.

The health professional is also in a position to provide an opportunity for family members to make contact with each other so that they may discuss fears, concerns, assumptions, hurt, and anger in a safe environment. Parents may especially need help with a disabled young person who is hostile, withdrawn, and setting up barriers. Defensive young people are often experiencing a loss of power over their lives, which can have a strong bearing on their sexuality and self-image.

Comprehensive Sexual-Counseling Programs

Specific counseling techniques are available for each disability group. For example, at the Bartimeus program (van'T Hooft & Heslinga, 1975)—described in detail in the excellent resource book titled: *Who Cares? A Handbook on Sex Education and Counseling Services for Disabled People*—emphasis is placed on sexual awareness within a residential setting. This program deals with both social and biological aspects of human sexuality. Married supervisors live together in an apartment within the facility, thus providing a "mother" and "father" role. Social interaction with persons of the opposite sex is encouraged. Because the residents are visually impaired, biological information is relayed verbally as well as tactually. Torso models used in medical training are provided to the children during nonschool hours. Other sexuality-related articles such as sanitary napkins, condoms, and birth control pills are also presented for tactual "seeing" by students. This program encourages both group discussions and private conversations with teachers and doctors. Attempts are made to deal openly with both social and biological issues raised by the children.

Another program described in *Who Cares?* is the Illinois Braille and Sight Saving School, where elementary through senior high school students are given formal coeducational sexuality training that utilizes films, tactile life-sized models, and books transcribed into Braille by the school. The major areas of training are interpersonal relationships, self-awareness, and body processes, including reproduction and heredity. Group discussions are encouraged. The sex-education program in this school is considered to be the communal responsibility of all staff members, including teachers, social service providers, supervisors, doctors, and psychologists. There are other programs that are custom-made for specific disability groups, but many program components are similar for all disabilities.

Helping the Allied Professional Feel Comfortable about Sex

The health professional's level of sexual comfort is often a key issue in sexual counseling. Many cities offer Sexual Attitudes Reassessment Seminars (SARS), which provide health professionals with new information, understanding of human sexuality, comfort and knowledge about their own sexuality, sensitivity to sexual concerns of persons with disabilities, and an opportunity to experience a desensitization process with regard to sexual issues. SARS are often sponsored by local universities. Examples of some departments that might offer these seminars at the university level are: family and community development; human sexuality; counseling and personnel; departments of social work, psychiatry, psychology, and the medical schools. Rehabilitation-hospital centers offer SARS in some states. An excellent reference on SARS is *Who Cares? A Handbook on Sex Education and Counseling Services for Disabled People* (Chipouras et al., 1982). The seminars focus on the individual trainee's own experience. This program has been very effective in assisting trainees dispel stereotypes and myths associated with sexuality. This approach can be adapted to use with a wide variety of people. Through the process of desensitization and resensitization, trainees learn to approach the topic of sexuality with a more open-minded attitude. If the health professional is unable to take such a training program, and if there are not other people in the facility who can assist the young person with sexual concerns, there are excellent books available to assist the professional (see reference list).

CONCLUSION

It has been said that "most teenagers feel a jumble of crazy, beautiful, frightening mixed-up emotions" (Bell, 1980, p. 133). Adolescents are full of conflicting feelings. On the one hand they want to grow up, and on the other hand they are frightened of the future. With a disability, the future is a difficult and at times overwhelming road on which to travel. There has to be a delicate balance between helping youngsters adjust to the disability and encouraging them to take risks. With the support and respect of understanding counselors, health professionals, and parents who are available but are also willing to allow the youngster to take the necessary risks, that road can be smoother.

RESOURCES

Short Term Counseling of Sexual Concerns: A self instructional manual (1982). T. Beresford, G. Beresford & J. Mogul. Planned Parenthood of Maryland, 610 N. Howard Street, Baltimore, MD 21201.

This is an excellent manual to use with physically disabled youth who need to have some vital questions answered with regard to their sexual needs and concerns. The manual is designed to assist helping professionals in responding to sexual questions, concerns and problems raised by their clients. A knowledge of basic counseling skills on the part of the reader is assumed.

Sexuality and the Spinal Cord Injured Woman (1975). Sue Bregman. Sister Kenny Institute, Minneapolis, MI.

This booklet describes interviews with 31 spinal cord injured women focusing on sexual adjustment and social development. It can be extremely helpful to the new female spinal injured individual who is seeking information about sexuality.

Sexuality and Physical Disability Personal Perspectives (1981). Edited by D. G. Bullard and S. E. Knight. C. V. Mosby Company, 111830 Westline Industrial Drive, St. Louis, MO 63141.

Who Cares? A Handbook on Sex Education and Counseling Services for Disabled People (2nd edition) (1982). D. A. Cornelius, S. Chipouras, E. Makas, and S. M. Daniels, University Park Press, Baltimore.

This handbook is organized into sections providing the reader with information and resources (including films, tapes, books and training programs) for a variety of physical disabilities and mental retardation.

The Regional Rehabilitation Research Institute on Attitudinal, Legal and Leisure Barriers has developed many excellent and highly usable publications to address issues concerning sexuality and disability.

Write to: Rehabilitation Research Institute, George Washington University, T-605 Academic Center, Washington, DC 20052.

For mentally retarded adolescents, Sol Gordon and Roger Conant provide excellent, inexpensive comic books on sex, love, V.D., birth control, etc.

Write to: Ed. U. Press, 123 Fourth St., N.W., Charlottesville, VA 22901.

For information on sexuality and visual disabilities, there are books available on cassette tape and in braille.

Write to: Library for the Blind and Physically Handicapped, 919 Walnut Street, Philadelphia, PA 19107. Phone (215) WA5-3213.

Family Planning Services for Disabled People (1980). The Department of Human and Health Services. Available from the National Clearinghouse for Family Planning Information, P.O. Box 2225, Rockville, MD 20852.

A manual for service providers offering information on a large variety of disabilities and mental retardation. Topics covered are: Contraceptive methods choice broken down by disability, counseling laboratory procedures, patient education, staff training, community outreach, architectural access, and medical aspects of specific disabilities.

The Source Book for the Disabled (1979). Edited by Glorya Hale and available through Paddington Press, Ltd., New York, distributed by Grosset and Dunlap.

An illustrated guide to easier more independent living for physically disabled people, their families and friends, provides a section which addresses sexual issues.

Sex Education for Persons with Disabilities that Hinder Learning – A Teacher's Guide by Winifred Kempton. Order from Planned Parenthood of Southeastern Pennsylvania.

An excellent book for both mentally retarded individuals and developmentally disabled people.

Sexual Counseling for Ostomates (1980). E. A. Shipes and S. T. Lehr. Charles C. Thomas, Springfield, IL.

For youngsters who are dealing with adjustment to ostomy surgery (colostomies, urostomies, ileostomies). This is a resource book for Health Care Professionals.

REFERENCES

Abramson, M., Ash, M. J., & Nash, W. R. (1979). Handicapped adolescents: A time for reflection. *Adolescence, 14*, 557–566.

Alcorn, D. A. (1974). Parental views on sexual development and education of the trainable mentally retarded. *Journal of Special Education, 8*, 119–130.

Annon, J. S. (1976). *The Behavioral treatment of sexual problems: Brief therapy*. New York: Harper & Row.

Bell, R. (1980). *Changing bodies, changing lives*. New York: Random House.

Bregman, S. (1975). *Sexuality and the spinal cord injured woman*. Minneapolis, MN: Sister Kenny Institute.

Buscaglia, L. (1975). *The disabled and their parents: A counseling challenge.* Thorofare, NJ: Charles B. Slack.

Campling, J. (Ed.). (1981). *Images of ourselves, women with disabilities talking.* London: Routeledge & Kegan Paul.

Castles, E. E., & Glass, C. R. (1986). The empirical generation of measures of social competence for mentally retarded adults. *Behavioral Assessment, 8*(4).

Chipouras, S., Cornelius, D., Daniels, S. M., & Makas, E. (1979). *Who cares? A handbook on sex education and counseling services for disabled people.* Washington, DC: George Washington University Press.

Dalton, J. (1977, July). Sexual and menstrual problems in the blind. *Israel Rehabilitation Annual, Special Issue on Sex and the Disabled, 14,* 89–91.

de la Cruz, F., & LaVeck, G. (Eds.). (1973). Human sexuality and the mentally retarded. New York: Brunner/Mazel.

Edmondson, B., McCombs, K., & Wish,, J. (1979). What retarded adults believe about sex. *American Journal of Mental Deficiency, 84,* 11–18.

Edmondson, B., & Wish, W. J. (1975). Sex knowledge and attitudes of mentally retarded males. *American Journal of Mental Deficiency, 80,* 172–179.

Foxx, R. M., McMorrow, M. J., Storey, K., & Rogers, B. M. (1984). Teaching social/sexual skills to mentally retarded adults. *American Journal of Mental Deficiency, 89,* 9–15.

Gordon, S. (1973). Sex education for neglected youth: Retarded, handicapped, emotionally disturbed, and learning disabled. In N. Scituati (Ed.), *The sexual adolescent.* Duxbury Press.

Greengross, W. (1976). *Entitled to love.* London: Malaby.

Hall, J. E., Morris, H. L., & Barker, H. R. (1973). Sexual knowledge and attitudes of mentally retarded adolescents. *American Journal of Mental Deficiency, 77,* 706–709.

Heshusius, L. (1982). Sexuality, intimacy, and persons we label mentally retarded: What they think—What we think. *Mental Retardation, 20,* 166–169.

Johnson, W. R., & Kempton, W. (1981). *Sex education and counseling of special groups.* Springfield, IL: Charles C. Thomas.

Katz, E. (1968). *The adult mentally retarded in the community.* Springfield, IL: Charles C. Thomas.

Kempton, W. (1975). *Sex education for persons with disabilities that hinder learning: A teacher's guide.* Philadelphia: Planned Parenthood of Southeastern Pennsylvania.

Library for the Blind and Physically Handicapped (1980, May). *Sexuality and visual disabilities.* Philadelphia: Author.

Linkowski, D. C., & Dunn, M. A. (1974). Self-concept and acceptance of disability. *Rehabilitation Counseling Bulletin, 14,* 28–32.

Mitchell, L., Doctor, R. M., & Butler, D. C. (1978). Attitudes of caretakers toward the sexual behavior of mentally retarded persons. *American Journal of Mental Deficiency, 83,* 289–296.

Mooney, T. O., Cole, T. M., & Chilgren, R. A. (1975). *Sexual options for paraplegics and quadriplegics.* Boston: Little, Brown.

Mosier, H. D., Grossman, H. G., & Dingman, H. F. (1962). Secondary sex development in mentally deficient individuals. *Child Development, 33*, 273–286.

Mulhern, T. J. (1975). Survey of reported sexual behavior and policies characterizing residential facilities for retarded citizens. *American Journal of Mental Deficiency, 79*, 670–673.

Nordquist, I. (1972). *Life together, the situation of the handicapped.* Stockholm, Sweden: E. Olofssons Boktryckeri AB.

Perske, R. (1973). About sexual development: An attempt to be human with the mentally retarded. *Mental Retardation, 11*(1), 6–8.

Pinkerton, P. (1971). The psychomatic approach in child psychiatry. In J. G. Howells (Ed.), *Modern perspectives in child psychiatry* (Vol. 1, pp. 306–335). New York: Brunner/Mazel.

Reuter, M. W. (1969). The father-son relationship and the personality adjustment of the late adolescent male. *Dissertation Abstracts International, 70*, 5237.

Rosenberg, M. (1979). *Conceiving the self.* New York: Basic Books.

Smith, D. C., Valenti-Heim, D., & Heller, T. (1985). Interpersonal competence and community adjustment of retarded adults. In M. Sigman (Ed.), *Children with emotional disorders and developmental disabilities* (71–94). New York: Grune & Stratton.

Szymanski, L. S., & Jansen, P. E. (1980). Assessment of sexuality and sexual vulnerability of retarded persons. In L. S. Szymanski & P. E. Tanquay (Eds.), *Emotional disorders of mentally retarded persons* (pp. 112–125). Baltimore: University Park Press.

van'T Hooft, F., & Heslinga, K. (1975). Sex education of blind-born children. In F. van'T Hooft & K. Heslinga (Eds.), *Sex education for the visually handicapped in schools and agencies—Selected papers* (pp. 1–7). New York: American Foundation for the Blind.

Zetlin, A. G., & Turner, J. L. (1985). Transition from adolescence to adulthood: Perspectives of mentally retarded individuals and their families. *American Journal of Mental Deficiency, 89*, 570–579.

Zisfein, L., & Rosen, M. (1974). Effects of a personal adjustment training group counseling program. *Mental Retardation, 12*(3), 50–53.

9 The Impact of a Handicapped Child on Adolescent Siblings: Implications for Professional Intervention

Carol Keydel

One of the most complex of the developmental stages is adolescence, and certain aspects of adolescence are complicated by the presence of a handicapped sibling. Until recently, little had been written about the effect on nondisabled siblings of having a handicapped brother or sister in the family, and there is currently little if any research that examines the differential effects of a handicapped sibling on the various developmental stages of the normal siblings. Interest in exploring this topic was generated by a meeting I attended in which mothers with both retarded and normal children discussed the problems they encountered in their children's relationships. A common theme that emerged was their awareness of an exacerbation of negative feelings toward the retarded child as the normal siblings approached adolescence. Several mothers remarked that prior to adolescence, negative responses were minimal. One mother astutely added that the relationships between her normal siblings became more estranged and conflictual as they entered the adolescent years, and she wondered if this negativism was not an attitude that was normal and expected in adolescence. She agreed, nonetheless, that the impact of her retarded child on her adolescent siblings was problematic.

In order to understand this issue, it is essential to provide a perspective that can explain why the adolescent may be threatened by the disabled sibling. Although the focus of this chapter is the effect of handicapped children on nonhandicapped adolescent siblings, the underlying concern is the well-being of the total family as well as of the disabled family member. It is from this perspective that the chapter discusses how nondisabled siblings are affected by the disabling experience. The chapter concludes with suggestions for intervention to create a healthy sibling interaction that can be a rewarding and positive experience for both disabled and nondisabled siblings. Thus, this chapter will first examine the normal developmental tasks of the adolescent and then discuss how the disabled sibling might affect their accomplishment. The resources used will include relevant literature and research as well as interview material gathered from the meeting with the previously mentioned mothers' group. Additional resource material is from interviews with nondisabled adolescents who have handicapped siblings.

THE NEEDS AND TASKS OF ADOLESCENCE

It is well established that a major task of the adolescent is to establish an ego identity. Erikson (1963), in *Childhood and Society*, describes this as a developmental crisis that is neither fatal nor pathological, but rather a turning point that is unavoidable and may be resolved by integrating various roles; the lack of a resolution will result in role confusion (Maier, 1978). Adolescence is a time of tremendous physical, emotional, and social change; the changes are both welcome and disturbing. Physiologically, adolescence is a period of body growth that is equal in rate to that of early childhood. Whatever trust adolescents previously established in their physical capabilities is temporarily shaken. They look to their peers for assurance and affirmation regarding their body image. Part of the body image is the addition of genital maturity and, particularly significant for this discussion, a sense of reproductive capability.

Emotionally, adolescents are beginning to separate from the adults upon whom they were previously dependent. There is a return to the original doubt regarding the trustworthiness of the training adults (Maier, 1978). It is the normal task of the adolescent to move from the exclusive commitment of the family group to membership in the larger community beyond the family. Separation is characterized by a struggle for power and frequently involves rebellion against parental rules with which the child has complied. This struggle may include behavior changes particularly significant for the interaction between the normal child and the handicapped sibling. If the family communication is satisfactory before the child becomes an adolescent, it usually becomes less open and more selective during this period. It is important to keep in mind that many of the changes that appear to be negative are the normal adolescent's attempts to establish a separate identity. Socially, adolescents must integrate various roles and begin to establish a place for themselves in society. The future becomes an imminent reality and the choices available are vast. It becomes imperative that they achieve a sense of skills mastery for future interpersonal relationships and for the work that they will ultimately choose to do as adults. The search for identity is a search for certainty, security, wholeness, and competence. Adolescents begin to prepare for the day when they will move from the family arena into their own emotional, social, and occupational arena.

Before discussing the impact of the handicapped child on the adolescent sibling's socioemotional development, it is essential to mention the developmental task of the family in the adolescent socialization process. In a functional family system, adolescent children are aided by the parents in the process of emancipation (Goldenberg & Goldenberg, 1980). They are helped to undertake more lasting peer relationships so that they may ultimately establish their own family and be an independent member of the larger society. Despite the adolescent's increased desire for privacy and exclusivity, the family must maintain good, clear communication channels. In a functional family system, the reciprocity of effect is recognized by the family members. In other words, family members acknowledge their effect on each other, even when one or more members are disabled. Any discussion of impact and intervention must consider the influence of the family environment as a factor in sibling interaction and developmental adaptation (Vadasy, Fewell, Meyer, & Schell, 1984).

Impact of a Handicapped Child on Adolescent Siblings

Most research on the impact of the handicapped child on siblings has focused on the correlation between demographic characteristics and impact. For example, a number of studies (Breslau, Weitzman, & Messenger, 1981; Cleveland & Miller, 1977; Farber, 1960; Farber & Jenne, 1963; Graliker, Fishler, & Koch, 1962; Grossman, 1972; McCallum, 1981; Miller, 1974) have dealt with individual characteristics of siblings, such as age, sex, birth order, socioeconomic status (SES), and have related these to differential impact. None of these researchers has looked at the effects on developmental tasks of the sibling and, in particular, the effect on identity formation and emancipation in the adolescent sibling. Furthemore, little has been done to examine the correlation between the function of the family interactional network and the adaptation of the adolescent sibling.

One recent investigation conducted by Wasserman (1983) identified the needs of siblings with retarded brothers and sisters. Wasserman (1983) examined the material that Grossman (1972), and that Schreiber and Freely (1965), had obtained from the self-reports of the adolescents in two discussion groups; she organized the information into four areas of need: (1) the need for information; (2) the need to understand and work through emotional reactions; (3) the need for self-identity and distinct roles; and (4) the need for effective coping strategies. All these needs have significance for the adolescent task of establishing an identity separate from the family and moving toward emancipation.

Having a disabled sibling appears to create considerable confusion about one's own identity. According to Helen Featherstone (1981), a few common themes run through children's responses to their sibling's disabilities: embarrassment, identification, and confusion. These themes are sibling rather than parental themes. Very young children express confusion about the cause of the disability and the fear of catching it. As they grow older, the nature of their reactions changes. Older children report that their sibling's disability compromises their own normality and sets them apart from normal peers.

For the adolescents who are struggling with their physiological changes, body image becomes a matter of tremendous concern. Grossman (1972) reported that the adolescents (college students) who had retarded siblings had real anxieties about their similarities to these siblings. Some even expressed the irrational fear that they might also be retarded. Identification with retarded siblings was a major component in the embarrassment reported by the adolescents in Grossman's groups. In particular, those students with retarded siblings of the same sex expressed considerable embarrassment. A critical and sensitive need in the adolescent's identity search is the need to feel sexually and reproductively normal. Having a disabled sibling raises terrifying and frequently realistic doubts about one's potential for having normal children. If the disability is hereditary, this may have a significant impact on dating relationships. One mother in the mothers' group attempted to allay her daughter's anxieties about how boyfriends would react to the knowledge that she might also bear a retarded child by pointing out that whoever married her would be a very special person. The mother of 15-year-old Deborah, whose older sister Lisa is retarded, reassured her that when she was ready to have children she could have a genetic evaluation. Neither of these two responses could possibly relieve the doubts that these adolescents have, and although they are well-intentioned, both responses reveal parental discomfort with their children's fears.

A very important outlet for overcoming doubts about identity is the adolescent's acceptance into and identity with the peer group. Having a disabled sibling is a difference that sets adolescents apart from their peers and makes the task of establishing an identity that is separate from the family much more difficult. Featherstone (1981, p. 148) quotes one young woman: "All the members of my family are disabled, but most people recognize only the disability of my deaf sister" (p. 148). The picture is further complicated because adolescents are uncomfortable with and intolerant of differences. The mothers in the mothers' group expressed the concern that when their children reached their teens, they stopped bringing their friends to the house; and when friends did come, they were uncomfortable around the disabled sibling. This frequently puts the normal siblings in a position of divided loyalty, in which they are embarrassed by and sensitive to their friends' discomfort on the one hand, and protective toward their disabled sibling on the other. The adolescents' feelings may be misinterpreted by family and friends who see their reluctance to include the sibling as rejection. An alternative explanation for excluding her disabled sibling, Wendy, was given by 16-year-old Jennifer when she was interviewed by the author:

> The reason I don't take Wendy along is because when I go places, I'm afraid I'll get angry when kids stare at her or make fun of her. I might lose control and say something which I'll be embarrassed about afterward.

Normal siblings are hurt and angered by the rejection of their disabled sibling, which, in a real sense, is a rejection of themselves.

For many siblings, in particular those with disabled brothers and sisters who will never be totally independent of the help of family members, the thought of true emancipation from the family may seem an impossible task. Of the adolescents interviewed by this author, all anticipated that they and their other well siblings would be responsible for their disabled siblings when their parents were no longer able to care for them. When asked if financial arrangements had been made for that eventuality, all but one had never specifically asked their parents about it. In this small sample, none of the adolescents expected to ever be completely free from responsibility for their disabled sibling but had neither confirmed nor negated the assumption. The literature supports the observation that in many families, the disabled sibling's future is not explicitly discussed among its members. In addition, in younger siblings, there is the feeling that the disabled sibling will always be a part of their lives because there has never been a time that they can remember not having a disabled sibling. In the previously mentioned interview, Jennifer contrasted her experience with her mother's when she said, "She has had 25 years without Wendy and I've had none."

One of the important aids for coping with a stressful circumstance is having accurate information about it. Unfortunately, many adolescents struggle with inadequate or distorted information about their handicapped sibling. All the subjects in Grossman's (1972) group reported a surprising lack of information and a great deal of confusion about the manifestations and limitations of their sibling's disabilities, In addition to a lack of information, many of the students did not feel that they had ever understood or worked through their emotional reactions to their disabled siblings. In many families, for various reasons, siblings do not feel that it is permissible to express their feelings of embarrassment, resentment, and, in some cases, hatred toward the disabled sibling. Grossman (1972) found that many of the students in her groups felt guilty about their own health and normalcy, and even more guilty about their negative feelings toward their disabled siblings. The guilt stems most often from their perception that their parents would not be able to tolerate these feelings. Unfortunately, this perception is often correct.

FAMILY FACTORS THAT CONTRIBUTE TO THE IMPACT

Parents may unwittingly prohibit the adolescent's self-disclosure. From her perspective as the mother of a disabled child, Featherstone (1981) discusses some of the needs that cause parents to discourage their normal offsprings' expressions. The parents are emotionally invested in the physical and emotional health of their normal children because it makes them feel more normal themselves. They tend to be uncomfortable with the idea that their able-bodied children may or may not be adjusted to the handicapped sibling. Parents frequently depend on their normal children to maintain morale and to show that the family is not having trouble dealing with the disability. Parents feel responsible for whatever pain they have caused their normal children, and they feel even more guilty if they think that the normal children are unhappy. Finally, parents feel guilty that they are frequently preoccupied with their handicapped child to the neglect of the normal children. It is hard for them to hear the resentment and jealousy. They expect their normal children to be more selfless and understanding.

Parents consciously and unconsciously communicate their vulnerability to the stresses of rearing a disabled child; the normal children are sensitive to this, often at the expense of their own emotional well-being. Discussion of how the handicapped sibling's behavior, needs, and problems affect the other children is, in many families, as taboo a subject as sex. The adolescent often struggles alone with these concerns without the knowledge or support of family or peers.

Mitchell and Rizzo (1985) describe families that seem to manage adolescent disability best as being characterized by the following conditions. These conditions provide a useful framework for assessing how well a family will manage the needs of its adolescents in general. These families are described as having:

1. A clear separation of generations. The parental and sibling subsystems are separate with delineated boundaries, and the parental coalition provides leadership for the family and a strong model for relating to others. When this separation exists in a family, siblings do not manipulate or play one parent against the other. Family rules are appropriate, unambiguous, and negotiable.

2. Flexibility within and between roles. As circumstances change, roles change. In a parent's absence, an older child may assume a more authoritarian role. As children mature, power is increasingly shared among parents and children.

3. Tolerance of individuation. Each member's individuality is appreciated and supported. Boundaries between people are clear and there is respect for individual points of view. An adolescent's need for independence and separateness is not regarded as disloyal but as an expression of healthy autonomy. The transition from child to adult is accepted realistically.

4. Communication that is direct, consistent, and affirms self-esteem. Family members are free to express thoughts, feelings and expectations. Their words are congruent with their behavior. Individuals are listened to and their input considered to be important. Any issue that concerns the family is discussed among its members and transactions are empathic, trusting, and caring.

THE ROLE OF THE ALLIED HEALTH PROFESSIONAL

Intervention

Most professionals recognize that there are many issues and needs related to the impact of a child with a disability on both siblings and parents. However, few health care delivery systems are proactive in terms of intervention. The ideal would be that the intervention process would be automatically initiated during the adolescent developmental stage. Unfortunately this may not occur because many families never have contact with a helping professional until there is some kind of developmental, dispositional, or traumatic crisis. Another factor is that allied health professionals are not often involved in preventative work, and this is probably one reason that the impact of a handicapped child is so frequently a negative one. Many problems that normal adolescent siblings experience might be avoided or limited if professionals intervened early in the family life cycle. Nurses and social workers are frequently in strategic positions to enable families to make healthy adaptations to life with a handicapped child. When a family with a handicapped infant is referred to a hospital social service department, services need to be extended beyond the initial period of birth and infancy. Moreover, intervention should be family focused and should include siblings in the process.

An assessment model is presented in Chapter 1. An integral part of that model is the exploration of selected family dynamics at critical points in the person's treatment and/or rehabilitation. The professional should be able to conduct a family interview both analytically and sensitively. In order to help adolescents make a satisfactory adjustment and transition when there is a handicapped sibling in the family, it will be important to make a comprehensive family assessment to determine how facilitative the family environment will be.

The goals of intervention should be to ameliorate present stresses, facilitate adaptation, prevent future stresses, and promote positive gains. Although every family has its unique intervention needs, it is nonetheless possible to develop an intervention framework that addresses many of the needs shared by families in similar circumstances. Thus, interventions are suggested that can be helpful to families with handicapped children and nonhandicapped adolescent siblings. Interventions are aimed at minimizing as much as possible the negative impact of a handicapped sibling and enabling family members to gain something positive from the experience. The focus is definitely a family focus, and the ultimate objective is a rehabilitation objective; if the family can function effectively, then the adjustment of its disabled member will be maximized. When the family is viewed in systems terms, it can be seen that the impact of siblings on each other is reciprocal. If there are problems in their relationship, both are affected and, conversely, if intervention helps one, the other is likely to benefit. It is very import for parents to realize this. One reason that parents are frequently less responsive to the feelings and needs of their able-bodied children is that they perceive their nonhandicapped children as meeting their needs at the expense of the defenseless, disabled sibling. It is essential for helping professionals to help parents understand that intervention will benefit both the nondisabled and disabled children. Perhaps this may be clearer as the professional keeps the focus on the family as a whole rather than on individual members.

Intervention is a multifaceted process. However, this discussion will be confined to those ingredients of intervention that address the needs of the adolescent with a disabled sibling, as identified by Wasserman (1983) and discussed previously in this chapter.

The Provision of Accurate Information

The importance of imparting information has been highlighted in Chapter 2. The information discussed with parents and their siblings can have a slightly different focus. Adolescent siblings should be encouraged to discuss their questions about the handicapped sibling's disability and its implications for the normal sibling's present and future. Parents and siblings need to discuss together the impact and significance of the disability, particularly if it is of a hereditary nature. Many young people carry around, as dreadful secrets, fears that are unfounded; these contaminate their identities and interfere with their abilities to cope. Even the most dreaded information loses its terrifying power once it is out in the open and can be dealt with. It is essential, however, that parents allow their adolescents to regulate the amount and kind of information they want. Information should be provided as the adolescent becomes ready for it. One young woman said that what she appreciated in her family was that she always knew that her parents were "askable."

It is important that counselors be alert to the possibility that the entire family's perception of the disability is inaccurate. Mitchell and Rizzo (1985) point out that, paradoxically, it is the family who is often responsible for the confusing and stereotypical perception of the disabled adolescent. For the majority of families, living with a disability has been like sailing in uncharted water. Parents have struggled to develop their own management model, and when a family enters treatment in the launching stage of the life cycle, many family structures are firmly entrenched and inflexible. Parents and children may discover through the intervention process that their disabled sibling has developmental capabilities not previously perceived by them. This information can be liberating for all concerned. An example of this was expressed by 16-year-old Greg, who when interviewed by the author described his disabled brother Ronnie's accomplishments.

> When I see him working at his job, I'm really proud of him, the same way I would be about any brother who is a responsible person. I never thought he would be able to do as well as he does. I now see the things that make him like other normal people and in a funny way, it makes me feel more normal.

The Improvement of Family Communication

As mentioned previously, it is not unusual or abnormal for adolescents to become less communicative as they begin to move away from the family. Therefore, it is all the more important for the family communication to be direct and receptive to individual feelings and differences. For the first time, the family can learn from the professional that it is not a threat for family members to express their resentments, embarrassments, jealousies, and so forth. Alex, whose mother was a participant in the mothers' group, recalled an incident that occurred when he was 14 and his autistic brother stripped during a family shopping trip.

> I turned around, and there was Brett without any clothes on. I remember feeling shocked and embarrassed, but I was also angry and jealous. How could my parents tolerate behavior in him that they would never tolerate in me? I wanted to tell them but I didn't have the words.

In the family interview, the counselor can help family members find the words to speak for themselves and to accept disagreements and differing perceptions of the same situation (Satir, 1967). The ultimate therapeutic goal is to help the family become effective in its communication without the presence of the counselor. An excellent vehicle for achieving this is the family council (Drei-kurs, 1955). The council, which should be incorporated into the family routine, meets weekly to air problems and find solutions through a democratic process. All decisions are majority decisions and are abided by until the next week's council when decisions may be amended or revoked. Major benefits of this approach are that all members speak for themselves, and every problem is addressed as a family problem.

Parents develop their own coping mechanisms for handling difficult behavior and may be so involved in day-to-day management that they simply do not see their adolescents' painful struggles. If adolescents are helped to work through some of their emotional reactions toward their disabled siblings, then both siblings can relate to each other more productively. For example, if embarrassing situations that arise can be discussed, they can perhaps be prevented in the future. And most important, adolescents will not have to struggle with their feelings alone, and the disabled sibling will not have to experience rejection.

The Development of Sibling Competency

Several mothers in the mothers' group mentioned in the beginning of this chapter reported that the nondisabled siblings felt the need to fight their retarded brother's or sister's battles. Featherstone (1981) recounted the poignant struggle of the adolescent boy who wanted to protect his retarded brother from the stares of the children on the playground where he was a counselor. He recalled, "On the one hand, I felt like saying—and it upsets me to think that I would say what I wanted to say—'Jim, hurry up and get out of here,' and at the same time, I wanted to say to all those little kids, 'If you don't move now, I'm going to throw you over the fence.' " Loneliness, anger, guilt, embarrassment, identification, and confusion merge and battle with one another (Featherstone, 1981). The nonhandicapped sibling needs behavioral strategies for coping with these situations. The ability to deal assertively with others who react ignorantly and cruelly toward the disabled sibling is a competency that few adolescents have and that all could use. Assertiveness training can be incorporated as an intervention strategy.

When the behavior of the disabled sibling is difficult for the family to handle and is particularly difficult for the adolescent, who is so conscious of his peer's intolerance of different or "odd" behavior, strategies for modifying behavior can be taught. Wasserman (1984) cites two projects in which siblings were trained in behavior-modification techniques so that they could modify the disabled sibling's unacceptable behavior. Shreibman, O'Neill, and Koegel (1983) report positive results from a program designed to teach normal siblings procedures to modify the behavior of their autistic siblings. Significant findings were that when the normal sibling developed a high level of training proficiency, there were observed improvements in the autistic sibling's behavior, and the reaction of the normal siblings to their handicapped brothers and sisters was more positive after training. A word of caution is indicated. Allied health professionals need to help parents understand that the training is intended to benefit the adolescent sibling and not to provide the parents with a parent aide. The goal is to modify the sibling's behavior so that it is socially acceptable, thus enabling both handicapped and normal siblings to interact comfortably with peers.

The Inclusion of Siblings in Planning for the Disabled Sibling

Social life, parental attention, available financial resources, and the future are all aspects of life that are changed because of the needs of the disabled sibling. Older children may resent what they perceive as unjust allocation of time and resources to the disabled sibling. They feel powerless to change anything because, in their families, they have little or no influence on parental decisions or plans. Many of their fears are either the result of uncertainty about how the disability will directly affect them, or from the certainty that it will affect them negatively. Jennifer expressed her frustration about her retarded sister's future:

> I didn't want to criticize the way my parents treated Wendy. They wanted to be sure that she knew that she wasn't a burden and that they enjoyed her company, but now she is so dependent on them that she'll never have a life of her own, and her dependency will be a burden to me someday. I wish I could have said that to them without feeling selfish.

The professional who is involved with the handicapped family member in school may be in the most advantageous position to engage the entire family in planning for the future. Heretofore it has been customary to involve only parents in discussions of this nature. Allied health professionals as they help the disabled adolescent make the transition to more independence need to broaden their focus and recognize the potential of sibling contributions to the process. Planning for the future is a logical item for the agenda of the family council mentioned previously. The opinions of all siblings should be solicited in regard to the decisions that affect their lives. Including adolescents in planning for the disabled child is a strategy that can have desirable outcomes for the entire family. Emotional involvement among siblings can be enhanced when they are taking responsibility for planning for each other's welfare. Parents can benefit from the often innovative ideas that adolescents may have about plans for their disabled sibling. Adolescents feel that they have some control over the decisions that affect them and consequently are less likely to feel resentful and unfairly treated. Featherstone (1981) adds another benefit to the list when she points out that when a family labors collectively on behalf of its handicapped member, it shares in the resultant successes, and its resultant pride enables it to cope with less pleasant aspects.

The Development and Utilization of Peer Support

Although most of the previous intervention strategies involve the whole family, it is important to remember that in this developmental stage, it is healthy and desirable for the adolescent siblings to establish their own support systems outside the family group. A great deal can be accomplished in a sibling peer group when its members share their emotional concerns and feelings. Grossman's (1972) discussion groups combined both education and counseling; participants received information and help from each other in coping with feelings, parental demands, outside peer reactions, and behavior of the disabled sibling. In one community mental health center, peer groups were used to help normal adolescents learn how to relate sensitively and helpfully to their disabled sibling (Churchill, 1974), and thus served a preventative as well as a supportive function. Because peer relationships are such an important part of the adolescent's development, the use of this kind of group is the most appropriate and effective support strategy to use. Featherstone (1981) tells us that most parents hope that their handicapped child will be able to join in activities with their able-bodied siblings on some kind of equal footing. The mothers in the mothers' group admitted their frustration and sadness when the handicapped child was excluded from the sibling peer group. They could see, however, that their temptation to "equalize their expectations" for all their siblings was unrealistic, often detrimental both to the handicapped and to the normal siblings, and likely to hurt their relationship. It is just as important, therefore, for the handicapped sibling, during adolescence, to also have a peer group with which to identify. Organizations for disability groups and schools for special education frequently set up such groups for disabled youngsters. Allied health professionals need to be familiar with such groups if they exist in their geographic area, and to advocate their establishment if they do not.

CONCLUSION

Professionals involved in helping a family with a handicapped child must broaden their focus to encompass the concerns of other family members. In order to assess the impact of having a handicapped sibling on the adolescent family members, the professional must first acknowledge that in any family, adolescence is a time of tumultuous change and is stressful for both parents and children. In a family with a handicapped child, the stress is often magnified. Even though parents may recognize their normal adolescents' needs to separate from the family, it may be difficult for them to encourage separation, particularly if they have depended on them for companionship and child care.

It is not surprising to hear that it is hard for families to see beyond their chronic pain and to recognize the positive aspects of having a disabled child. It is probably even harder for the adolescent siblings. For many of them, the realization may not occur until long after they have left the family. One mother in the mothers' group remarked that "the positives are often ignored and need to be reflected upon." Researchers (e.g., Grossman, 1972) discovered that there were positive effects for siblings. For example, many students in her groups were more tolerant of differences and were more aware of intolerance and prejudice. Jennifer exemplifies the acceptance of differences. A pretty, outgoing girl, who is popular with her peers, Jennifer dates a boy who has a visible handicap. Her acceptance of his disability has certainly been influenced by her experience with her retarded sister; this acceptance can, in turn, influence the attitude of her peers.

Further study is needed in order to know what determines whether the disabled sibling will have a positive or negative impact on the normal sibling. Researchers have theorized that the family structure, relationships, and parental attitudes are important determinants. Because adolescence is a time of transition—and a particularly difficult time when one has a disabled sibling—the adolescent and the family may be floundering and therefore receptive to intervention; that in itself may bring about positive effects. Intervention at an earlier stage might have been preventative, but it is never too late for families to change. As a result of intervention, family members may become more direct and empathic in their communication, more flexible in their expectations, and more adaptive to transition. Not only is it possible for the able-bodied adolescents to come to terms with their negative feelings about their "different" family members, but they may also attain insights and capabilities far more mature than those of their peers. Ann, a bright young woman now working as an advocate for retarded citizens, discussed her experiences with her autistic brother and underlined the gains.

> When I think about my life with my brother, I know it has been a challenge and a growth experience. As a result, I have some pretty neat tools in my toolbox for the rest of my life.

RESOURCES

Suggested Literature for Adolescent Siblings

Cleaver, V. (1973). *Me too.* New York: Lippincott.

Featherstone, H. (1980). *A difference in the family: Living with a disabled child.* New York: Penguin.

Keane, B. (1984). *Sex education coalition tips for parents.* Washington, DC: Sex Education Coalition.

Lynch, M. (1979). *Mary Fran and me.* New York: St. Martin's.

Information and Service Sources

Sibling Information Network
Department of Educational Psychology
Box U-64, The University of Connecticut
Storrs, CT 06268.

Siblings Helping Persons with Autism through Resources and Energy
c/o National Society for Children and Adults with Autism
1234 Massachusetts Avenue, N.W., Suite 1017
Washington, DC 20005-4599
(202) 783-0125

Siblings for Significant Change
823 United Nations Plaza, Room 808
New York, NY 10017

SIBS
123 Golden Lane
London, EC1Y ORT
England

REFERENCES

Breslau, N., Weitzman, N., & Messenger, K. (1981). Psychological functioning of siblings of disabled children. *Pediatrics, 67,* 344–353.

Churchill, S. (1974). Preventive, short-term groups for siblings of child mental hospital patients. In P. Glasser, R. Sarri, & R. Vinter (Eds.), *Individual change through small groups* (pp. 362–374). New York: Free Press.

Cleveland, D., & Miller, N. (1977). Attitudes and life commitments of older siblings of mentally retarded adults: An exploratory study. *Mental Retardation, 15,* 38–41.

Dreikurs, R., with Soltz, V. (1964). *Children: the challenge.* New York: Hawthorne.

Erikson, E. (1963). *Childhood and society.* New York: Norton.

Farber, B. (1960). Effects of a severely mentally retarded child on family integration. *Monographs of the Society for Research in Child Development, 21* (2, Serial No. 75).

Farber, B., & Jenne, W. C. (1963). Interaction with retarded siblings and life goals of children. *Marriage and Family Living, 25,* 96–98.

Featherstone, H. A. (1981). *A difference in the family: Living with a disabled child.* New York: Penguin.

Goldenberg, I., & Goldenberg, H. (1980). *Family therapy: An overview,* Monterey, CA: Brooks/Cole.

Graliker, B. V., Fishler, K., & Koch, R. (1962). Teenage reaction to a mentally retarded sibling. *American Journal of Mental Deficiency, 66,* 838–843.

Grossman, F. K. (1972). *Brothers and sisters of retarded children: An exploratory study.* Syracuse, NY: Syracuse University Press.

Maier, H. W. (1978). *Three theories of child development.* New York: Harper & Row.

McCallum, N. (1981, November). My brother Jon. *Sibling information Network Newsletter, 1*(3), 2.

Miller, S. G. (1974). An exploratory study of sibling relationships in families with retarded children (doctoral dissertation, Columbia University). *Dissertation Abstracts International, 35,* 2994B-2995B.

Mitchell, W., & Rizzo, S. (1985). The adolescent with special needs. In Mirken, M., & Koman, S. (Eds.), *Handbook of adolescents and family therapy.* New York: Gardner.

Satir, V. (1967). *Conjoint family therapy.* Palo Alto, CA: Science & Behavior Books.

Schreiber, M., & Freely, M. (1965). Siblings of the retarded: A guided group experience. *Children, 12*(6), 221-225.

Schreibman, L., O'Neill, R., & Koegel, R. (1983). Behavioral training for siblings of autistic children. *Journal of Applied Behavior Analysis, 16,* 129-138.

Vadasy, P., Fewell, R., Meyer, D. J., & Schell, G. (1984). Siblings of handicapped children: A developmental perspective on family interactions. *Family Relations, 33,* 155-157.

Wasserman, R. (1984). Identifying the counseling needs of the siblings of mentally retarded children. *The Personnel and Guidance Journal, 61,* 622-627.

10 Enabling the Family in Supporting Transition from School to Work

Edna Mora Szymanski,
David B. Hershenson,
and Paul W. Power

Transition from school to work for adolescents with disabilities has been a concern of professionals in education and rehabilitation since at least the 1940s (Szymanski, 1984). Interest has intensified in recent years as a result of legislation and federal program initiatives (Brown, Hallpern, Hasazi, & Wehman, 1987; Will, 1984; Wright, Emener, & Ashley, 1988). Concomitant with this intensified interest has been a recognition of the importance of family roles and interventions in career preparation and transition (Beckett, Chitwood, & Hayden, 1985; Benson & Turnbull, 1986; Kokaska & Brolin, 1985).

At the same time as an interest in transition was increasing, so too was recognition of the effect of the environment on individual behavior. This recognition, often referred to as the ecological approach, has been articulated in a variety of disability-related areas including: blindness and visual impairment (Scott, 1969); developmental disabilities (Chadsey-Rusch, 1985); independent living (DeJong, 1978); mental health (Hershenson & Power, 1987); rehabilitation counseling (Szymanski, Rubin, & Rubin, 1988); special education (Masters & Mori, 1986); and spinal cord injury (Treishman, 1980).

Two school-to-work transition models that include the environmental dimension were proposed by Szymanski and Danek (1985) and by Daniels (1987). Szymanski and Danek suggested that the process of school-to-work transition could be viewed from two types of reference points—individual and environmental. Individual factors included both personal characteristics and individual perception of the transition. Environmental factors included support networks, especially families, and available service delivery systems. These factors were seen as interactive with deficits in one area, such as individual ability, and potentially offset by strengths in another area, such as family support. The model proposed by Daniels used individual competence, environment, and discrepancy as the key constructs. Intervention plans resulted from analyses of individual competence, environmental demands, and resultant discrepancies. The goal of such interventions has been the enhancement of the congruence between the person and the environment.

The model presented herein combines the essential features of these two models and clarifies the family's place in the process. It also addresses, albeit in less detailed fashion due to its multidimensionality, the concept of planning for independence proposed by Corn (1985). A transition planning guide, based on the model, is provided to facilitate transition planning and intervention with adolescents with disabilities and their families (Tables 10.1 to 10.4).

FACTORS IN TRANSITIONING: A CONCEPTUAL MODEL

The salient factors of school-to-work transition can be conceptualized in a $3 \times 5 \times 3$ design. The principal dimensions are Client Variables, Environment, and Perceivers. The conceptual framework presented in Figure 10.1 depicts the interaction of these dimensions in influencing transition.

We shall now examine each of the elements in this figure.

Client Variables

Client variables in Figure 10.1 consist of two types: internal and manifest. The internal variables are the work-adjustment-related constructs of work personality, work competencies, and work goals. The manifest variables, which relate to performance in an actual job or training situation, are task performance and work role behavior.

The internal variables are derived from Hershenson's (1974, 1981) work-adjustment model. Hershenson described work adjustment for persons with and without disabilities as the result of the sequential, interactive development of three domains: (1) *work personality* (i.e., self-concept as a worker and a personal system of motivation for work); (2) *work competencies* (i.e., work habits, physical and mental skills applicable to jobs, and work-related interpersonal skills); and (3) appropriate crystallized *work goals*. Each of these domains becomes the focus of development in the sequence in which they are listed, but each domain also reciprocally influences the development of the other two. Thus, the development of work adjustment is a dynamic process: Each domain can only develop to a level supported by its predecessor, but the next focal domain to develop can subsequently affect that predecessor

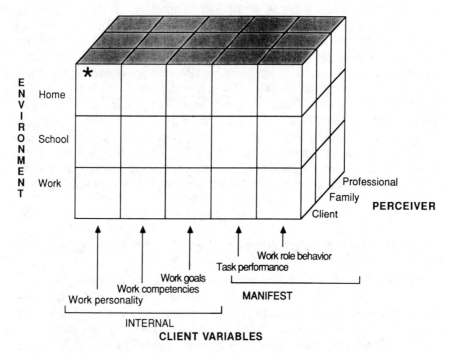

FIGURE 10.1 Client variables (Measures within each cell: satisfactoriness of resolution; satisfaction).

and thereby change the limits of its own further development. For example, the basic work-personality domain is fairly well established before the development of work competencies assumes primacy. But as work habits and skills develop or fail to develop, the configuration of the individual's self-concept as a worker and motivational system (i.e., the components of work personality) are necessarily affected. Similarly, the development of work goals influences the configuration of the other two domains. For instance, skills not relevant to the evolving goals may atrophy, and the individual's motivational system must become consistent with the goals that have been developed. The model also posits that, as long as the individual lives, all domains will continue to develop, although not as rapidly or dramatically as at the time they are focal. The three domains establish a dynamic balance, so that any change in one domain will necessitate changes in the other two in order to restore balance.

In this model, work personality develops primarily under family influence during the preschool years. Work competencies develop primarily as a result of successes and failures in school. Work goals reflect the influences of peer or reference groups (which, in turn, reflect the options provided by the school) as the person prepares to leave school and enter the world of work. The career-related behavioral output of this process at any point in the person's career is referred to as *work adjustment*.

The manifest client variables in Figure 10.1 represent observable measures of work adjustment. They are *task performance* (quality and quantity of production of the expected product or service) and *work role behavior* (e.g., promptness, neatness, cooperation, ability to follow directions, and ability to get along with coworkers and supervisors). Meeting or exceeding employer standards in both task performance and work role behavior is requisite for continued employment as well as for advancement in a specific job or career.

These elements and their interrelationships are diagrammed in the inner box (Individual Elements) in Figure 10.2. In this diagram the large arrowheads represent the directions of primary influence (e.g., work personality on work competencies, work competencies on work goals, all three on work adjustment), and the small arrowheads represent reciprocal feedback.

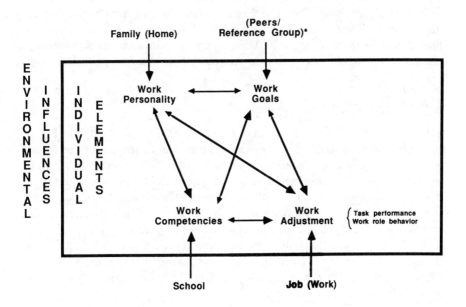

FIGURE 10.2 Components of the school-to-work transition.
*Largely determined by home and school

Environmental Influences

The environment and its interaction with the individual can substantially influence the extent of handicap resulting from a particular disabling condition (Bruininks & Lakin, 1985; DeJong, 1979; Hahn, 1985). It is therefore reasonable to suspect that environment should produce significant dimensions in a transition model for adolescents with disabilities.

The environmental dimensions of Figure 10.1 are home, school, and work. All are part of the larger sociocultural environment that can either reduce or exaggerate the handicap resulting from a particular disabling condition and can thereby either support or impede transition. A brief discussion of each of these environmental variables and their potential interaction with the other dimensions in the transition follows.

Home Environment

The family is a major influence of the environmental dimension. Not only does the family itself constitute a major part of the student's environment (home), but the family also chooses or limits exposure to other environments. As indicated in the outer portion of Figure 10.2, the family provides the values and reinforcement that shape work personality. The family selects (and possibly advocates within) the school environment in which competencies are initially established and in which a major peer reference is likely to influence the development of work goals. The quality of these areas of development will have substantial effect on how smoothly the school-to-work transition will be accomplished.

School Environment

School is another important environmental dimension represented in Figure 10.1. Many factors, including the family, influence the impact of the school environment on transition. Class placement, peer influences, type of training techniques, and characteristics of the school environment are just some of the important aspects. For students with developmental disabilities, there is a growing body of evidence suggesting that the training techniques and environment during the last few years of school may have a critical influence on acquisition, maintenance, and adaptability of work skills and work behaviors (Hanley-Maxwell, 1986; Stodden & Browder, 1986; Wacker & Berg, 1986). School environments can also represent transition goals, as in transitions from high school to college.

Work Environment(s).

An individual work environment has a variety of characteristics that can influence work adjustment. Such characteristics include expected work performance, physical accessibility of the workplace, naturally occurring cues and reinforcers, attitudes of coworkers and supervisors toward the worker, work tasks, and physical layout of the workplace. Factors in the work environment can either support or impede transition.

Fortunately, many factors in the work environment (as well as in college environments) are amenable to modification either directly, as in job modification, or indirectly, as in the provision of client support (e.g., supported employment), or through application of compensatory skills or devices (e.g., a calculator to aid in simple arithmetic). Additionally, decisions with respect to the feasibility or desirability of a particular work environment can be guided by examination of the potential interaction of that particular environment with the client variables and perceiver dimensions of Figure 10.1. Daniels and Wiederholt (1986) illustrated the importance of such comparisons with their discussion of functional competency. An individual may be seen as functionally competent in one work environment and functionally incompetent in another.

Perceivers

How the transition process is perceived is an important and often overlooked dimension in transition planning. The model in Figure 10.1 depicts three types of perceivers—the client, the family, and the professional. The intent of such depiction is to enable the professional to surface those discrepancies between student, family, and professional perceptions that frequently impede transition efforts. Following are brief discussions related to each of the three perceivers depicted in Figure 10.1.

Client

The student's perception of the transition may be influenced by a variety of surrounding events or situations. The extent to which the tasks of adolescence (separation, sexual identity, and independence) have been accomplished may influence students' perceptions of the tasks of transition and personal competence for accomplishment (Goldberg, 1981). McCarthy's (1983) discussion of the potential approach-avoidance conflicts that can characterize transition illustrated the complexity of student perception of transition. The student can eagerly anticipate the challenges, rewards, and independence of the work role. Simultaneously, however, the student may also dread the responsibilities and demands which accompany the change in role from student to worker. Previous experiences and environmental supports may affect the relative dominance of these or other themes with respect to the student's perception of transition goals and activities and thus, potentially, affect the level of success of the transition.

Family

A number of factors can affect the family's perception of the transition. Depending on the level of earlier resolution, the transition can trigger feelings associated with adjustment to their child's disability (e.g., grief). Adjustment may be required to changes in family roles, functions, and boundaries (Benson & Turnbull, 1986; Rehabilitation Brief, 1984). How they perceive their child's abilities and possibilities for successful entry into the world of work will have substantial effect on the degree to which they advocate for various employment opportunities.

Professional

The perceptions and attitudes of professionals can have significant impact for persons with disabilities. Professional need to be aware of and guard against their potential for negative attitudes that can influence their perceptions of transition possibilities for individual clients. Paternalistic attitudes, lowered or limited expectations, and limited understanding of disability on the part of the professional can have negative effects on the self-esteem of the individual with a disability (Rubenfeld, 1988; Tuttle, 1984). The expectations and perceptions of the professional when entering a relationship with the family can have significant impact on the nature of the relationship. "To enter into a helping relationship with a family with a prior expectation of pathology or deviance will create a sense of unjustifiable power in the helper, and a sense of dependence and helplessness in the 'recipient' " (Mallory, 1986, p. 318). Szymanski, Rubin, and Rubin (1988) suggest that the prevalent "functional limitations" of disability may predispose some rehabilitation professionals to such perceptions.

Within-Cell Measures

Within each cell in Figure 10.1 one may take two measures: satisfactoriness of resolution (i.e., how effectively the set of issues represented by that cell objectively appears to have been resolved) and satisfaction (i.e., how content the perceiver is with that resolution). For instance, clients may be meeting industrially acceptable levels of performance on the job (satisfactory outcome in the cell: work × task performance × client), but the client may not feel satisfied with his or her performance in that cell because he or she may wish to qualify for a promotion. Thus, discrepancies may exist between satisfactoriness and satisfaction within each cell. Moreover, discrepancies may exist across cells on satisfaction and satisfactoriness. For example, the family and the educator may disagree as to how satisfied they are with the client's work goals while the client is still in high school. Thus, there would be a discrepancy in satisfaction between cell: school × work goals × family, and cell: school × work goals × professional. Similarly, the client's work behavior (neatness, promptness, cooperativeness, etc.) may be satisfactory at home but may not be satisfactory on the job. In this case, there would be a discrepancy in satisfactoriness between cell: home × work role behavior × client, and cell: work role behavior × client.

A further illustration of the potential complexity of this situation is that there may be a number of potential school and work environments. The client's work role behavior could be seen as satisfactory in one work environment (e.g., a sheltered workshop) and not in another (e.g., a competitive food-service job). This situation would represent a discrepancy in satisfactoriness between cells: client × work role behavior × $work_1$, and client × work role behavior × $work_2$, where $work_1$ represented the sheltered work environment and $work_2$ represented the competitive work environment. There would also be a discrepancy in satisfaction between these cells if the client was satisfied with the situation and performance in the competitive situation ($work_2$) and dissatisfied with the situation and performance in the sheltered workshop ($work_1$).

The role of the counselor is to assist the client and family in locating and resolving discrepancies that impede successful transition. This is not meant to imply that each cell must attain total satisfactoriness or satisfaction, or that absolutely all discrepancies must be resolved. Rather, this model is intended to offer a framework for conceptualizing and locating the often multidimensional impediments to successful transition.

INTERVENTIONS

In this chapter interventions are conceptualized as (1) assisting a helping professional to follow a transition planning guide, based on the multidimensional transition model introduced in Figure 10.1; and (2) guiding the helping professional to develop one's own knowledge and skills to assist in the transitioning process.

A Transition Planning Guide

Tables 10.1 and 10.2 introduce a transition planning guide based on the multidimensional transition model introduced in Figure 10.1. Table 10.1 provides a structure for identification of perceptions and discrepancies with respect to the following areas: (1) target environment, (2) target activity, (3) success criteria (for that activity in that environment), (4) environmental barriers, and (5) individual needs. Table 10.2 is a planning aid based on target activities, environments, and success criteria that are mutually agreed upon by the client, family, and professional. Both tables use the perceiver dimension of Figure 10.1 as the starting point for examining and effecting change in both the individual and environmental dimensions.

TABLE 10.1 Transition Planning Guide

	Part 1: Discrepancy analysis	
Area/Perceiver	Perception	Discrepancy
Target activity Client Family Professional		
Target environment Client Family Professional		
Success criteria Client Family Professional		
Environmental Barriers Client Family Professional		
Individual needs Client Family Professional		

TABLE 10.2 Transition Planning Guide

Part 2: Enabling activities

Mutually-agreed transition goal

Target activity

Target environment

Success criteria

Enabling activities

Short-term activities
  Client
  Family
  Professional

Long-term activities
  Client
  Family
  Professional

The identification of discrepancies allows the professional to facilitate communication. Subsequently, information can be provided and options discussed to assist the student and family in identifying mutually agreed-upon goals and criteria for independent performance. At that point, enabling activities can be jointly planned.

This planning guide cuts across individual client variables and potential environments. It can be used by professionals in a variety of human service and allied health professions. The major focus is on surfacing and resolving discrepancies in order to enable focused transition planning.

The areas listed in Table 10.1 are likely to reveal some discrepancies in perception among students, families, and professionals involved in planning school-to-work transition. Other areas can be added to Table 10.1 depending on individual situations.

In order to examine the potential discrepancies in each area, the professional may ask the student and family a series of questions. For example, for target environment the initial question for the student might be, "Exactly what do you see yourself doing next year?" The time line of the question can be adjusted according to the circumstances of the particular transition. Comparable questions can be asked of students and involved family members in each of the areas listed in Table 10.1. Professionals may want to encourage students and family members to provide as much detail as possible on each area in order to fully illuminate potential discrepancies.

Subsequently, professionals are encouraged to consider their perceptions of the student's potential future activities, work (or school) environments, relevant success criteria, environmental barriers, and individual needs. This part of the exercise will help the professional in two ways. First, it will help to examine any underlying assumptions that the professional may have formed regarding the client's potential posttransition functioning. Second, it will illuminate areas where the professional's understanding of the requirements of a particular activity or environment differs substantially from that of the student and/or parents. Discrepancies can be indicated in the far right column by lines connecting the specific conflicting perceptions.

Without some vigilance on the part of the professional, subtle differences in perception or underlying assumptions can go unnoticed. If they remain unresolved, these differences can emerge as obstacles to successful transition.

Table 10.3 depicts a discrepancy analysis for the following situation. Both client and parent may have agreed on a goal of competitive placement in a fast-food restaurant. However, both client and parents may have had unrealistically low expectations regarding criteria for independent performance. Such perceptions, which would surface in a careful discussion of the criteria for success and independent functioning in the target activity and environment, could have led to significant difficulties in job retention.

Once discrepancies have been illuminated and mutually agreeable target activities, environments, and success criteria have been determined, transition planning can proceed. Clients should be encouraged to take as much responsibility as possible for individual planning activities. Such encouragement will facilitate the development of independence and personal responsibility. Table 10.2 provides a family-oriented planning framework.

Table 10.4 is an example of Part 2 of the Transition Planning Guide (Table 10.2), depicting planning of enabling activities for the following situation:

> The client, parents, and professional have agreed on a local college program. The client has a significant hearing loss and uses an amplification device that requires the lecturer or major speaker wear a microphone. The client also relies on preferential seating to facilitate lipreading, and on notes taken by classmates to fill in gaps. The severity of the client's hearing loss affects both communication and learning (Chapter 6 of this volume).

In summary, Part 1 of the Transition Planning Guide (Table 10.1) provides the professional with an organized framework from which to examine potential discrepancies in client, family, and professional perceptions regarding transition. Table 10.3 is an example of such a discrepancy analysis for a client who desires a food-service job. Once discrepancies have been identified, professionals can work with clients and families toward some resolution, which will

TABLE 10.3 Transition Planning Guide (Example)

	Part 1: Discrepancy analysis	
Area/Perceiver	Perception	Discrepancy
Target activity		
Client	Employment as a kitchen helper.	
Family	Employment as a kitchen helper.	
Professional	The client should be able to learn a variety of entry level, unskilled occupations.	
Target environment		
Client	Specific local restaurant.	↕ ↑
Family	Specific local restaurant.	↓
Professional	Any environment where the job has a reasonably stable work routine and a relatively slow pace of work. (The client has demonstrated excellent quality of work in past training experiences but has consistently worked at a slower than average pace).	
Success criteria		
Client	Wearing uniform and going to work every day.	↕
Family	Going to work every day.	↓ ↕
Professional	Good attendance and punctuality, and meeting the specific requirements for quality and quantity of work detailed in the job description on job analysis.	
Environmental barriers		
Client	None.	↕ ↕
Family	Transportation home from work.	↓ ↕
Professional	A very busy work environment with peaks of activity (e.g., lunch rush).	
Individual needs		
Client	Uniform and paycheck.	↕ ↕
Family	An understanding employer and transportation home from work each day.	↓ ↕
Professional	A job coach to teach specific job skills, help client learn to monitor and increase speed, and teach client to use available public transportation.	

TABLE 10.4 Transition Planning Guide (Example)

Part 2: Enabling activities
Mutually-agreed transition goal

Target activity	Completion of 4-year degree (most likely in accounting).
Target environment	Local college. College is a small school with very little experience with students with special needs.
Success criteria	Completion of required coursework with at least a C average.

Enabling activities

Short-term activities

Client
1. Completion of all necessary admission requirements.
2. Meet with students special-services counselor to discuss necessary accommodations (e.g., preferential seating, use of special amplification device, note-taking arrangements, potential reduced course load, and other accessibility or accommodation needs.

Family
1. Complete necessary financial-aid forms.
2. Arrange to make quiet study space available.
3. Plan with client regarding transportation needs.

Professional
1. Meet periodically with client to discuss results of enabling activities and to alter plans as necessary.
2. Discuss additional potential vocational-rehabilitative services.

Long-term activities

Client
1. Obtain and become familiar with course materials before beginning of semester.
2. Arrange to meet individually with professors before classes begin to discuss special accommodation needs.
3. Either arrange to photocopy a classmate's notes after each class or arrange for a classmate to use special carbonless note-taking pads to provide instant copies.
4. Plan to participate in at least one extracurricular social or sports activity.

Family
1. Provide assistance with tuition.
2. Provide support and encouragement.

Professional
1. Assist student and family in resolving problems on an as-needed basis.
2. Meet with the student periodically to review progress toward goals.
3. Assist student in learning appropriate ways to get accessibility and accommodation needs met.

then lay the groundwork for focused transition planning. Part 2 of the Transition-Planning Guide (Table 10.4) provides a framework for planning enabling transition activities with clients and their families, once mutually agreed upon goals have been reached. Table 10.4 is an example of such planning with a client attending a local 4-year college program.

The tools of the Transition Planning Guide focus on all three dimensions of the transition process depicted in Figure 10.1: perceivers, environment, and client variables. The direct focus on client variables is, however, limited to the manifest variables of work role behavior and task performance, along with the internal variable of work goal. The internal variables of work personality and work competencies are addressed indirectly. The process of transition, by its multidimensional and interactive nature, will necessarily affect and be affected by both work personality and work competencies.

With the utilization of a transition planning guide, there are specific skills needed by the helper to enhance its implementation. These skills are also applicable in many situations involving assisting an adolescent from school to work. Mendelsohn and Mendelsohn (1986) encourage the following:

1. Development of mutual respect.
2. Open attitude.
3. Availability.
4. Perseverance. Long-standing parent-professional relationships make the best transitional alliances.
5. Early intervention. Become acquainted with the family when the client is in his or her teens. If that is not possible, review the social, medical, and educational history as extensively as possible. Talk to parents, teachers, sibs, and so on in order to get a deeper understanding of the potentials of the client.
6. See the disabled adolescent in real situations. Visit the classroom. Watch social interactions. Have the family meet as a unit with you; visit the home.
7. Set up vocational-counseling groups in the schools. Listen to what young people have to say about their interests, their fears. Encourage kids to talk about their handicaps and how they will affect their ability to work, and to live independently.
8. Involve disabled adults. There is no better model for success than a success story in the flesh. Bring disabled adults together with disabled adolescents. Use adults as consultants to the family. Enlist their aid in advocacy efforts.

Moreover, there are general suggestions that focus on the development of the client variables of work personality, work competencies, and work goals.

These are general suggestions for professionals working to create conditions favorable to eventual positive work adjustment.

1. Share information with the family in such a way as to emphasize the student's strengths and competencies while not ignoring deficit areas.
2. Seek information from the family about the student's strengths, learning styles, preferred environments, and so forth.
3. Encourage normalized and positive expectations and activities (e.g., chores).
4. Discuss and encourage planning for independence in a variety of activities.
5. Discuss age-appropriate behaviors and peer-group expectations.
6. Encourage choices and allow clients to experience consequences of making wrong choices.
7. Suggest that parents discuss their role and responsibilities as workers with their son or daughter.
8. Encourage the family to begin to think of their son or daughter as a worker who must meet certain expectations in order to remain employed.
9. Discuss planning for normalized social and leisure-time pursuits (e.g., participation in extracurricular activities).

SUMMARY

School-to-work transition is a difficult time for adolescents with disabilities and for their families. They are confronted with changing roles, environments, and expectations. Families have been major parts of the young person's life through childhood and adolescence. In order to focus the potent resources offered by families, professionals will need to form respectful relationships that are centered around enablement of the individual with a disability. The family provides the best opportunity for growth and fulfillment, and the home is the place where young people can best express their natural potentialities and satisfy their career and creative needs.

A multidimensional approach to transitions, such as that presented in Figure 10.1, will be necessary in order to address the multiple, interactive dimensions of the transition process. Again, due to the complexity of transition, an organized framework, such as that presented in Tables 10.1 and 10.2, can enhance communication and promote effective transition planning. Actual completion of forms such as those of Tables 10.1 and 10.2 is not necessary although some professionals may find this practice helpful for case recording and for planning intervention.

REFERENCES

Beckett, C., Chitwood, S., & Hayden, D. (1985). The parent role in the transition from school to work. In S. Moon, P. Goodall, & P. Wehman (Eds.), *Critical issues related to supported competitive employment: Proceedings from the first RRTC symposium on employment for citizens who are mentally retarded* (pp. 129–140). Richmond, VA: Rehabilitation Research and Training Center, Virginia Commonwealth University.

Benson, H. A., & Turnbull, A. P. (1986). Approaching families from an individualized perspective. In R. H. Horner, L. H. Meyer, & H. D. Fredericks (Eds.), *Education of learners with severe handicaps* (pp. 127–157). Baltimore: Brookes.

Brown, L., Halpern, A., Hasazi, S. B., & Wehman, P. (1987). From school to adult living. A forum on issues and trends. *Exceptional Children, 53*, 546–554.

Bruininks, R. H., & Lakin, K. C. (Eds.). (1985). *Living and learning in the least restrictive environment*. Baltimore: Brookes.

Chadsey-Rusch, J. G. (1985). Community integration and mental retardation: The ecobehavioral approach to service provision and assessment. In R. H. Bruininks & K. C. Lakin (Eds.), *Living and learning in the least restrictive environment* (pp. 245–260). Baltimore: Brookes.

Corn, A. L. (1985). An independence matrix for visually impaired learners. *Education of the Visually Handicapped, 18*(1), 3–10.

Daniels, J. L. (1987). Transition from school to work. In R. M. Parker (Ed.), *Rehabilitation counseling: Basics and beyond* (pp. 283–317). Austin, TX: Pro-Ed.

Daniels, J. L., & Wiederholt, J. L. (1986). Preparing problem learners for independent living. In D. D. Hammill & N. R. Bartel (Eds.), *Teaching students with learning and behavior problems* (4th ed.). Newton, MA: Allyn & Bacon.

DeJong, G. (1979). Independent living: From social movement to analytic paradigm. *Archives of Physical Medicine and Rehabilitation, 60*, 435–446.

Goldberg, R. T. (1981). Toward an understanding of the rehabilitation of the disabled adolescent. *Rehabilitation Literature, 42*(3–4), 66–74.

Hahn, H. (1985). Changing perception of disability and the future of rehabilitation. In L. G. Perlman & G. F. Austin (Eds.), *Social influences in rehabilitation planning: Blueprint for the 21st century (pp. 53–*64). Report of the Ninth Mary E. Switzer Memorial Seminar, in Nov. 1984. Alexandria, VA: National Rehabilitation Association.

Hanley-Maxwell, C. (1986). Curriculum development. In F. R. Rusch (Ed.), *Competitive employment issues and strategies* (pp. 187–197). Baltimore: Brookes.

Hershenson, D. B. (1974). Vocational guidance and the handicapped. In E. Herr (Ed.), *Vocational guidance and human development*. Boston: Houghton Mifflin.

Hershenson, D. B. (1981). Work adjustment, disability, and the three r's of vocational rehabilitation: A concept model. *Rehabilitation Counseling Bulletin, 25*, 91–97.

Hershenson, D. B., & Power P. W. (1987). *Mental health counseling: Theory and practice*. NY: Pergamon.

Kiernan, W. E., & Stark, J. A. (Eds.). (1986). *Pathways to employment for adults with developmental disabilities*. Baltimore: Brookes.

Kokaska, C. J., & Brolin, D. E. (1985). *Career education for handicapped individuals* (2nd ed.). Columbus, OH: Merrill.

Mallory, B. L. (1986). Interactions between community agencies and families over the life cycle. In R. R. Fewell & P. F. Vadasy (Eds.), *Families of handicapped children: Needs and supports across the life span* (pp. 317–356). Austin, TX: Pro-Ed.

Masters, L. F., & Mori, A. A. (1986). *Teaching secondary students with mild learning and behavior problems.* Rockville, MD: Aspen.

McCarthy, H. (1983). Understanding motives of use in transition to work: A taxonomy for rehabilitation counselors and educators. *Journal of Applied Rehabilitation Counseling, 14*(1), 51–61.

Mendolsohn, B., & Mendolsohn, B. (1986). Families in the transition process: Important partners. In L. Perlman & G. Austin (Eds.), *The transition to work and independence for youth with disabilities.* A Report of the Tenth Mary E. Switzer Memorial Seminar, May 1986. Alexandria, VA: National Rehabilitation Association.

Rehabilitation Brief. (1984). Disability and families: A family systems approach. *Rehabilitation Brief, 7*(9). Washington DC: National Institute of Handicapped Research, Office of Special Education and Rehabilitation Services, U.S. Department of Education.

Rubenfeld, P. (1988). The rehabilitation counselor and the disabled client: Is a partnership of equals possible? In S. E. Rubin & N. Rubin (Eds.), *Contemporary challenges to the rehabilitation counseling profession* (pp. 31–44). Baltimore: Brookes.

Scott, R. A. (1969). *The making of blind men: A study of adult socialization.* New York: Russell Sage.

Stodden, R. A., & Browder, P. M. (1986). Community based competitive employment preparation of developmentally disabled persons: A program description and evaluation. *Education and Training of the Mentally Retarded, 21*(1), 43–53.

Szymanski, E. M. (1984). Rehabilitation counselors in school settings. *Journal of Applied Rehabilitation Counseling, 15*(4), 10–18.

Szymanski, E. M., & Danek, M. M. (1985). School to work transition for students with disabilities: Historical, current, and conceptual issues. *Rehabilitation Counseling Bulletin, 29*(2), 81–89.

Szymanski, E. M., Rubin, S. E., & Rubin, N. M. (1988). Contemporary challenges: An introduction. In S. E. Rubin & N. Rubin (Eds.), *Contemporary challenges to the rehabilitation counseling profession* (pp. 1–14). Baltimore: Brookes.

Trieschmann, R. B. (1980). *Spinal cord injuries: Psychological, social, and vocational adjustment.* New York: Pergamon.

Tuttle, D. W. (1984). *Self esteem and adjusting with blindness.* Springfield, IL: Charles C. Thomas.

Wacker, D. P., & Berg, W. K. (1986). Generalizing and maintaining work behavior. In F. R. Rusch (Ed.), *Competitive employment issues and strategies* (pp. 129–140). Baltimore: Brookes.

Will, M. (1984). OSERS programming for the transition of youth with severe disabilities: Bridges from school to working life. Washington, DC: Office of Special Education and Rehabilitative Services, U.S. Department of Education.

Wright, B. A. (1983). *Physical disability—A psychosocial approach* (2nd ed.). New York: Harper & Row.

Wright, T. J., Emener, W. G., & Ashley, J. M. (1988). Rehabilitation counseling and client transition from school to work. In S. E. Rubin & N. Rubin (Eds.), *Contemporary challenges to the rehabilitation counseling profession* (pp. 135-151). Baltimore: Brookes.

11 Family Involvement in Mental Health Interventions for Women with Physical Disabilities

Kay Harris Kriegsman and Beverly Celotta

When a woman is disabled, her physical rehabilitation needs are usually adequately addressed. If she incurred the disability as a youngster, her parents and teachers taught her ways to overcome her physical deficits and to work with her strengths. If she incurred the disability in adulthood, a team of physicians, nurses and rehabilitation specialists, and family members saw to it that she relearned ways to accomplish normal tasks. Quite frequently, however, her mental health needs were ignored.

In the past decade, increasing attention has been paid to the mental health needs of women with physical disabilities. Recently, national forums (e.g., The International Rehabilitation conference in 1985; the Sixth Margaret Switzer Memorial Seminar: Women in Rehabilitation, 1981), research efforts, and services have focused on the mental health needs of this population (Fine & Asch, 1981; Vash, 1982).

In thinking about ways to better serve these women, rehabilitation professionals looked to the family as one very important but relatively ignored resource for change (Lindenberg, 1980; Power & Dell Orto, 1980). This chapter explores the issue of family involvement in mental health interventions for women with physical disabilities by first examining the mental health needs of these women, then the interventions designed to meet these needs, and finally some optimal family roles for each intervention. The chapter concludes with some selected suggestions for the preparation of families for a more active role.

MENTAL HEALTH NEEDS OF WOMEN WITH PHYSICAL DISABILITIES

Studies to date of women with physical disabilities suggest that this population has a variety of mental health needs. The women need to feel that they are able to share their problems with others in an understanding and supportive environment (Blandford, 1968; Celotta & Kriegsman, 1980; Henkle, 1975; Oradei & Waite, 1974; Power & Rogers, 1979). They need to become aware of their present status, behavior, and feelings (Celotta & Kriegsman, 1980; Henkle, 1975; Oradei & Waite, 1974). They need to increase their self-acceptance (Atkins,, 1982; Banik & Mendelson, 1978; Celotta & Kriegsman, 1980; Fine & Asch, 1981; Guggenheim & O'Hara, 1976; Henkle, 1975; Hollingsworth & Harris, 1980; Kriegsman & Bregman, 1985) and their acceptance of others (Celotta & Kriegsman, 1980). They need to set new, more adaptive goals (Banik & Mendelson, 1978; Celotta & Kriegsman, 1980; Danek & Lawrence, 1985; Guggenheim & O'Hara, 1976; Roessler, Milligan, & Ohlson, 1968) and to learn new behaviors to meet these goals (Carrick & Bibb, 1982; Celotta & Kriegsman, 1980; Harris & Hollingsworth, 1980; Kriegsman & Bregman, 1985; Kubler-Ross & Anderson, 1968; Roessler, Milligan, & Ohlson, 1979).

Based upon research concerned with women's mental health needs, and our extensive experience working with this population, a needs hierarchy has been developed. Included in this hierarchy are all of the need categories listed above with the exception of the first need listed: the need to share problems in an understanding and supportive environment. This is not listed as a mental health need because it is instead considered a condition for effective interventions. There is also an additional need category not found in the literature, but encountered by us: environmental mastery needs.

Table 11.1 shows the three main need categories arranged in hierarchical order. They are: basic mental health needs, and environmental mastery needs. Basic mental health needs deal with issues of self-awareness, self-acceptance, and acceptance of others. Women with these needs are usually in a great deal of distress and have problems in many or all areas of their lives. An example is the blind woman who was taught that she would always need to be dependent upon others for her survival, thus creating feelings of her being unacceptable in some important ways. The basic mental health needs are critical fundamental needs, and they must be met before adequate progress in other areas is possible.

Problem-solving needs deal with issues of setting goals and learning goal-related skills. A woman with needs in this category usually has one or two problems that are causing her concern, but she is able to function well in most other areas of her life. Often these needs can be met without the aid of a professional. Examples are the deaf woman who must select a career or the newly paraplegic woman who must learn how to cook while remaining in a wheelchair.

Finally, environmental mastery needs deal with issues of goal actualization. At this point we assume that the woman is mentally healthy and has all the skills she needs to survive in a hospitable environment. The problem here is that psychological and physical barriers in that environment make it difficult for her to use the skills she has. An example is the woman with multiple sclerosis who is being shunned by her fellow employees.

TABLE 11.1 Mental Health Needs of Women with Physical Disabilities and Suggested Interventions

Basic mental health needs	
Need area 1:	The need to be self-aware.
Need area 2:	The need to accept oneself.
Need area 3:	The need to accept others.
Suggested strategies:	Individual counseling, family counseling.
Problem-solving needs	
Need area 5:	The need to set new, realistic goals.
Need area 6:	The need to learn skills to reach these goals.
Suggested strategies:	Peer-support groups, focused counseling.
Environmental mastery needs	
Need area 7:	The need to actualize goals.
Suggested strategies:	Organizational consultation.

Note that these needs are shared by many men and women who seek mental health counseling. In fact, research has shown that among women who have participated in support groups, many of the needs of women with physical disabilities are similar to those of women in general (Warren, 1976; Whitely, 1978). In our experience, what separates these women from the population in general as well as from men with disabilities is not the type of basic needs but rather the expression of those needs under the influence of both disability and sex factors.

Both disability and sex factors can determine the extent of the need as well as influence the intervention process. For example, a woman with cerebral palsy may have a more severe self-acceptance problem when compared with an able-bodied woman, due to society's reaction to her in the course of her growing up. Or a blind woman, trying to set realistic career goals, may need to take her disability into consideration when exploring possible careers, schools, and transportation. She may have to take her gender into consideration when she is examining the possibility of combining a career and motherhood.

At any one time, a woman may be placed in different need categories for different areas of her life. Take the case of the newly paraplegic wife and mother of two, who had been a successful accountant. After months of physical and psychological readjustment she finds that she can no longer discipline her children nor move comfortably about her old office. In the parenting area she has a problem-solving need to learn techniques for "disciplining with a disability." In the career area, she has an environmental-mastery need to redesign the office space to accommodate her wheelchair.

For any particular problem, the needs can be arranged in a hierarchical order, with lower order needs assuming precedence over higher order needs. One example of the hierarchical nature of these need categories is seen by looking at the woman who cannot set realistic academic goals because she has not developed adequate self-acceptance. Another example is the woman who cannot keep a job because she has not set realistic career goals.

Factors that Create Needs

We have just discussed mental health need categories that apply to women with physical disabilities. It is also important to try to understand what factors create the needs in the first place. Some preliminary ideas about major factors are considered here. These factors include (1) personality, (2) life experiences, (3) the nature of the specific disability, (4) the age and life stage of occurrence of disability, and (5) the current age and life stage. Each is discussed briefly below.

The first factor, personality, greatly affects the way in which life challenges are met. For example, a woman who is by nature shy may find it difficult to deal with situations that require asking for help, and therefore may have problems accomplishing tasks both at home and at work.

The second factor, life experiences, concerns the types of people and events in the life of the woman. Certain experience, such as abuse in childhood, negative societal attitudes toward disabilities, and physical barriers can create numerous mental health needs.

The third factor is the nature of the specific disability. Disabilities can range from hidden ones, such as chronic pain or epilepsy, to visible ones, such as spinal cord injury or cerebral palsy. They can also range from marginally disabling conditions, such as slight hearing loss, to major disabling conditions, such as paraplegia. Each disability creates its own set of challenges. For example, chronic pain may cause a woman to be irritable in her dealing with others; a spinal cord injury (causing one to be wheelchair bound), may cause a woman to have a problem with physical barriers.

The fourth factor is the age and life stage of incurrence of the disability. Some disabilities, such as cerebral palsy, may appear at birth; others start in childhood or adolescence, such as those due to accidents. In the middle years, disabilities such as those due to diabetes or heart problems may be incurred. In the later years, conditions such as chronic disabling arthritis are more common. A disability incurred in childhood may disrupt or slow down the normal developmental process, creating an assortment of mental health needs. A disability incurred in the teen years may cause needs related to self and other acceptance and career goals. A disability incurred in midlife may cause needs related to maintaining or finding a new career. Finally, a disability incurred in old age may create needs related to social and financial goals.

The fifth factor is the current age and life stage of the woman. A college student may need to learn how to maintain independent living arrangements, whereas a wife and mother may need to learn new techniques for managing her home and children.

Women with physical disabilities have a variety of needs created by a number of factors, only some of which we have begun to explore here. It is hoped that future research efforts will be directed toward understanding the roots of mental health needs. Next we turn to those mental health interventions that can best address these needs.

MENTAL HEALTH INTERVENTIONS FOR WOMEN WITH PHYSICAL DISABILITIES

The interventions discussed next have been selected as appropriate for women with physical disabilities, who have needs for which the disability is a factor, and who for one reason or another require the help of a mental health service provider.

There are two important concepts, however, that must be explained before the interventions are described. First, professionals often assume that women with physical disabilities always have problems with a disability component, when in fact they may not. For example, one might begin to work with a young woman who has a marked facial disfiguration and assume that the counseling issue would be disability related, such as poor self-acceptance or being afraid of social interactions. The woman might really be concerned about a disagreement with her husband, related to the adoption of another child. For many women, the disability will not be an issue at all, while other concerns, such as how to communicate more effectively with a spouse, may be. This chapter deals only with those needs that are affected by the disability. Non-disability related mental health problems can be addressed by the typical mental health interventions available to the general population.

Second, many women with mental health needs will not require the help of a mental health service provider. Women who have both their basic mental health needs met and a supportive environment may well be able to work out problems on their own. Sometimes support groups, run without the aid of a professional, can be helpful.

There are a number of mental health interventions that have been available to women with physical disabilities (Vash, 1982), which are described below. Not included in this list are interventions that are either physical (e.g., physical rehabilitation) or political/economic (e.g., legislation) because they do not directly address mental health concerns. But these latter types of intervention are crucial and powerful interventions nevertheless, and must be considered when developing an exhaustive list of interventions that affect mental health. For example, teaching a woman to walk with the aid of crutches is a critical physical intervention; working to increase the number of women with physical disabilities who are hired is an extremely important political/economic intervention. Both of these interventions have an impact on the mental health needs of the women, but they do so indirectly, and are therefore not taken up in the following discussion.

A basic consideration underlying the selection of mental health interventions is that for each situation, some methods will be more cost-effective than others. In other words, the selected intervention should produce the greatest therapeutic gain for the least cost in terms of money, time, and emotional pain. As with medical treatments, there are preferred interventions, given the current needs of the woman, her personal preferences, strengths and resources, the support available to her, and the resources in the agency and community. The need area, however, remains the primary selection factor; although one must keep in mind all of these parameters when selecting interventions.

Although the current state of research is inadequate to indicate the best interventions given the needs, we suggest the following selections based both upon our experience and research and that of others, as well as upon logical analysis. These interventions are grouped by the three need categories described previously.

All of the interventions discussed below require the provision of a good deal of support, encouragement, and understanding, especially concerning the impact of a disability. In addition, the addressing of basic mental health needs requires an intense, supportive relationship with the mental health services provider, one that is of long-term duration. This is necessary in order to tackle pervasive problems that have been present for many years. The addressing of problem-solving needs requires the presentation of opportunities to explore various goal options and to learn new skills. Finally, the addressing of environmental mastery needs requires the provision of disability related information to others in the client's environment. These concepts will be further elaborated upon in the following sections.

Interventions for Basic Mental Health Needs

Two interventions are optimally suited to meeting basic mental health needs for this population; they are individual and family counseling. We consider these to be the interventions of choice because they have the power to address problems that are pervasive and deeply rooted. The power derived from these interventions is because of their intense focus on the woman and/or her family, and because there is sufficient time for significant growth to occur. Because of these factors, the mental health professional will be able to establish a good deal of trust. This will allow for a deep understanding of the forces operating on the woman and her family, and will enable the necessary role modeling, "reparenting," and reeducating.

Individual Counseling

Individual counseling, under the supervision of a mental health service provider, has long been an intervention of choice for women with physical disabilities. Often it is the only intervention available. Because of the nature of the needs addressed in individual counseling, the intervention time span may be from several months to years.

Many clients come to both individual and family counseling with hidden agendas that require surfacing and addressing. The presenting concern is often an issue (such as a disagreement with a friend) that may be worked through within a short period of time. Once the initial issue is resolved, and the woman is convinced of the therapist's concern, understanding, and competence, the therapist and client may renegotiate counseling objectives. The new objective is typically one of more fundamental concern, such as poor self-acceptance.

Individual counseling for women with physical disabilities may differ somewhat from counseling for a nondisabled population. Because some women with disabilities have had limited life opportunities, the therapist may find it necessary to work on some basic issues, such as teaching (primarily through example) about human relationships, rights, and responsibilities. Therapy may take longer because these women frequently spend much of their physical and emotional energy in physical challenges, and therefore often have fewer resources available for them to digest sessions and to practice new skills.

Family Counseling

In family counseling (Atkins, 1982; Shapiro & Harris, 1971), the woman with the disability and all or some of the family members (including, at times grandparents and other pivotal relations) are directly involved in the counseling process (Huberty, 1980). Family counseling is conducted by a mental health service provider who is trained to work not only with disabilities, but with families as well. As in individual counseling, issues may at first be obscured, and sessions may last from months to years. As trust develops, the therapist will help the family to look at its old behavior and communication patterns and to learn to change those that are unproductive.

In contrast to individual counseling, the family members must be willing to change themselves as well as provide support and encouragement. In the next section we move on to problem-solving needs and the interventions best suited to meeting them.

Interventions for Problem-Solving Needs

Two interventions are optimally suited to dealing with problem-solving needs of women with physical disabilities: peer support groups and focused counseling. These are the interventions of choice because they can offer the women support and encouragement along with practical, goal-related suggestions and opportunities to practice new, goal-related skills. These interventions have a heavy educational component and do not depend upon the development of a very close relationship with the counselor or on delving into the past. The mental health professional must be careful to screen out those women for whom individual or family counseling would be more appropriate.

Peer Support Groups

In the peer support group, a woman with a disability is joined by other women, or women and men with similar needs (Kriegsman & Celotta, 1981). This type of support group is facilitated by a mental health service provider with expertise both in disabilities and in leading groups (Kriegsman & Celotta, 1981). The groups may have from 5 or 6 to 10 members and usually have a time limit of 8 to 12 sessions.

The strengths of these groups are many. Group members feel at home rather quickly as they realize they do not have to explain themselves to the other members. The members can see that many of their concerns are shared by others; this "normalizing" effect is very comforting and motivating. Because members of these groups are usually in a variety of life stages, group members can use each other as role models (Atkins, 1982). There are opportunities to practice new skills with a variety of different people. As time goes on, members of the group act as resources for each other, further enhancing their self-acceptance and competence. Members often remain friends after the group dissolves and can thus depend upon one another when new problems arise.

Focused Counseling

Another type of intervention for problem-solving needs is focused counseling. Sessions are best facilitated by a mental health service provider who has both expertise with disabilities and with specific counseling areas, such as phobias, stress management or career development. Sessions in focused counseling are usually of short duration. The techniques used in focused counseling are often more informational and directive than are the interventions previously described. The mental health counselor may give lots of information and advice about specific areas. Reading assignments are frequently given.

Interventions for Environmental Mastery Needs

The final category of needs, environmental mastery needs, concerns the actualization of goals. Organizational consultation is the intervention of choice, because at this point, although a woman will have most of the competencies necessary for success, the environment might not be ready to physically or psychologically accommodate her. It is the organizational consultant's task to help prepare environments for the woman's entry or reentry.

Organizational Consultation

There are two basic types of organizational consultation: work/school consultation and community-group consultation. A mental health service provider who understands both disability issues as well as work/school organizations and/or communities is best suited to conduct this type of intervention. We have found that interventions are most effective when conducted by a person with a disability.

Interventions are usually of very short duration; sometimes one session is sufficient for change. What is required here are physical, behavioral, informational, and/or attitudinal changes in the organization. These usually come about through an open and honest interaction with the consultant and through the provision of information.

It is crucial that the consultant be prepared to deal with the emotional impact of the disability on those in the woman's environment. A number of feelings are expected to surface; there may be feelings of concern, loss, helplessness, guilt, and anger. Coworkers or friends may worry about incurring a disability themselves. They may feel embarrassed and uncomfortable in the presence of the woman and not know how to handle social interactions. Stereotypes must be elicited, if they exist, and must be gently confronted.

In work/school consultation, the mental health consultant works with people and/or the physical environment in the work/school setting to aid women who are either newly disabled, starting a job in a new setting, or who are going to school (Kriegsman & Bregman, 1985). In the work setting, the consultant advises employers about tasks that might be difficult for newly disabled women returning to work. The consultant may also work with employees who have questions or concerns about their new coworker. In addition, the consultant will advise the employer about removal of physical barriers. In the school setting, the consultant works with administrators, faculty, and/or students to help them understand the abilities and needs of the women and, again, to offer advice about how to deal with physical barriers.

Working with administrators and others in positions to effect change is a challenging prospect. The problems and practical concerns of administrators must be kept in mind. In addition, because administrators usually feel competent to deal with work-related problems, they must be approached as equals, albeit equals with different sets of skills. Working as a team, the administrator and consultant find ways to encourage employees to go along with suggested changes.

In community-group consultation, the consultant works with a woman's social community. The consultant facilitates community attitude change toward the disability and advises on physical barriers through group support sessions with friends and neighbors. These sessions allow individuals to vent their sadness, fear, or concerns, to ask questions, and to learn strategies for reincorporating the woman into the life of the community.

Additional Thoughts About Interventions

In some situations interventions may be flexible enough to encompass more than one need category. We have found, for example, that peer groups, although structured to help women with problem-solving issues, have sometimes been instrumental in increasing self-acceptance. These groups are not the optimal forum for increasing self-acceptance, however, and whenever possible should not be selected as the modality of choice for this problem. As was mentioned above, self-acceptance problems are deeply rooted and need a great deal of time and energy on the part of the client and professional for resolution; peer groups cannot provide this. Some women, in fact, with severe self-acceptance problems can become acutely distressed in peer groups and will need to be referred for individual or family counseling.

In other situations, an intervention that is not ideally suited for a particular need may have to be used as a compromise when it is the only alternative available. This can occur due to such restraints as money, time, and/or agency personnel, or due to a woman's preferences. Although a blind woman, for example, would benefit most from a peer group when tackling such issues as managing a first apartment, a group may not be available. She could receive some help from individual counseling, however, if necessary. In addition to the added expense of individual counseling, this intervention, as compared with a peer group, would most likely provide fewer solutions to this or related problems and therefore would not ordinarily be selected as the intervention of choice.

It is important to be alert to interventions that are not meeting the woman's needs and to make recommendations for change should this occur. The mental health service provider should watch for one or more of the following signals that point to a problem with the selected intervention. The most telling signal is that a woman will be absent from many sessions without a reasonable explanation or will drop out of the sessions altogether. Another signal is lack of progress on the part of a woman who comes to sessions. A final signal is the frustration and/or anger felt, but often ignored, by the mental health service provider when working with a particular woman. Instead of blaming either themselves or their client for a perceived failure, they must first consider whether a reasonable intervention was selected.

A mistake frequently occurs when an intervention is selected based upon an initial but cursory assessment of the woman's needs. A reassessment of those needs will have to be done in order to find the most appropriate intervention. As we have suggested, clients will often present an issue to be worked on that is put out as a test case. Once resolved, the therapist must see if the next problem presented is amenable to the same intervention. If it is not, the therapist must either change interventions or refer.

THE FAMILY'S ROLE IN MENTAL HEALTH INTERVENTIONS

The needs of women with physical disabilities and the interventions designed to meet those needs have been considered. The family's vital role in these interventions is discussed next.

The family can have a profound effect on the course and outcome of an intervention. Family members have strong emotional ties to each other, and these ties can be used to offer support in numerous ways. We believe that the degree and appropriateness of that support may often determine the efficacy of any mental health intervention.

As will be shown below, the type and degree of family support varies with the interventions. Interventions designed to meet basic mental health needs will require the greatest support from family members, followed by interventions designed to meet problem-solving and environmental-mastery needs.

When either individual or family counseling is selected as an intervention for meeting basic mental health needs, the family plays a highly significant role (Cook & Ferritor, 1985). There are a number of activities the family can engage in throughout the course of either individual or family counseling.

One or more of the following supportive roles may be needed in all interventions that follow, but these roles are of primary importance for individual and family counseling.

First, the family may initiate the referral process for counseling and help gather a list of competent mental health professionals who have experience working with women who have similar needs. The family might get this list from a family physician, from a rehabilitation hospital, or from an advocate group for women with physical disabilities.

Decreasing the woman's anxiety about getting help may be very important at this stage too. Most advocacy groups for persons with disabilities have volunteers who will make home visits or provide telephone conversations. These volunteers have disabilities themselves and speak from experience. Many of the advocacy groups have provided their volunteers with training in paraprofessional peer counseling. This initial, nonthreatening encounter often helps the woman consider the possibility of getting professional counseling. Family members can also help by listening to and acknowledging the woman's fears about counseling and by asking her how they can best assist.

In addition, the family may provide financial support and transportation to sessions. This will depend upon the age of the woman and her circumstances, the sense of responsibility the family feels toward individual members, and the family's own resources. If the woman is in need, but the family cannot manage to provide support, they can help by looking for alternative sources of support. It is most important to allow the woman with the disability as much independence as is possible. Financial aid and transportation should not be provided if the woman can reasonably provide these for herself.

If family counseling is selected, the family must commit themselves to the counseling process and attend sessions regularly. Most importantly, the family members must be prepared to change themselves, for as one member of a unit changes significantly, all other members will be affected (Bray, 1977). This means that they may have to change some attitudes and behaviors of their own in order to help facilitate change in their relative. For example, many parents will have to give up their understandable yet unproductive overprotectiveness or undeserved guilt. A husband may have to acknowledge his fear, anger, sadness and/or guilt. Children may have to assume more responsibility at home.

Once the woman has begun counseling, the family should be available to listen and to support her for her courage, growth, and increasing independence. The family members must be prepared to accept new attitudes and behaviors on her behalf, even though this may provoke some initial discomfort. For example, a severely physically disabled woman may want to dress herself, although the process may require 2 hours. Family members may find it difficult to accept this new, time-consuming behavior. Understanding the woman's "obstinance" as "determination" may require growth on the part of the family as well.

The family should also be sensitive to the woman's need for both physical and emotional privacy. Often the woman may require a great deal of personal care by family members and others. Those giving the care may feel unappreciated and hurt if the woman asks them to leave so that she may be alone. The woman may not want to share some of what she has discussed in counseling. Her privacy in this area, too, must be respected.

When counseling is terminated, the family may need to continue to provide support and encouragment. They may suggest interventions for problem-solving needs if the woman seems ready. Should there be significant regression, or should new issues emerge, the family must deal with them too, perhaps by tactfully suggesting that the woman consider follow-up help and/or by being prepared to reenter family counseling themselves.

Some women may not agree to seek professional help although they are in need. The family members must find ways to assist in promoting self-awareness when such needs are apparent. This can be done by letting the woman know how proud they are of her and of her efforts at growth. They might suggest that if she gets help she may reach some of her own important goals. The family must let the woman know that they will join with her in counseling if that becomes necessary. Using the services of volunteers from advocacy groups might help her as well. When all else fails, the family should seek help from a mental health provider experienced with these issues, and work with the provider on ways to assist the woman's self-development. As a last resort, it may be necessary to withdraw some support, such as financial assistance, until such time as the woman agrees to enter counseling.

The role of the family is still vital, but usually less intense when the intervention deals with meeting problem-solving needs. The family can help with the referral process, and provide support and encouragement during the intervention and termination stages.

When organizational strategies are selected to help women operationalize their goals, the family is less active than in the previous interventions. As the women are ready to set their goals in motion, it is important to work with the social, business, or academic communities, preparing them for the entering or reentering woman. Family members need to support the woman in her attempts to find a niche in the real world by being available to listen to the frustrations that are a predictable part of such endeavors. The family may also help arrange for an organizational consultant and come to meetings when appropriate.

Although the type and degree of support varies with the intervention, it is nevertheless true that the family's role is a critical one. Next we discuss the unfortunate situation that arises when families cannot act as a resource.

WHEN FAMILIES CANNOT HELP

Realistically, it is not always possible for families to assist the women. For instance, the family may not be available due to distance, death, or alienation. Some families may not know how to help, and community resources to assist them in this role may be nonexistent. Still other families may be dealing with needs of economic survival, precluding participation. Other families might have such severe psychopathology that they are unable to help.

The minimal involvement or noninvolvement of family members may in some cases prevent or slow progress. But for many women growth will occur in spite of a lack of family support. A woman with strong inner resources, a strong network of friends, and a counselor on whom she can depend, may still be able to make considerable progress. She may need to have internal dialogues with family members from time to time, if they are unavailable to her. Other techniques to use with unavailable family members are psychodrama, talking to an empty chair, and writing letters to unavailable family members. These techniques can often help a woman gain understanding and sometimes resolve differences.

Ideally we would hope that the family members were available to help. The next section explores those competencies families need to provide appropriate support.

SUGGESTED COMPETENCIES FOR FAMILIES

Some professionals have stated that families often lack the competencies necessary to be of help to women with physical disabilities (Lindenberg, 1980; Power & Dell Orto, 1980). What are some of the competencies needed by family members to provide effective support?

An often-overlooked but crucial family competence is the ability to acknowledge and attempt to meet all family members' needs, not just the needs of the woman with the disability. If all members do not feel supported, the family unit will not be strong enough to help the woman with the disability.

Another basic requirement for all families is to learn to accept the woman as a whole, unique person, despite the disability. This may require the realigning of values concerning physical abilities, with emphasis on what a woman *can* do rather than on what she is unable to do. For example, instead of focusing on a house that is no longer compulsively clean, family members should appreciate that their wife and mother is now working as a volunteer to help newly disabled teenagers.

Families must try to understand the thoughts and feelings of the woman with a disability. To do this, family members must learn active listening techniques. Family members must try to suspend judgment and listen for and accept the hidden meanings and feelings that often lie beneath the words because the woman herself may not be aware of these initially. They may gain increased understanding by attending family support groups, by imagining themselves in the woman's place, by reading books written by persons with disabilities, by talking to others with disabilities, and by watching honest portrayals of persons with disabilities in movies, plays, and television productions. One of the most supportive steps might be to work with a counselor familiar with disability issues who can explain the processes involved in the adjustment to a disability and teach the family productive communication skills.

Families need to be realistic about the woman's limitations. Because these may be difficult to assess, it is often best to allow the woman herself to be the determiner of what she is physically and/or psychologically prepared to do. Most importantly, families must refrain from limiting the woman's potential.

Families need to allow the woman as much independence as possible. Home management responsibilities may be dealt with creatively by the reassignment of chores, by the use of special adaptive devices, by the employment of extra household help, or by a move to a more accessible environment.

Families also need to be aware of the vital roles they play in the intervention process and be motivated to play that role. They need to understand how their roles may vary with the intervention selected. They need to learn when to support and when to challenge, when to intercede and when to withdraw.

Individual family members may need to change. They must be flexible and willing to grow individually and as a family unit. Finally, family members need the knowledge and the ability to make use of available resources for women with disabilities. This competency enables family members, when it is appropriate, to assist the woman to make better decisions.

ENABLING FAMILIES TO HELP

How can we help families to develop the competencies they need to provide optimal support to the woman with the disability? The mental health service provider can encourage their involvement in a number of ways (Shellhase & Shellhase, 1980). The provider may actually play one or more of four key roles: coach, educator, counselor, and advocate.

When a woman is newly disabled, the mental health professional may play the role of coach. At this time, it is very important to motivate families to become involved. They can do this by establishing a caring, supportive relationship with all members of the family. They must encourage family members to speak about their concerns and must take extraordinary care not to create or reinforce any guilt. They must demonstrate through words and actions that they feel the family plays a critical role in the growth process.

As they begin to work with the woman and her family, mental health providers may find themselves in the role of educator. In this role they may inform family members about disabilities in general and their own relative's specific disability. They must also help family members understand the nature of the intervention, how long it will take, what can be accomplished and how family members can help.

Information can be provided through the use of printed materials, phone conversations, or information sessions with family members. In addition, the mental health professional might recommend that family members join an educational class or group where one or more families attend sessions together. This type of group is found primarily in hospitals or rehabilitation centers (Huberty, 1980).

Sometimes family members will need more than information alone. They may need to get some counseling themselves. In their roles as counselors, mental health service providers can work, upon request, with family members in counseling sessions, or refer them to other helping professionals. There are family-support resources for helping family members cope with the disability of a relative.

Two commonly used types of family-support interventions are relations' support groups and families' support groups. In relations' support groups, the children, siblings, spouses or parents of the women meet primarily to support each other. These groups are facilitated by a professional with expertise both in disabilities and in working with relations' groups. The group size may range from 5 or 6 members to 10 or more. The issues discussed in these groups usually lend themselves to a limited number of sessions.

In the families' support group, one or more families meet to address the personal needs and concerns of family members, rather than the needs of the woman. The groups may be facilitated by a mental health service provider with expertise both in specific aspects of a variety of disabilities and in working with families. There are no set number of sessions in most groups, with many groups having rotating membership. Usually located in a rehabilitation center, these groups respond to the concerns members have at the time the group meets; typically there is no preset agenda. Group members, as they gain experience and sophistication through the sessions, reach out to newer members. They offer hope that the current hurts "shall also pass." They share techniques that have worked for coping with the disability and its effects.

Mental health providers frequently work as advocates when they help the community learn about and support women with physical disabilities. They can make themselves available to speak before community groups about the needs of these women. They can help create a speakers' bureau and enlist the women with disabilities to speak to such groups as community-service organizations, schools and other youth organizations, radio and TV talk shows, and special community events. They can prepare lists of resources and other written materials for those dealing with the everyday needs of a person with a disability. These can be distributed in libraries, supermarkets, doctors' offices, churches, schools and colleges, public-assistance distribution locations, lodges, and at county and state fairs and any other public facility where people may seek information. They can also lend their support to legal and economic policies that will assist the women and their families.

We have come to see that women with physical disabilities have a variety of mental health needs that must be met. If we select interventions judiciously, and if we train and involve families to assist in those interventions, we will be enabling these women to take their rightful places in society.

RESOURCES

Information

Contact: City and county governments' offices for handicapped persons.

Social work departments, local hospitals.

State/local office dealing with vocational rehabilitation. Provides financial aid for education and training for persons with disabilities.

Handicapped Organization for Women, Inc. (HOW, Inc.)
P.O. Box 35481
Charlotte, NC 28235

Nonprofit support group for women with physical disabilities, in the process of developing into a national organization.

Network for Equality of Women with Disabilities
Community Service Centers
1295 University Avenue
San Diego, CA 92103

Provides information nationwide on women's groups and needs.

Filmstrip

Mimi: This Is Who I Am. (1977).

Filmstrip showing the useful, productive, creative life of a woman with a physical disability; she also shares her past and current concerns.

Discussion guide by Peter J. Ketchum also available.

Guidance Associates
757 Third Avenue
New York, NY 10017

REFERENCES

Atkins, B. J. (1982). Women as members of special populations in rehabilitation. In L. Perlman (Ed.), *Women in rehabilitation: The sixth Mary E. Switzer memorial seminar and monograph* (pp. 38–43). Alexandria, VA: National Rehabilitation Association.

Banik, S. N., & Mendelson, M. A. (1978). Group psychotherapy with a paraplegic group, with an emphasis on specific problems of sexuality. *International Journal of Group Psychotherapy, 28*, 123–128.

Blandford, B. R. (1968). Peer group membership of young women with cancer. *Journal of Chronic Diseases, 21*, 325–322.

Bray, G. P. (1977). Reactive patterns in families of the severely disabled. *Rehabilitation Counseling Bulletin, 20*(3), 236–239.

Carrick, M. M., & Bibb, T. (1982). Disabled women and access to benefits and services. In L. Perlman (Ed.), *Women in rehabilitation: The sixth Mary E. Switzer memorial seminar and monograph* (pp. 25–35). Alexandria, VA: National Rehabilitation Association.

Celotta, B. (1979). The systems approach: A technique for developing counseling and guidance programs. *The Personnel and Guidance Journal, 57*, 412–414.

Celotta, B., & Kriegsman, K. H. (1980). Creative coping: An evaluation of counseling groups for women with physical disabilities. Paper presented at the American Personnel and Guidance Association meeting, Atlanta, GA.

Cook, D., & Ferritor, D. (1985). The family: A potential resource in the provision of rehabilitation services. *The Journal of Applied Rehabilitation Counseling, 16*(2), 52–53.

Danek, M. M., & Lawrence, R. E. (1985). Women in rehabilitation: An analysis of state agency services to disabled women. *Journal of Rehabilitation Counseling, 16*, 16–18.

Dimsdale, J. (1981). Aiding families' coping in cardiac rehabilitation programs. *Rehabilitation Counseling Bulletin, 24*(3), 256–257.

Fine, M., & Asch, A. (1981). Disabled women: Sexism without the pedestal. *Journal of Sociology and Social Welfare, 8*(2), 233–248.

Guggenheim, F. G., & O'Hara, S. (1976). Peer counseling in a general hospital. *American Journal of Psychiatry, 133*, 1197–1199.

Harris, R. N., & Hollingsworth, D. (1980). Locus of control and work limitations of disabled women. *Journal of Applied Rehabilitation Counseling, 11*(1), 140–143.

Henkle, C. (1975). Social work as a treatment modality for hospitalized people with rheumatoid arthritis. *Rehabilitation Literature, 36*(11), 334–341.

Hollingsworth, D., & Harris, R. N. (1980). Chronic low back pain and the rehabilitation process. *Journal of Applied Rehabilitation Counseling, 11*(2), 90–93.

Huberty, D. J. (1980). Adapting to illness through family groups. In P. W. Power & A. E. Dell Orto (Eds.), *Role of the family in the rehabilitation of the physically disabled* (pp. 433–443). Austin, TX: Pro Ed.

Kriegsman, K. H., & Bregman, S. (1985). Women with disabilities at midlife. *Rehabilitation Counseling Bulletin, 29*(2), 112–122.

Kriegsman, K. H., & Celotta, B. (1981). A program of group counseling for women with physical disabilities. *Journal of Rehabilitation, 47*, 36–39.

Kubler-Ross, E., & Anderson, J. R. (1968). Psychotherapy with the least expected: Modified group therapy with blind clients. *Rehabilitation Literature, 29*(3), 73–76.

Lindenberg, R. E. (1980). Work with families in rehabilitation. In P. W. Power & A. E. Dell Orto (Eds.), *Role of the family in the rehabilitation of the physically disabled* (pp. 516–525). Baltimore: University Park Press.

Oradei, D. M., & Waite, N. S. (1974). Group psychotherapy with stroke patients during the immediate recovery phase. *American Journal of Orthopsychiatry, 44*(3), 368–395.

Power, P. W., & Dell Orto, A. E. (1980). Approaches to family interventions. In P. W. Power & A. E. Dell Orto (Eds.), *Role of the family in the rehabilitation of the physically disabled* (pp. 321–330). Austin, TX: Pro Ed.

Power, P. W., & Rogers, S. (1979). Group counseling for multiple sclerosis patients: A preferred mode of treatment for unique adaptive problems. In R. G. Lasky & A. E. Dell Orto (Eds.), *Group counseling and physical disability* (pp. 115–127). North Scituate, MA: Duxbury Press.

Roessler, R., Milligan, T., & Ohlson, A. (1979). A personal adjustment training for the spinal cord injured. *Rehabilitation Counseling Bulletin, 19*(4), 554–555.

Rosin, A. J. (1975, August). Group discussions: A therapeutic tool in a chronic diseases hospital. *Geriatrics*, pp. 45–48.

Shapiro, R. J., & Harris, R. I. (1971). Family therapy in treatment of the deaf: A case report. *Family Process, 15*, 83–96.

Shellhase, L. J., & Shellhase, F. E. (1980). Role of the family in rehabilitation. In P. W. Power & A. E. Dell Orto (Eds.), *Role of the family in the rehabilitation of the physically disabled* (pp. 526–535). Austin, TX: Pro Ed.

Vash, C. (1982). Women and employment. In L. Perlman (Ed.), *Women in rehabilitation: The sixth Mary E. Switzer memorial seminar and monograph* (pp. 15–24). Alexandria, VA: National Rehabilitation Association.

Warren, L. (1976, May). The therapeutic status of consciousness raising groups. *Professional Psychology*, pp. 132–140.

Whiteley, R. M. (1978). Women in groups. In H. W. Harmen & J. M. Birk (Eds.), *Counseling women* (pp. 34–48). Monterey, CA: Brooks/Cole.

Personal Statement: Living in Spite of Multiple Sclerosis

Tosca Appel

Multiple sclerosis (MS) was something I knew nothing about or even considered being part of my life. Even if I did, it was more an illness for those who were young adults. However, I was one of those rare cases of MS that occur before age of 20—I was 11 years, 9 months old when my first symptom occurred.

My first attack of MS took the form of a lack of motor coordination of my right hand. I was unable to hold utensils and my hand was turned inward; my parents in their concern rushed me to the emergency room of the hospital. The intern who saw me at the emergency room told my parents without any exam that I had a brain tumor. Needless to say, this shocked my parents because, other than this attack, limited to my right hand, I was otherwise normal and healthy. I was admitted to the hospital, where I stayed for 12 days. Ten days after the initial attack the symptoms abated. Twelve days later I was discharged from the hospital and was totally back to normal. The doctors had put the blame of the attack on a bad case of nerves. Before the attack I was enrolled in Grove Lenton School of Boston. This was a very high-pressured school. From my A average in grammar school, my grades had dropped to roughly a B− average. I was worried, and I spent many sleepless nights crying myself back to sleep. I could not handle the pressure of going to a private school. Consequently, I transferred to a public junior high school. Without the pressure, my grades went up to an A− average. I was happier and everything was fine.

My second attack occurred when I was 16 years old and in the 11th grade. My mother and I were planning my sweet-16 birthday party. My mother rented a room in a nightclub. I was all excited, planning who I was going to invite, what it was going to be, and what the room was going to be like. One day before the party, my history teacher asked me a question. I stood up to answer and my speech came out all garbled. I was unable to string the words into a sentence. I was even unable to utter words. All that came out were sounds. I clutched my throat to help the words come out easier. At times they did, but at times it came out a garbled mess. I remembered the teacher's look. He looked at me in utter surprise and a little bit helplessly. In total utter shock, my attempts at speech sounded so ludicrous to me—so totally as if it did not belong to my head, and so totally foreign that I started laughing hysterically. I couldn't be serious about the sounds I was making. Again, my parents rushed me to the hospital where again another intern did his initial workup on me. However, the sounds that came out of me were so funny that I again started laughing almost hysterically, because I was well aware of what I wanted to say and I was also well aware that it was not coming out of my mouth right. The intern, in his wisdom, thought that this behavior was an attention-getter. He thought I was faking the whole thing.

After the first attack my mother had decided that she would not let me be admitted to the hospital. I was then not admitted, but I was instead seen on an outpatient basis. The inability to speak lasted roughly 2 weeks. I had the party and had a good time. But pictures were taken during this time, and I hated them. Why? My smile came out cockeyed. I smiled with the left half of my mouth, without moving the right side. To me it was quite ugly. After my speech returned, the doctors said that the right side of my mouth and tongue were numb, paralyzed, thus making it very hard for me to talk. Overall, I do not remember the attack. After 2 weeks of this attack, I again went into complete remission.

In 1967, at the age of 19, I applied to and was accepted at Northeastern University. However, during the fall term I started having trouble seeing. My father drove me to the train station so that I would be able to take the trolley to school. But after I got on the trolley, I took it beyond my stop, and went to the Massachusetts Eye and Ear Infirmary to have my eyes checked out. I did not tell my family about my concerns because I did not want to worry anybody. A doctor put me through a whole eye workup, and he said that he could not promise how much sight I would get back in my eye but that he would do all he could. Considering that I was an English major and I loved to read, this freaked me out. I asked him if glasses would help, and he said no, that he might be able to get all my sight back or none of it, but that he could not promise me anything. I had to call my mother after I left him. I first went into the restroom and cried. I controlled myself long enough to call my mother. I got off the phone with my mother as quickly as possible, and left for school on the train.

During the ride, I was attempting to figure out if it would have been better to have been born blind and never have seen anything than to lose sight after having it and know what you are missing. As a result of this thinking process, I came to the conclusion that it would have been better for me to have been born blind, because I now knew the beauties of a sunset, of reading, of a flower, of all the things that people who have sight take totally for granted. I do not know how I would rationalize it now.

When I got to school I went into the cafeteria, sat with my friends, and began crying. Once I stopped crying, I got it all out of my system and my friends and I decided that crying would not solve anything, and the best thing I could do was to go home, take some medication, and see if my sight returned. When I returned home, I did not initially tell my parents of what the doctor had said about the possibility that my sight might not return. I decided that my parents always got very nervous when something happened to me and that there was no need to worry them about me.

So, I did not say anything until my mother mentioned that she had spoken to my neurologist. At this time, unbeknownst to me, I was diagnosed as having MS. My neurologist had told my mother of the diagnosis and told her to tell me. My mother had refused. The doctor then told her that I would never forgive her if she did not tell me. She said that was something that she would have to deal with and did not want to tell me. Consequently, following my mother's wishes, the doctor naturally did not tell me.

The loss of sight in my left eye lasted 3 weeks, and then I went back to college and continued the daily routine of living. Still my mother had not told me about the MS. She bore it alone and did not tell anyone for 6 months after she knew. The only person she spoke to about my MS was my older sister, who is 6 years older than I am. When my mother would become depressed, she would call my sister and cry about the injustice of its having happened to me rather than to herself.

My mother's rationale for not telling me was basically twofold. First, she felt that she should not burden me with the knowledge of my chronic degenerative disease because the knowledge of MS could deter me from doing what I wished to do. Second, when my mother saw me running out of the house to go on a date or to a party, she would get scared and sad, thinking about the day that I would not be able to go out and enjoy myself. My mother felt that the knowledge would hang like a cloud over my head, so she made it her responsibility that I was not to know.

However, this conspiracy of silence put my doctors in a difficult position when I went to see them. I would beg the doctor to tell me what was wrong, but he could not because of a promise made to my mother. Because I remembered when a doctor had told me I might have had a brain tumor, which was incorrect, I asked my neurologist if I was going to die of a brain tumor—to which he said, "You can only die of a brain tumor if you have a brain." This may have been a joke to him; it was not for me! The worry about the brain tumor was a preoccupation of mine. My fingers would tingle, or I would feel something go wrong with my balance, and I would be worried that it might be caused by a brain tumor. I was really worried about dying. I found no comfort in the silly remark that I would need a brain to have a brain tumor. At the time, I told the doctor that I was not kidding and that I was very worried. To that, he replied that they did not know what was wrong with me, but when they discovered a pill for it they would rush it to me. I left his office feeling very depressed, very alone, and not understood.

Finally, when my mother told me I had MS I was sad and confused, but also very much relieved. Now there was a basis for my physical concerns. Because I had long periods of remission over the next 10 years, there were the low points of exacerbation but the long periods of life, living, and the pursuit of happiness. It was great to be a young adult who was living life and running ahead of the long-reaching shadow of MS.

At age 28, I reached a major crisis point in my life. I was faced with the reality of ongoing deterioration. My sight reached the point where I was not able to read the newspaper. In addition, I lost what functional use I had in my left hand. Although these losses may not seem to be catastrophic issues to the nondisabled, they were catastrophic to me. The reason was that they reaffirmed the reality that I had little control of my body and of what was happening to it.

The feeling intensified when I had to resign myself to the fact that I needed to use a wheelchair. To me, this was an admission of defeat and that my disease was getting the best of me. While I made the cognitive decision to continue to struggle, it was very difficult when the little physical control I had was slowly eroding away. As a result, I made the choice to live, rather than to deteriorate or die. Although this is easy to verbalize, it is often not easy to implement. I can choose to actualize myself, but I am limited by physical and emotional resources to follow through completely in that process.

My unique situation is that I was dependent upon my family, with whom I lived. I was also dependent upon my mother to provide me with the assistance I needed, such as cooking and partial dressing. Even though I wanted to live independently, I had to accept that I had a wonderful home life, caring parents, and a loyal brother.

The next major transition was when my father and mother died, both within the same year. While initially having to deal with the impact of the loss of people I care about, I also had to face the question of what would happen to me. Fortunately, when my parents became ill I made the choice to get an apartment and to develop the independent-living support systems I would need. Another possibility for me was to extend the relationship with my boyfriend, to whom I was once engaged and whom I had been dating for 15 years. However, this possibility is questionable, for there were reasons we did not get married and they are still real concerns.

This is my response to the disease that has plagued me for 24 years and has altered the course of my life. I will not let it beat me. What motivates me is the memory of my parents and the knowledge of my heritage. My mother and father spent years in a concentration camp, and many of my other family members perished there. I feel the obligation to make the best of my situation and draw on the strength of those persons who suffered far more than I am suffering. As I see it, the key to my ability to survive is the memory, support, and encouragement of others. They have made the difference, accepting me as I am and helping me to resolve my feelings about not being what I was or could have been.

PART III: Study Questions and Suggested Activities

1. Identify the critical issues in the case of a young woman who has had an experience similar to that of Robert Neumann as related in his personal statement.
2. What was your reaction to the statement by Neumann: "Self-esteem is most enhanced when one's positive expectations converge with the reality of one's experience."
3. How is an adolescent's search for self-identity complicated by spina bifida?
4. How can the family facilitate the process of grieving and acceptance for adolescents with spina bifida?
5. Who should be responsible for sex-education programs for adolescents coping with disabilities?
6. What role has society played in the formulation of attitudes toward the sexuality of persons with disabilities?
7. How has the AIDS issue created additional concerns for families of adolescents with special needs?
8. What is the role of the health professional in working with parents concerned about the sexuality of their children?
9. How can the family be a liability in the school-to-work transition for an adolescent with a disability?
10. What role does birth order play for the disabled adolescent in the area of sibling rivalry?
11. What role do sibling play in the developmental process of a disabled sibling?
12. Do you think that the mental health needs of women with disabilities are different from those of men with disabilities? If so, please explain in what way(s).
13. How do societal roles and expectations for women create stress for women with disabilities?

14. If you were in Tosca's situation, after reading her personal statement, would you consider marriage or having a child?
15. What are the family issues with Tosca that helping professionals should be aware of?
16. What is your reaction to how Tosca was told about MS?

IV
Selected Challenges of the Later Years

Introduction

The goals of this section are to emphasize the relationship between the person with an illness or disability and the family environment, to provide the reader with insights into how the family can be assisted to achieve its own adjustment in a disability or illness situation, and to explain how family members can become significant factors for the patient's treatment and eventual rehabilitation. Each chapter was selected because of the increased public attention to a particular disease, trauma, or service delivery system and because of the importance of exploring how the family can make a difference when intervention efforts are planned. The material in this section illustrates how a particular disease or trauma stimulates unique family needs. When these needs are responded to by the helping professional, intervention and rehabilitation strategies are considerably enhanced.

A critical issue for all families that deal with the demands of the illness and disability experience is the availability and accessibility of respite-care services. Respite care has been a topic of rapidly emerging interest because of the increased incidence of the chronically ill and the severely disabled person who is being cared for by family members, either by choice or by default due to limited feasible alternatives. Respite care itself represents a valuable, needed resource for families coping with continued stress that is created by intense caregiving efforts. In Chapter 12, Arthur E. Dell Orto focuses attention on the accruing need for respite care from his perspective as a rehabilitation psychologist working with families that are stressed by the illness experience. Also within Chapter 12 is a discussion of existing respite-care models and how they can be applied to persons and families affected by a severe disabling condition.

Chapter 13, "Alzheimer's Disease: Impact on Family and Caregivers," notes that at least 2 million adults in the United States are affected by Alzheimer's disease and 13 billion dollars per year is spent on maintaining Alzheimer patients in nursing homes. Yet, the preponderance of care for impaired elderly persons is provided by the family. One of the authors of this chapter, Rennie Golec, was for many years a caregiver for her elderly father, and both authors, Rennie Rogers Golec and Ann D. Lassalle, high-light the role of the family in the care of the Alzheimer's patient. They also explain different roles both for family members and helping professionals when caring for the ill person.

The personal statement by Judy Teplow confronts the reader with many critical issues related to caring for a parent with amyotrophic lateral sclerosis (ALS). This powerful statement indicates that family needs must be consid-ered when treatment plans are developed. The account of what it was like to care for a chronically ill person emphasizes to the reader that families are crucial for the patient's well-being. The statement conveys the message that helping professionals have a unique opportunity to enhance their interven-tion efforts and that they must consider the changing needs of family members.

Not only does this personal statement address the enormity of the issues relative to amyotrophic lateral sclerosis, but it illustrates the cumulative stres-sors associated with caregiver issues of elderly ill parents. Part IV concludes with study questions and suggested activities designed to facilitate the per-sonalization of the topics addressed in Part IV.

12 Respite Care: A Vehicle for Hope, the Buffer Against Desperation

Arthur E. Dell Orto

The ultimate tradegy in health care today is that most of the problems associated with the illness experience (e.g., pain, stress, heartaches, inconvenience, and aggrivation) are not necessary. The irony is that these problems are caused not only by the disease, illness, or disability, but are also often caused by the health care system that is supposed to help but that often does not. This situation is created more by default than by intent. Frequently, the health care system is designed to provide treatment based on the assumption that at some point the person, the family, or significant others will be able to develop the physical and emotional resources necessary to contain the ravages of illness while facilitating the process of restoration and rehabilitation.

Although this is fine in theory, the reality is that most people do not have the family or significant others who are ready, willing, and able to respond to the evolving challenges of the illness experience. Therefore, when discussing, designing, and implementing comprehensive health care programs, it is imperative that the respite-care needs of the individuals as well as families be taken into consideration.

In order to develop a perspective on respite care, there must be an understanding of how respite care has been defined, an awareness of the need for respite care, an exploration of existing models and a presentation of its application to persons and families affected by selected illness and disabilities. Discussion of these areas also necessitates that other issues, such as caregiver stress, rejuvenation needs, quality of life and creative interventions, be addressed.

Any discussion of respite care should include a recognition of the pioneering efforts of the groups and organizations that conceptualized and implemented respite-care programs for the developmentally disabled (DeJong, 1977; Loop, 1979; Pullo & Hahn, 1979; Shoob, 1978; Warren, 1979). Although these efforts are reflected in the following definitions of respite care, the principles and philosophy of respite care have become applicable to many populations, such as the physically disabled (Frankel, 1984; Goethe & Levin, 1984; Huberty, 1974; Livsey, 1972; Power & Sax, 1978; Scheinbert & Kaplan, 1983; Yalom & Greaves, 1977), the elderly (Heckler, 1985; Jones & Vetter, 1984; Osborne, 1985; Ware & Carper, 1982), and the mentally ill (Carter, 1984; McCubbin, 1979; Ryglewicz, 1985; Spaniol & Zipple, 1986).

DEFINITIONS

Because of the mission of respite care, it is important to consider how it is defined. Just as there is variability in the populations served, there are differences among the definitions of respite care.

In their outstanding book, *Respite Care*, Cohen and Warren provide the following statement:

> The definition of respite care as "the temporary care of a disabled individual for the purpose of providing relief to the primary caregiver" seems straightforward and noncontroversial. However, in practice, there is considerable variation in the interpretation of the scope of services to be called respite care. One of these variations concerns the distinction between intermittent and ongoing services. Virtually all definitions of respite care include the idea of temporary services. (Cohen & Warren, 1985, p. 26)

The major problem with a time-limited definition of respite care is that the needs, problems and concerns of both the patient and family may be fluctuating in nature and exist over a lifetime.

Pullo and Hahn have presented another definition of respite care:

> The temporary and periodic provision of a range of services which prevent individual and family breakdown by relieving the caretaker of stress resulting by giving continuous support and/or care to a dependent individual. These services are not meant to replace other specialized services provided to an individual in need of care. (Pullo & Hahn, 1979, p. 1)

What is significant about this definition is that it conveys a sensitivity to the consequences of unchecked demands made on the family of an ill member and recognizes that illness and disability can overwhelm the family if consistent help is not provided.

Another definition which is more open-ended but population specific, is that of the New York State's Chapter 548, 1982:

"Respite" shall mean the provision of intermittent temporary substitute care of mentally retarded or developmentally disabled persons on behalf of and in the absence of the parent or legal guardian of the mentally retarded or developmentally disabled person, for the purpose of providing relief from the stresses of responsibilities concomitant with providing continued care. (Cohen & Warren, 1985, p. 26)

This definition is limited to the developmentally disabled, but it is sensitive to the need for intermittent care and recognizes the stressors associated with continued care.

The State of California's definition of respite care identifies the factor of constant care, and also identifies the need for both in-home and out-of-home services.

Respite care is the provision of intermittent and/or regular temporary care to persons with developmental disabilities on an in-home or out-of-home basis. It is designed to relieve families of the constant responsibility of caring for a member with a developmental disability. (Raub, 1982, p. 2)

Although the definitions of respite care focus upon the importance of providing relief for the consumers, family, and/or caregiver, they also address the *need* for viable and accessible respite care programs.

Theoretically, the availability of such programs should reflect a match between need and resources. Unfortunately, the *need* most often is in excess of the resources, which in turn may create stress and frustration on the part of those caregivers who are in need of and most often are desperate for such services.

NEED

In order to better understand the family's need for respite care, it is important to recognize the developmental process associated with the illness experience. Because illness and disability do not affect everyone at the same point in the developmental process or in the same manner, it is imperative that respite-care programs have the potential to respond to a changing needs system. Although the nature of the illness plays a major role in the determination of need, consideration must also be given to the complexities surrounding the emerging interaction between the family and the patient.

The need for respite care has been well documented in the literature (Cacioppo & Andrews, 1979; Featherstone, 1980; Greenfeld, 1972; Kenney, 1982; McCubbin et al., 1980; Upshur, 1983; Winkler, 1981). The commonality of these need statements is that they are multidimensional in both theory and application. First, there are the needs of the family member who is directly challenged by illness and/or disability. These needs vary according to the physical and emotional aspects of the illness as well as the age of the person, the person's position in the family, and the person's potential to assume a degree of self-determination and independence. Second, the needs of the family vary according to its structure, resources, traditions, developmental stage, and its ability to access and use support. These individual and familial needs, however, do not exist in isolation from the community, society, or the health care system, which in fact may not see need from the same frames of reference as the patient or family. In fact, perhaps they should not because the roles and functions of these systems are distinct from those of the client and the family. However, these systems should be complementary to the respite-care goals and familial needs of the family and not adversarial to them. Unfortunately, most health care and political systems are burdened with primary concern in the areas of policy and finances, whereas consumers of respite care and their families are often concerned about more basic concerns, such as emotional survival and quality of life.

For some families, the issue of respite care is cast in the shadow of a life-or-death reality, whereas some families are faced with a chronic situation that is stable, deteriorating, or in flux. In these situations, there is an intensification of the responsibilities and consequences of care. Therefore, some families are caught between being stressed and being resentful during the illness experience, as well as feeling guilty about anticipated relief consequent to the institutionalization or death of a loved one.

In exploring the life-or-death issues surrounding severely disabled infants (Head, Head, & Head, 1985), consider not only the stress faced by families during the process of decision making, but also the long-term implications of decisions. For example, some spouses may be put in a position of having to choose between their marriage or the care of an ill child because one spouse may want to keep the child at home, whereas the other wants to institutionalize the child.

Recently problems have arisen for families due to the impact of deinstitutionalization, which has taken away options for families who want to "place" a family member. As Cohen points out, "many families are not capable of coping with the awesome responsibility of caring for a severely disabled child day after day, without considerable help" (Cohen, 1982, p. 8).

MODELS

Respite care exists today because there were people who recognized the need, developed the concepts, and evolved the models with which to respond to those patients and families terrorized by the illness experience. These models are recent developments in the health care delivery system: The first national conference on temporary family-support systems and community-based respite services for developmentally disabled persons and their families took place in 1978 (Taylor & Loop, 1978). Since 1978, there has been a dramatic increase in the awareness of the need for and the potential of respite care. Consequently, there has been an emergence of various models that have unique assets and limitations reflective of the variability of the problems they attempt to address. In discussing the need for programmatic variability, Upshur states, "A variety of approaches to providing respite care have developed each with its particular advantages and disadvantages" (Upshur, 1983, p. 19).

An example of the pros and cons of a respite-care model is presented by Macourt and Southam (1983). This particular approach employs "regular intermittent admissions," which is helpful because the family can count on a planned program of respite care on a proactive rather than a reactive basis. The limitation of this planned program is that services may be used regardless of whether they are needed. Also focusing on scheduled respite, Macourt and Southam (1983) discussed an alternative approach that includes a once-per-year or once-per-month option as well as a holiday relief period. Similarly, following the philosophy that respite care should be accessible as well as flexible, some models employ a full respite system as well as intermittent respite, such as a weekend per month, or scheduled annual respite periods (Dunn, MacBeath, & Robertson, 1983).

However, although respite-care programs may have varying structures, philosophies and resources, they may not meet the specific needs of individual families. When this occurs, families are often forced to develop new programs or to modify existing ones. An example of this is the response of parents of severely disabled children who could not use respite services as they existed, and who therefore established a cooperative program among themselves (Ferguson, Lindsay, & McNees, 1983). The advantages of this "respite-care-co-op" model were that the families had similar problems, appreciation of the needs of the patient, as well as an awareness of the resources required to respond in a helpful way. This model stresses the importance of mutual peer-group support, not only in areas of information, but also in the development of specific skills needed to work with a child. By matching resources with needs, families have the opportunity to develop a system of care that is stable and responsive to ongoing need through peer support, education, and encouragement.

When we consider the needs of the sick and disabled, and the untapped resources of this country, we must recognize that there must be a better way to conceptualize and deliver respite care that can make coping with illness more reasonable, bearable and survivable. This is an especially crucial aspect when dealing with the unique needs of specific illnesses and their impact on the person and family.

SPECIFIC ILLNESSES

Even though there is a commonality of need for persons and families challenged by the demands and stressors of illness and disability, there is also a uniqueness relative to each illness experience. The contributions of respite care to the treatment and rehabilitation processes have been recognized for many illnesses, such as stroke (Kinsella & Duffy, 1979; Livsey, 1972; New, Ruscio, & Priest, 1968; Power & Sax, 1978; Stroker, 1983; Travis, 1976), multiple sclerosis (Frankel, 1984, p. 282; Scheinberg & Kaplan, 1983), head injury (Ben-Yishay et al., 1981; Chadwick et al., 1981; Goethe & Levin, 1984; Hayden et al., 1982; Lezak, 1978; Long & Webb, 1983; Lynch, 1983; Najenson, 1974; Romano, 1974), cancer (Berger, 1985; Huberty, 1984; Yalom & Greaves, 1977), mental illness (Carter, 1984; Grad & Sansbury, 1963; McCubbin, 1979; Ryglewicz, 1985; Spaniol & Zipple, 1986; Thompson & Doll, 1982) and Alzheimer's disease. The complexity of the problem and the potential of respite care is readily seen in the needs of Alzheimer patients who manifest physical as well as intense emotional needs.

ALZHEIMER'S DISEASE AND RESPITE CARE

Because approximately 5 million older people are able to live in the community with some help, the added dimension of 2.5 million Alzheimer victims creates an emergency situation that will make respite care more of a necessity than a luxury (Osborne, 1985). In addressing the problems faced by families challenged by Alzheimer's disease, Heckler points out the severe and chronic stress that exists, the need to support caregivers, and the importance of respite-care programs that reduce the need for hospitalization (Heckler, 1985).

This support and respite care are needed because families of Alzheimer patients are challenged by a long-term situation that may last 5 to 10 years following diagnosis. This time frame accentuates the differences between acute and chronic situations. Acute illness has a built-in respite due to the time limitation, compared with the expanding and long-term demands of chronic conditions that can intensify the need for respite care as well as models of effective long-term coping.

Although home care for a loved one is difficult in most situations, it is intensified particularly when the elderly person's disability is affected by dementia (Ballard, 1984). Presenting dementia as a complex process that requires complex interventions, Zarit & Zarit (1982) feel that interventions with the family can be helpful by reducing stress to a manageable level. A major factor in the stress reaction of families of Alzheimer patients is that the medical community has little to offer in terms of a cure or arresting the process; consequently, families are often forced to accept the reality of deterioration rather than to continue to rely on the hope for a cure. For some, this facilitates the decision for a nursing-home placement. For others, it is a motivation to attempt home care, due to the prognosis of a limited life span for their loved one. However, no matter what the choice, nursing home or home placement, the burden is still there, but different (Zarit & Zarit, 1982).

There is an added stressor for families when their loved one's behavior becomes destructive, aggressive, and dangerous. This occurs when the elderly person is perceived to be a stranger whose behavior makes hospitalization more attractive and home care more impossible. An explanation for this reaction is that families are so burdened and frustrated that they burnout, thus forcing institutionalization—not by choice, but out of frustration and desperation. One problem common to families of Alzheimer patients is the reluctance to seek help until they are at the point of physical, financial, and emotional exhaustion. Often at this point great damage has been done, and an intensive and comprehensive intervention program must be instituted to try to stabilize the patient as well as the family. Often this can be achieved through a combination of direct services as well as seminars that provide information, skills, and peer support.

Not only does respite care help families to cope with aging parents. It also helps the elderly person by creating an opportunity to have basic needs met periodically by the respite-care process, which in turn affords a chance for nonmaintenance interaction with the family.

The priority is to maintain elderly in the community with their families; however, there are problems inasmuch as all communities are not in positions to provide significant support, and some families do not want to, or feel that they cannot, take care of an elderly ill member. Given that support systems and familial resources may vary, there is a commonality of caregiver and patient need as reflected in the work of Jones and Vetter, who concluded:

> The family is the main source of assistance to dependent elderly and usually it is the woman in the family who is the primary caregiver. With very little assistance, either informal or formal received by the carers, there was a great deal of distress and psychological morbidity among the carers. (Jones & Vetter, 1984, p. 511)

Although recognizing that the family is the primary support system for the elderly (Eggert et al., 1977; Hasselkus & Brown, 1983), a problematic situation is created in which older persons without families are often the ones who are institutionalized because there are limited alternatives (Fengler & Goodrich, 1979; Shanas, 1979). Given the increasing number of older persons in need of services, the option of institutional respite care may not be available to those persons with a family. This is an ironic situation because those persons who have had families and have made an effort to maintain and sustain family bonds are often forced to deplete their emotional and financial resources because they "cared too much." However, being an outstanding parent and making lifelong sacrifices does not necessarily mean that the children will be willing to take care of their elderly ill parents. The following case synopses illustrate an example of two responses to a family crisis. The first case synopsis illustrates how one family had as part of its tradition to take care of family members in sickness and health.

> The family consisted of a mother, father, three sons and a daughter. The parents immigrated to the United States in the 1920s. They pursued the American Dream through total parental sacrifice and focused on the well-being of their children and on the desire that they become educated and productive members of society. However, their cultural background valued education for the sons, whereas the daughter's role was to stay home to take care of the family.
>
> Eventually, the sons got married and started families and careers of their own. At this point, it was possible for the daughter to begin to develop a life of her own. However, the illness of her mother created the situation where she was expected to care for her mother because (1) she was a woman, (2) she was at home, (3) she was not married, and (4) this was the way it was traditionally done. More importantly, this was what she wanted to do and was happy about it. Therefore, her role emerged as caretaker for her ill mother, who suffered a stroke, and father who had Alzheimer's disease. Her mother began to deteriorate and needed continuous care, which tested the resiliency of the family and its ability to provide respite care. Not only did all the sons share in the financial aspects of sustaining their sister and parents, but their wives equally divided the tasks of caring for the patient. They worked from the framework of a family conference, designated the tasks, and identified who would be responsible for specific tasks. What was most impressive about this family is that even considering that they had the advantages of geographically centralized living arrangements, they had a functional attitude that was demonstrated in the willingness to do more than was expected or designated as their tasks. An example was how one daughter-in-law provided constant care for 3 weeks while another daughter-in-law cared for a sick child. She did not think to expect that the time should be made up and did not accept it when the offer was made.
>
> This high level of functioning continued for 7 years at which time the mother died, and then for another 5 years, when the father died. This created a situation where the daughter was left alone without a job or income. A family meet-

ing was held and the decision was made to give the family home to the daughter and to provide her with a weekly income for the years she sacrificed for the family. Unfortunately, this was a short-lived pause, because the wife of one of the brothers became ill and the daughter resumed her role as caregiver. When her sister-in-law died, her brother moved in with her and stayed 2 years until he died. At this point, the daughter became ill and was cared for by her sister-in-law until her death.

This unique example of self-provided family respite care demonstrates what can be accomplished, However, not all families are able to respond at this level, as the following case example illustrates:

There were 12 children and their spouses living within 2 miles of each other. As a consultant to the family, the present author initially thought that designing and implementing a functional respite-care system would be very possible. Unfortunately, the family relegated care to an unmarried daughter, and the only participation was at a primitive level. The other children would insist that their mother receive the best care and only from the daughter, because no stranger should be allowed to take care of their mother. Regrettably and predictably, the primary caregiver became ill herself. The mother was placed in a nursing home and the family reached a state of dysfunction by not speaking to each other.

Quantitatively, this family had the structure and resources to provide an effective and efficient family-based respite-care system. However, due to their inability to make the transition from a physically healthy family to a family with a sick parent, they were stuck at a level of disassociation due to a lack of commitment and a history of dysfunctional interaction. Even when supportive services and other options were presented, they refused to accept them because it would increase their responsibility—when it was a way for them to reduce chaos and to minimize dysfunction. But, as it often occurs, severely dysfunctional families are unable to mobilize their resources and do what may be in everyone's best interests.

ROLE FATIGUE AND STRESS

Respite care is often the primary focus of programmatic models, but attention must also be given to the multidimensional problems that families may face, such as role fatigue, stress, the need for rejuvenation, and the importance of quality of life.

Frequently, the major stressor in the illness process is the dramatic change of roles. These role shifts can occur when the affectionate, responsible spouse becomes a demanding, irresponsible patient, and the loving, caring wife or husband becomes a resentful caregiver with a role that is seen more as a curse than an opportunity. The following examples may provide a perspective on the stressors that could warrant or require respite care:

1. An infant with brain damage who could not regulate body temperature and had to be fed every two hours. Enormous stress was placed upon the parents, who are refusing help because they previously had another child with a similar condition who aspirated food and died while in the hospital. In this situation, both parents had desperately wanted respite care but the highly specialized nature of the condition precluded traditional help. Home respite care was made possible when several highly skilled persons earned the trust of the parents and demonstrated their skills in caring for the child.

2. A person with a spinal cord injury who had to be moved every four hours. Respite care had been possible prior to the emotional collapse of the spouse, who felt totally trapped by the disability and had spent 411 consecutive days being the primary caregiver. This spouse refused all help because she felt responsible for the disability because she was driving the car when the accident that caused the injury to her husband occurred.

3. The elderly parent who had two retarded children, aged 56 and 51, who had been able to manage with the help of her husband. When the husband suddenly died she was left in a difficult situation in a remote rural area with limited options for help.

4. A woman who had multiple sclerosis and could not get the help from her elderly husband who was very ill and unable to provide the care she needed. This situation was complicated by the constant turnover of workers who could not work with the woman, due to her incessant demands and abrasive personality characteristics.

What these examples have in common is the intensity of a situation that was left without intervention and resulted in increased family stress and accelerated familial deterioration. Respite care in such situations provides the patient and family with an opportunity to take a pause in the illness process and create a different frame of mind that can benefit all involved. This also enables family members to renegotiate their familial roles, as well as to establish new ones more conducive to coping and rejuvenation.

In a comprehensive examination of the needs of caregivers, Bader (1985, p. 48) concluded it may be more practical and cost-effective to invest in caregiver's physical, financial, and emotional well-being, rather than providing this help only when the caregiver becomes "the patient." Key points made by Bader in reference to respite care are as follows:

1. Caregivers' needs should be recognized through provision of adequate community services, including day care for disabled spouses.
2. Allocations should be made on the level of functional disability rather than on arbitrary means-tested eligibility requirements.
3. Incentives should be available for caregivers in order to facilitate home care.
4. Families and government should be seen as partners, not as adversaries. Government-supported services should supplement spousal care and should not be withdrawn when a wife is present.
5. The importance of support groups should be stressed. They can provide emotional respite as well as a focal point for advocacy initiatives.
6. In order to mitigate the pressures and pain of the caregiving spouse, there must be adequate support in all the areas of need: financial, physical and emotional.

In exploring the issues relative to caretakers' role fatigue, Goldstein, Regnery, and Wellin (1981, p. 25) express concern regarding the limited awareness about the economic, physical, psychological, or social costs and benefits to a family involved in long-term care. The conclusion was that caretakers' role fatigue affects all aspects of the caretakers' life and they identified four variables that were particularly important:

1. Patients' level of disability and dependence.
2. Caretakers' own health and functional mobility.
3. Presence or absence of other assistance.
4. Caretakers' other roles and responsibilities.

Examination of these variables indicate the individuality of each family situation as well as that these variables are subject to change. For example, when considering the patient's level of disability and dependence, we can readily see how change in the patients' health could increase or decrease the stress and strain on the caregiver. This is especially important in cases that involve progressive illness such as multiple sclerosis, Alzheimer's disease, or amyotrophic lateral sclerosis. Similarly, variables of the health and functional mobility of the caregiver can create unique problems, especially when home care is dependent upon a spouse or significant other who can physically and emotionally provide care as needed in the present and in the future. This is a critical issue for elderly persons who depend on a spouse who, due to cardiac, orthopedic, or emotional factors, cannot provide care even though they had done so in the past. For the patient, the physical and/or emotional problems of the caregiver may be perceived as an additional rejection by the significant other. Frequently, the quality of the pre-illness relationship determines the ability of caregivers and patients to negotiate such role change in a constructive or destructive manner.

Interestingly, the third variable, presence or absence of other assistance, is determined by the two variables listed previously. Unfortunately, as needs and stress increase, the caregivers may find themselves abandoned by significant others. The final variable, caretakers' other roles and responsibility, is also in flux, sometimes by choice, and at other times out of necessity. For example, a spouse may have to work in order to fill the financial void created by the loss of income, or the illness of other family members may require a further redefinition of roles and responsibilities and in turn create more stress and strain.

REJUVENATION

An awareness of the pervasive stress that accompanies illness increases the importance of personal and familial rejuvenation. Halpern (1985) explored the impact of respite care on the regenerative power of the family, particularly on its ability to recover from a stressor. This study indicated the value of respite care in facilitating the development of coping skills, which are major elements in the adaptation process. Discussing the resources needed by the caregiver and family to meet the needs of the severely disabled, Warren and Cohen (1985, p. 67) identify the following:

1. Good physical health and stamina.
2. Good mental health.
3. An emotionally strong marriage.
4. Healthy family interaction.
5. A support network of family and friends.
6. Time and skill in negotiating the service system.
7. Financial resources.

These are important and desirable elements for families and persons challenged by illness and disability to have, but they are elusive to most families and subject to flux. Even if a family system has all of these resources, the illness-disability experience can rapidly reduce these resources to memories.

In discussing the demands and challenges of child rearing, Cohen (1982) makes an interesting point when she states that a basic coping mechanism for families not faced with the demands and needs of an ill family member is to have time away. For families having a severely ill family member, time away may be impossible, due to their abandonment of other family and friends as well as limited financial and emotional resources.

Pointing out the direct benefits of respite care, Cohen (1982, p. 9) identifies benefits to families in the following areas:

- Satisfaction with life
- Hopefulness about the future
- Ability to cope with a disabled child
- More positive attitude toward the child

When combined with improvement in areas such as emotional and physical well-being of parents, it is apparent that respite care can increase the likelihood of coping with illness rather than of being overwhelmed by it.

Another critical factor to consider when discussing the proactive impact of respite care is how many persons are placed in residential facilities because programs are not available or because if they were, they did not meet the specialized needs of the patient or the family. This contrast between theoretical models and real-life needs is addressed by Cacioppo and Andrews (1979) when they point out that many parents find it difficult to find baby-sitters for well children—not to mention the challenge of a child who may have a combination of problems in behavioral, intellectual, motor, sensory, and social problems. In these situations, the demands on the family can be very intense, thus creating a chronic situation that depletes emotional, physical, and financial resources.

In response to potential caregivers' burn-out, Morse (1979) discusses a programmatic model that has as its goal the prevention of family breakdown through a combination of respite care, training, and community-resources development. Specifically, those families faced with extraordinary care giving requirements are targeted as priority recipients of support to facilitate care in the natural home (Salisbury, 1985).

This is an important issue because the stress created by long waiting lists for residential care results in families not being able to cope effectively and efficiently. This is a critical situation for the health care system to address because it is evolving into a pattern of responding only to the most desperate and to those in a state of crisis (Rogerson, 1984). This approach of waiting until the situation is almost out of control is short-sighted at best because it creates a reactive response to families in crisis and creates a system of respite-care management by default.

The outcome of this process is that those in need are further victimized, not by the illness, but by the system designed to provide help.

QUALITY OF LIFE

Discussing the need for and benefits of respite care and home-based alternatives, a frequent approach to justify their use has been that it is more cost-effective. However, for families of the ill and disabled as well as the person in need, the question is not whether the costs are effective, but whether they are helpful in improving the quality of life.

When discussing respite care or any health care issue, the concept of the quality of life should be addressed because it can be the pivotal issue for families considering maintaining a loved one in the home. Investigating the impact of respite care on the quality of life, Joyce, Senger, and Isralowitz (1983) found that there was a positive impact in areas such as family relations, social activities, and reduction in emotional and physical strain. The cumulative effect was that the basic quality of live was improved.

Health care professionals must attend to the issue of quality of life. If, however, they do not consider it as an important element in their treatment plan, the patient may not stabilize, and the family may be faced with a deterioration of its resources. This places the total system at risk and in turn may force a family cutoff, premature institutionalization, or increased occurrence of neglect and abuse directed toward both patient and caregiver.

It is clear that we are addressing a quality-of-life issue that has impact on the family not only for the present but also for the future. If most of the energy of the family is expended on the needs of an ill member, a result may well be the emotional and physical neglect of individuals or the entire system, often with disastrous results. In a presentation focusing on respite care, Cutler (1979) presented this issue from the frames of reference both of a mother of a child with special needs and as a professional. Her focus is that respite care is an *essential* service based on the following rationale:

> Parents make *extraordinary* sacrifices to keep their disabled children at home. Health care professionals, mental health systems, and health care policy must recognize these personal sacrifices and extraordinary commitments by providing moments of ordinary living which most people take for granted. (Cutler, 1979)

An explanation for the lack of awareness with people in general and health care professionals in particular regarding the stress created by illness is that there is little or no exposure to the day-to-day stress faced by families in a health care process. Awareness of the impact of illness on patients and families is important for health care workers in general and medical students in particular (Hunsdon & Clarke, 1984).

CONCLUSION

A major contribution of respite care is the ability to replace desperation with hope, nothingness with dreams, and isolation with support.

No child, adolescent, adult, or family should have to deal with the ravages of illness or disability. Unfortunately, life does not always conform to our hopes or aspirations. When severe illness occurs, it is often an unending, familial nightmare that depletes resources, insults dignity, and often pushes the family to the brink of desperation. Sometimes the families survive. Other times, however, the outcome is more disappointing.

Illness or disability, however, is so pervasive, powerful, and all-encompassing that coping with it should not be the sole responsibility of the family. Therefore, it is imperative that health care professionals be aware of and in tune with the complexities surrounding the illness or disability experience and how it affects the family. In discussing respite care, there are several principles that must be considered:

- No one is completely prepared for illness or disability.
- Illness changes a family and challenges its resources.
- The illness process brings out the best and worst in families.
- Disability can deplete family resources as well as create them.
- Often the only support is the family.
- All people do not have families they can rely on.
- Not all families are capable of responding to the illness and disability of a family member.
- New skills are needed by the family to meet the new challenges created by illness.
- Coping with chronic disability is an ongoing developmental process for the patient as well as the family.
- Existing health care resources can help as well as hinder adjustment.
- Respite care is often the difference between coping and deteriorating.

These points are made as selected examples of issues that must be expanded, explored, understood, and attended to if the family and friends of people with disabilities are to renegotiate a position of survival, development, enrichment, and attainment for themselves and their loved ones.

When discussing the differential impact of disability, we must be aware that the resources, problems, needs, hopes, and dreams of people are as different as snowflakes. Although the element of individuality is the key to emotional survival, it must be fueled by the commonality that all challenged people and their families share. This commonality is the active ingredient that can enable people to negotiate the perils of the physical and emotional rehabilitation process by recognizing they are not alone and that respite-care services are available to them.

The real value of respite care is that it helps families to maximize their chances for survival when faced with illness and disability. Why should persons with disabling conditions feel isolated? Can they not learn from each other, share mutual strengths, and create an environment that models success?

Illness has the power to limit those affected by it, as well as to fragment the family. Respite care has the potential of putting illness into perspective and creating an option for the family to live as fully as possible. The harsh reality of the illness and disability experience may be impossible to change, but it certainly can be made more bearable!

RESOURCES

Home Aid Resources Program
Division of Developmental Disabilities
Department of Social and Health
  Services
Olympia, WA 98504

Respite Care Coordinator
Time Out for Parents
Easter Seal Society of Greater
  Cleveland
Suite 300, 2728 Euclid Ave.
Cleveland, OH 44115

Parent Respite Care Co-op
c/o Kalamazoo Association for
  Retarded Citizens
132 West South St., Suite 305
Kalamazoo, MI 49006

Extend-a-Family
Box 122
Postal Station K
Toronto, Ontario M4P2EO
Canada

The Hartford Regional Center
Connecticut Department of Mental
  Health
Office of Mental Retardation
71 Mountain Rd.
Newington, CT 06111

Director of Program/Services
United Cerebral Palsy Association of
  Sacramento-Yolo Counties, Inc.
Sacramento, CA 95816

National HomeCaring Council
235 Park Ave. South
New York, NY 10003

Care Co-op Consultants
2324 West Main St.
Kalamazoo, MI 49007

Extend-a-Family
416 West Onondaga St.
Syracuse, NY 13202

Additional resources are listed in *Respite Care* by S. Cohen and S. Warren, 1985, Austin, TX: Pro-Ed.

REFERENCES

Bader, J. (1985). Respite care: Temporary relief for caregivers. In Miller, R., & Rehr, H. (Eds.), *Health needs of women as they age* (pp. 39–51). New York: Haworth.

Ballard, R. (1984). Respite care: Welcome help for the disabled elderly and their caregivers. *Post Graduate Medicine, 75*(5), 15–18.

Ben-Yishay, Y., et al. (1981). Working approaches to remediation of cognitive deficits in brain damaged persons. *Rehabilitation Monograph* (No. 61). New York: Institute of Rehabilitation Medicine, New York University Medical Center.

Berger, J. (1985). Crisis intervention: A drop-in support group for cancer patients and their families. *Social Work in Health Care, 10*(2), 81–92.

Cacioppo, B., & Andrews, S. (1979). Respite care for parents of handicapped children. *Social Work in Health Care, 5*(1), 97–101.

Carter, G. (1984). Why are the mentally handicapped admitted to hospitals? *British Journal of Psychiatry, 145*, 283–288.

Chadwick, O. (1981). A prospective study of children with head injuries. *Psychological Medicine, 11*, 49–61.

Cohen, S. (1982). Supporting families through respite care. *Rehabilitation Literature, 43*(1–2), 7–11.

Cohen, S., & Warren, R. (1985). *Respite care.* Austin, TX: Pro-Ed.

Cutler, B. (1979). *Respite care and parents.* Unpublished presentation, Boston: Massachusetts Developmental Disabilities Conference, June.

DeJong, G. (1977). *The need for personal care services by severely physically disabled citizens of Massachusetts.* Waltham, MA: Levinson Policy Institute, Brandeis University.

Dunn, R., MacBeath, L., & Robertson, D. (1983). Respite admissions and the disabled elderly. *Journal of the American Geriatric Society, 31*(10), 613.

Eggert, G. (1977). Caring for the patient with long-term disability. *Geriatrics, 32*, 102–114.

Featherstone, H. (1980). *A difference in the family: Life with a disabled child.* New York: Basic Books.

Fengler, A., & Goodrich, N. (1979). Wives of elderly disabled men: The hidden patients. *Gerontology, 19*, 175–183.

Ferguson, J., Lindsay, S., & McNees, M. (1983, February). Respite care co-op: Parents helping parents. *The Exceptional Parent*, pp. 9–15.

Frankel, D. (1984). Long term care issues in multiple sclerosis. *Rehabilitation Literature, 45*(9–10), 282–285.

Goethe, K., & Levin, H. (1984). Behavioral manifestations during the early and long term stages of recovering after closed head injury. *Psychological Annals, 14*, 7.

Grad, R., & Sansbury, L. (1963). Mental illness and the family. *Lancet, 1*, 544–547.

Goldstein V., Regnery, G., & Wellin, C. (1981, January). Caretaker's role in fatigue. *Nursing Outlook*, pp. 24–30.

Greenfield, J. (1972). *A child called Noah.* New York: Holt, Rinehart, & Winston.

Halpern, P. (1985). Respite care and family functioning in families with retarded children. *Health and Social Work, 19*, 138–150.

Hasselkus, B., & Brown, M. (1983). Respite care for community elderly. *The American Journal of Occupational Therapy, 37*(2), 83–88.

Hayden, M. (1982). Neuropsychological sequence of closed head injury. *Archives of Physical Medicine and Rehabilitation, 62,* 522–526.

Head, D. W., Head, B., & Head, J. (1985). Life or death of severely disabled infants: A counseling issue. *Journal of Counseling and Development, 63,* 621–624.

Heckler, M. M. (1985). The fight against Alzheimer's disease. *American Psychologist, 40*(11), 1240–1244.

Huberty, D. J. (1974). Adapting to illness through family groups. *International Journal of Psychiatry in Medicine, 5*(3), 231–242.

Hunsdon, S., & Clarke, S. (1984). The impact of illness on patients and families: Social workers teach medical students. *Social Work in Health Care, 102,* 41–52.

Jones, D. A., & Vetter, N. (1984). A survey of those who care for the elderly at home: Their problems and their needs. *Social Sciences Medicine, 19*(5), 511–514.

Joyce, K., Senger, M., & Isralowitz, R. (1983). Impact of respite care on patient's perceptions of quality of life. *Mental Retardation, 21*(4), 153–156.

Kenney, M. (1982). *Giving families a break: Strategies for respite care.* Omaha: University of Nebraska Medical Center.

Kinsella, G., & Duffy, D. (1979). Psychosocial readjustment in the spouses of aphasic patients. *Scandinavian Journal of Rehabilitation, 11,* 129–132.

Lezak, M. D. (1978). Living with the characterologically altered brain injured patient. *Journal of Clinical Psychiatry, 39,* 592–598.

Livsey, C. (1972). Physical illness and family dynamics. *Advances in Psychosomatic Medicine, 8,* 237–251.

Long, C. J., & Webb, W. L. (1983). Psychological sequelae of head trauma. In R. C. W. Hall (Ed.), *Psychiatric medicine* (pp. 35–77). New York: S. P. Medical and Scientific Books.

Loop, B. (1979). *Family resource services and support systems for families with handicapped children.* Omaha: University of Nebraska Medical Center, Meyer Children's Rehabilitation Institute.

Lynch, R. (1983). Traumatic head injury: Implications for rehabilitation counseling. *Journal of Applied Rehabilitation Counseling, 14*(3), 72–79.

Macourt, P., & Southam, M. (1983, December). Respite care provides relief for caregivers. *Dimensions,* pp. 18–19.

McCubbin, H. (1979). Integrating coping behavior on family stress theory. *Journal of Marriage and the Family, 41,* 237–244.

McCubbin, H. I., Joy, C. B., Cauble, A. E., Comeau, J. K., Patterson, J. M., & Needle, R. H. (1980). Family stress and coping: A decade review. *Journal of Marriage and the Family, 42,* 855–871.

Morse, J. (1979). A program for family management of the multiply handicapped child. *Rehabilitation Literature, 40,* 134–145.

Najenson, T. (1974). Rehabilitation after severe head injury. *Scandinavian Journal of Rehabilitation Medicine, 6,* 5–14.

New, P., Ruscio, H., & Priest, R. (1968). The support structure of heart and stroke patients: A study of the role of significant others in patient rehabilitation. *Social Science Medicine, 2,* 185-200.

Osborne, L. (1985, Novermber 13). Sharing the caring. *Washington Post,* pp. 12-13.

Power, P. W., & Sax, D. (1978). The communication of information to the neurological patient: Some implications for family coping. *Journal of Chronic Disease, 31,* 57-65.

Pullo, M. L., & Hahn, S. (1979). *Respite care: A family support service.* Madison, WI: United Cerebral Palsy of Wisconsin, Inc.

Raub, M. J. (1982). *How to start a respite program.* Sacramento: California State Council on Developmental Disabilities.

Rogerson, B. (1984, December). Ignore them at your peril. *Nursing Times,* pp. 436-439.

Romano, M. (1974). Family response to traumatic head injury. *Scandinavian Journal of Rehabilitation Medicine, 6,* 1-4.

Ryglewicz, H. (1985). How can professionals help families and patients?: Issues and approaches. *Tie Lines, 2*(1), 1-4.

Salisbury, C. (1985). Young children with severe handicaps in community residential facilities. *Journal of the Association of Severe Handicaps, 10*(3), 164-167.

Scheinberg, L., & Kaplan, R. (1983). *Medical Rehabilitation Research and Training Center for Multiple Sclerosis' progress report.* Washington, DC: National Rehabilitation Information Center.

Shanas, E. (1979). The family as a social support system in old age. *Gerontology, 19,* 169-174.

Shoob, D. (1978). *A community respite care program for the mentally retarded and/or physically handicapped.* Springfield, VA: Childcare Assistance Program for Special Children.

Spaniol, L., & Zipple, A. (1986). Families with a chronically mentally ill member: A review of the research finding. In J. P. Bowker & A. Rubin (Eds.), *Studies on chronic mental illness* (pp. 52-82). Washington, DC: Council on Social Work Education.

Stroker, R. (1983). Impact of disability on families of stroke clients. *Journal of Neurosurgical Nursing, 15*(6), 360-365.

Taylor, T., & Loop, B. (1978). The First National Conference on Temporary Family Support Systems and Community-Based Respite Services for Developmentally Disabled Persons and their Families. Omaha, NB: University of Nebraska Medical Center.

Thompson, E., & Doll, W. (1982). The burden of families coping with the mentally ill: An invisible crisis. *Family Relations, 31,* 379-388.

Travis, G. (1976). Chronic illness in children, its impact on child and family. Stanford, CA: Stanford University Press.

Upshur, C. (1983). Developing respite care: A support service for families with disabled members. *Family Relations, 32,* 13-20.

Ware, L. A., & Carper, M. (1982). Living with Alzheimer's disease: Family stresses and coping mechanisms. *Psychotherapy: Theory, Research and Practice, 19*(4), 472-481.

Warren, R. (1979). Demonstrating continua of respite care and parent training services for families of persons with developmental disabilities—Project Visit No.
5, UCP of Northeastern Maine. New York: United Cerebral Palsy Association,
December 4–6.

Warren, R., & Cohen, S. (1985). Respite care. *Rehabilitation Literature, 46*(3–4), 66–71.

Winkler, L. (1981). Chronic stress of families of mentally retarded children. *Family
Relations, 30,* 281–288.

Yalom, I., & Greaves, M. (1977). Group therapy with the terminally ill. *American Journal of Psychiatry, 134,* 396–400.

Zarit, S., & Zarit, J. (1982). Families under stress: Interventions for caregivers of senile
dementia patients. *Psychotherapy: Theory, Research, and Practice, 19*(4), 461–471.

13 Alzheimer's Disease: Impact on Families and Caregivers

Rennie Rogers Golec and Ann D. Lassalle

There is no true "living" in the full sense of the word for the family of an Alzheimer's victim. We merely *cope* as best as we can. Each day, we, as caregivers, face the full gamut of the more tragic human emotions: grief and loneliness, frustration, anger, bitterness and sometimes guilt and depression. I found no joy or happiness, no anticipation or enthusiasm for what tomorrow may bring, no contentment or peace of mind. How to cope with it? Who can tell? (Alzheimer's Disease and Related Disorder Association, 1985, p. 1)

Alzheimer's disease (AD) is an organic brain disorder, characterized by the progressive and irreversible loss of intellectual and social functional capabilities, with an eventual physical deterioration leading to death. Its effect has been described (Rovner, 1986) as the loss of one's uniqueness, the loss of the personality. Although a number of causal factors have been proposed, including biological or genetic defects, viral infections, incorrect metabolization of aluminum, and immunological deficiency, its cause is unknown (Goldberg, 1985).

AD affects 6% of those aged 65 or older, 10% of those aged 75 and over, and 20% of those aged 85 and over (Roach, 1985). It is estimated that over 2 million adults in the United States today are affected by AD. By the year 2000, it is expected that this number will double to over 4 million, with the cost of institutionalization rising to $78 billion annually. At the present time, over $13 billion per year is spent on maintaining AD patients in nursing homes (Heckler, 1985), and these costs tend to pose particular difficulties for the middle class. Expenses range from $20,000 to $35,000 annually. Generally, those who can afford to use nursing homes have assets in excess of $500,000 or are the indigent, whose costs are paid by Medicaid.

A recent study by Harvard School of Public Health (Ross, 1986) reports that 9 out of 10 nursing-home residents exhaust their resources within 2 years,

This creates a hardship for the surviving family members, particularly the postretirement spouse who is left impoverished, with a lifetime of savings depleted in order for the afflicted spouse to become eligible for Medicaid assistance. The prevalence of this situation has led to the coining of the term *spending-down* to describe the process people must go through in order to obtain financial aid. An AD victim's husband recounts his experience with the system:

> There are various agencies and institutions funded (at least in part) by the government for the care and treatment of other victims, including illnesses such as alcoholism and drug abuse. But when Alzheimer's disease strikes a member of a family, I feel there is no relief or assistance for the hard-working, God-loving family. All we get is "Sorry, your policy doesn't cover that," or, "No, we don't have facilities for care of that kind of patient." So the family pays, and pays and pays because we will not give up trying to provide the best care possible for our stricken loved one. (Alzheimer's Disease and Related Disorders Association [ADRDA], 1985, p. 2)

The preponderance of care for impaired elderly persons including AD victims is thus provided by the family. The Traveler's Corporation of Hartford, Connecticut surveyed their employees and found that "28% of their full-time employees spent an average of 10.2 hours per week in caregiving activities; 8% spent 40 hours or more; and some devoted as much as 80 hours per week, beyond family and work responsibilities, to caring for elderly family or friends" (U.S. Congress, 1986).

The magnitude of this issue is such that The Honorable Olympia Snowe, of the U. S. House of Representatives, has proposed that there be a declared Family-Caregiver Day in recognition of this silent labor force. The ultimate purpose of such a day would be twofold. It would serve as a form of consciousness-raising for the general public and it would give caregivers some recognition of the importance of their efforts in maintaining family and intergenerational ties in the face of enormous responsibilities (U.S. Congress, 1986).

Among caregivers of AD patients, many needs have been identified and many strategies following from these needs have been suggested. These range from medical advancements (particularly better diagnostic techniques) and services designed to assist the individual caregiver (including improved information about the disease process, psychological and legal counseling, and respite care) to more global policy changes (such as revisions to Medicaid and mandatory insurance coverage for long-term care needs). Although these proposed reforms are well founded, obtaining them will be both expensive and time consuming.

Professionals faced with the immediate responsibility of working with caregivers and victims of AD need readily accessible strategies to facilitate the process of helping family and caregivers to cope with the symptoms of the disease. In this chapter, we discuss the progressive nature of Alzheimer's disease, the needs of caregivers associated with the different stages of decline, and strategies to facilitate coping.

CHARACTERISTICS OF ALZHEIMER'S DISEASE

> My husband and I went to our grandson's birthday party. He didn't want to go, but I said "We're going," and I didn't give him an alternative. At the party, he had fun, he laughed and joked; he has a terrific sense of humor, and he remembers things that happened years and years ago. He had a good time. On the way home he admitted that. The next day I mentioned some of the nice people that were at the party. He said, "What party?" I was stunned. I couldn't believe it. He had totally forgotten about the party as if he'd never been there. (Powell, 1985, p. 56)

Although Alzheimer's disease is a physiological disorder, it is manifest through the loss of behavioral and affective functional capabilities. This includes but is not limited to restlessness, disorientation, forgetfulness, delusional thoughts, and irrational accusations often directed toward the caregiver (Rovner, 1986). In the early stages, this decline can be represented by memory impairment and subtle personality changes including apathy, withdrawal, and loss of spontaneity. In the middle stages, inability to care for oneself becomes apparent, and the intellectual decline becomes more severe (Heckler, 1985; Powell, 1984, 1985). In the advanced stages, the person becomes virtually incompetent.

While AD victims have been known to survive for over 15 years after diagnosis, the average life span is 6 to 8 years and a significant reduction in overall life span of up to one-third has been observed (Powell, 1984; Heckler, 1985). There is no known effective treatment to stop the progress of AD or to reverse the effects that it has had on the patient, nor is there any known way of preventing this disease. Further, a diagnosis of Alzheimer's disease is made after eliminating other treatable conditions, such as depression, chemical imbalance, vitamin deficiency, and certain brain disorders—conditions that can masquerade as AD. The definitive diagnosis is obtained only through autopsy. In recent years, the medical community has begun to address the perplexing problem of diagnosing and staging a disease that does not initially have any physical symptoms.

Reisberg, Ferris, deLeon, and Crook (1982, 1985) have characterized AD as the progressive loss of cognitive functioning, and have devised a model for behaviorally assessing the progress of the disease. Their assessment of behavior demonstrates that the behavior we see is a reflection of cognitive ability. Their research has revealed that AD patients lose skills and abilities in an order opposite from that in which they are acquired.

Piaget (1952), well known for his conceptualization of cognitive development in children, proposed a sequential and hierarchical model that orders the tasks of infant and child development. The observable behavior organized in Piaget's model implies a parallel or corollary progression in cognitive development. In much the same way, Reisberg et al. (1982, 1985) infer cognitive decline from observable behavior. The Global Deterioration Scale (Reisberg et al., 1982) provides a way to stage the progress of AD by assessing this loss of ability through behavioral observation. The process of decline associated with Alzheimer's disease is thus construed as a mirror image of the developmental process (see Figure 13.1).

Reisberg et al. (1982, 1985) are basically assessing functional capability with an inference of cognitive decline, but in fact we consider their model to be a behavioral diagnosis of Alzheimer's disease. The levels of decline are predictable in sequence but unpredictable in terms of duration and tend to overlap as well. Consequently they are represented as points on a continuum rather than as discrete stages. The model is useful as a general characterization of the decline associated with AD as opposed to the specific process representative of the experience of some individuals.

Vitaliano, Russo, Breen, Vitiello, and Prinz (1986) report on their work in the assessment of "staging" in AD patients. They were able to differentiate two domains of "functional competence—maintenance (e.g., feeding,

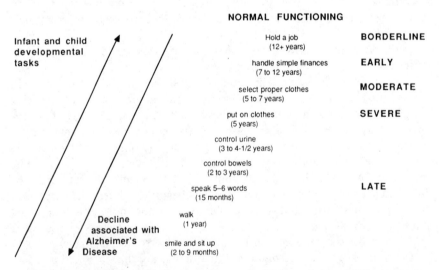

FIGURE 13.1 Global Deterioration Scale (Reisberg et at., 1982) reconceptualized as a continuum.

toileting, dressing) and higher functioning (e.g., hobbies, writing, reading)" (p. 41). By observing the performance of individuals diagnosed in different stages of the disease, they discovered that persons they identified as being in the early stages of AD did in fact later exhibit the characteristic decline in both areas of functioning. One conclusion of this study was that persons with AD can be identified early in the disease process using behavioral criteria.

Vitaliano et al. (1986) examine both maintenance and higher functioning activities, whereas Reisberg et al. (1982, 1985) appear to be observing maintenance functions alone. Because the progression of AD affects the integrity of the cortical tissue, the higher functioning activities are the first to be impaired. The research of Vitaliano et al. (1986) suggests that an earlier diagnosis might be achieved through more direct cognitive assessment. Both strategies, however, propose the structure for a method of diagnosing Alzheimer's disease. In addition, it is thought that prediction of the course of the disease will serve a dual role. For professionals, it should facilitate patient management. For family members, the anticipation of change should enable, at the least, more adequate coping responses if not a significant reduction in the overall level of family stress resulting from the rigors of contending with the behavior patterns of AD that have previously been characterized as unpredictable.

ISSUES OF CONCERN TO CAREGIVERS

Although some people assume that caregiving in the family is a fairly new phenomenon, associated with our aging society, in fact the family has always assumed this role. Hagestad (1986) discusses the historical importance of caregiving. In the past, it was extended to family members of all ages rather than to only the very young or the very old, as it is today.

There are three major demographic trends of relevance to family caregiving (Hagestad, 1986): increased longevity, smaller families and closer spacing of children, and the increased disparity in longevity between men and women (with women's life expectancies now being 7 years greater than those of men). Because we now live longer, we have come to expect long life as the norm. We anticipate that our parents will live autonomously through our middle age and that our children will outlive us. Disruption of this assumed pattern becomes a major life transition, because it is unexpected and uncommon among our peers. We are shocked and we are taken by surprise when our children die, if our parents die in our early adulthood, or if our parents become dependent on us.

Hagestad (1986, p. 119) refers to this set of expectations as "the rectangularization of survival curves." With 75% of all deaths occurring in those beyond age 65, implicit in this curve is the assumption that most deaths occur among the very young or the very old. Figure 13.2 is a graphic conceptualization of this curve, with a plateau between infancy and retirement age.

One consequence of this curve is that the relationship between parents and children goes beyond the child's childhood into the child's adulthood. This, coupled with a trend toward smaller families, leads us to a situation where parents and children share many adult experiences, resulting in a new and more intensive kind of relationship than was characteristic in the past. However, Hagestad (1986) adds that this is the first time in history that we have associated death and frailty with old age, and in the case of the family it is particularly heartbreaking when it is the parents. Those whom we have always associated with strength and with comfort are the ones we have lost or are losing.

The disparity in life span between men and women means that women tend to outlive their husbands. Therefore, wives are often the caregivers for men, yet often they need care as well, because more women than men are victims of AD (Powell, 1984). It is the daughters and daughter-in-laws, however, who generally assume the responsibility for eldercare. In Norway, the care that women provide to family members has come to be called "the hidden welfare state" (Waerness, 1978). It has commonly been believed that when women take on roles in the world of work the amount of time spent in caregiving activities is reduced. She cites evidence that women, in fact, change their work routines to enable them to care for aging parents. This stands in stark contrast to men, whose work responsibilities often tend to take priority over caring for aging parents.

A study conducted by the Governor's Task Force on Alzheimer's Disease and Related Disorders in the State of Maryland indicated that twice as many wives care for husbands who are victims of AD, yet four times more mothers are being cared for than are fathers (Kirkland, 1985). Even though the effects of AD appear to be an issue of particular relevance to women, diagnosis of

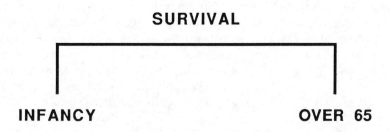

SURVIVAL

INFANCY   **OVER 65**

FIGURE 13.2 Rectangularized survival curve.

AD in a family member represents a critical ongoing life transition, regardless of who is doing the caregiving.

Kirkland (1985, p. 4) quotes the wife of an AD patient:

> I am the wife of a man who has Alzheimer's Disease. I run a one-bed nursing home. . . . My husband must be fed, diapered, washed, dressed; he cannot walk without help; and he cannot talk. . . . I spend over $500 for diapers . . . if you want to care for your family member you need training. I had never seen a bed-sore in my life before this, or dealt with someone else's constipation, or seen anyone hallucinate.

Another respondent:

> I feel like a prisoner in my own home. . . . I am a single person and this is a tremendous burden on me financially, socially, and emotionally.

Because the primary responsibility for care of AD patients is provided by their families, the level of family stress and the impact of the disease on the caregiver is an important consideration. For many people, an AD patient is disconcerting to be around. Friends and neighbors often stop making contact, and the healthy spouse finds his or her social circle greatly reduced. This can lead to a sense of isolation and is true of family members as well as friends (Kirkland, 1986). "Caregivers sometimes feel like 'married widows or widowers'" (Powell, 1985, p. 61).

> Recent memory loss is the most prevalent symptom of Alzheimer's Disease. The tragedy of the illness is that without memory, time is a meaningless abstraction and every routine experience becomes a venture into the unknown. Without memory we don't know if we have loved or felt pleasure, sorrow, or regret. We also don't know if *we* are loved and our sense of security and reliability is so shaken that we become anxious and afraid, even of those on whom we once could depend. Both victims of the illness, the patient and the caregiver, feel alone, abandoned and frightened. (Powell, 1984, p. 5)

The problems family and caregivers face can be directly inferred from the levels of functioning identified on the continuum of development (see Table 13.1). As capabilities are lost, family and caregivers must assume increasing degrees of responsibility for the maintenance and support of the Alzheimer patient. They must cope with their own affective responses to these changes as well.

What is often even more difficult than these pragmatic problems, however, is the violation of the assumptions that have been made regarding the way people expect the rest of their lives to be. Everything we do in life is based

TABLE 13.1 Issues of Concern for the Caregiver, Associated with the Global Deteriorioration Scale (Reisberg et al., 1982)

Level of disease	Functional ability	Behavioral manifestation	Caregiver/family response
Normal functioning			
Borderline	Hold a job (12+ years)	Forgetfulness, social withdrawal.	Uncertainty; confusion over unexplained changes; anger at irrational behavior; suspicion of alcoholism or extramarital affair; denial.
Early	Handle simple finances (7 to 12 years)	Anger, confusion related to loss of autonomy.	Anger at situation and victim; loss of income results in fear about future financial situation; denial; search for alternate diagnosis, if diagnosed; search for cure.
Moderate	Select proper clothes (5 to 7 years)	Inability to participate in household decision making; increasing disorientation.	Increased responsibility for household decision making and maintenance; sense of loss; confusion and despair—do not know where to turn.
Severe	Put on clothes (5 years)	Increasing disorientation; flattening of affect; withdrawal; unsafe to be left alone.	Inability to meet home care demands; may need assistance— semiskilled aide or day care to continue work outside of home, for social activities, and for respite.
	Control urine (3 to 4½ years) Control bowels (2 to 3 years)	Incontinence; hygiene problems requiring semiskilled care.	Maintenance in home increasingly difficult; anger and despair at lack of control over process.

(continued)

TABLE 13.1 (continued)

Late	Speak 5–6 words (15 months) Walk (1 year) Smile and sit up (2 to 9 months)	Virtual incompetence; loss of basic psychomotor skills.	Necessity for skilled care, special diet, and feeding needs may require placement in a nursing home; anger, despair, and fear at loss of independence and mobility.

on the assumptions we make about the world. For many, the retirement years are anticipated as a reward for years of hard work, careful saving, and planning for "the twilight years." The myth is destroyed when one partner can no longer participate in life and is forced into a position of childlike dependency—with savings depleted almost overnight and the healthy partner faced with the necessity of spending down to qualify for Medicaid funding.

The needs of family and caregivers of Alzheimer's disease patients thus arise from the responsibilities of home care, coupled with the expense of professional care both in the home and in residential facilities. Other potential sources of stress include a perception of role reversal by the caregiver, the frustration associated with the difficult nature of diagnosing this disease, and the lack of informed medical personnel (Roach, 1985).

USING THEORY TO DEVELOP COPING STRATEGIES

When a family member is diagnosed as having Alzheimer's disease, the changes in family roles and structure tend to be complex and problematic. This involves loss on a number of levels—of personality and companionship, of financial assets, of a way of life, of control, and of one's expectations regarding the future. At the same time, it involves a gain of new responsibilities in terms of roles, financial obligations, and time commitments. The insidious onset of AD tends to minimize the reality of this transition. As one family recalls, their initial response to a diagnosis of AD was disbelief:

When my father was diagnosed with Alzheimer's, his physician gave my mother the title of a book about AD and said, "Buy it and read it. It will tell you what you need to know. There's nothing more I can do." and went on to his next patient. He made no referrals to other resources and didn't even offer to be available if she had any questions. . . . At the time, Daddy was reticent and slightly disoriented but at home [he was retired] he was functional. The book discussed incontinence, wandering behavior, all of the worst case scenarios. We didn't know whether to believe the doctor or look for a second opinion and we had no idea what we should do.

The usual support systems that can facilitate adaptation are often unavailable or needing support themselves. There is no hope for medical intervention, and public policy offers no relief.

With AD, these changes are additionally problematic because the disease is manifest through an overtly observable process of incremental decline of the personality, with the inevitability of death overshadowed by the outward absence of physical disability. Many AD patients appear, on the surface, to be younger and healthier than their caregivers. In our conversations with caregivers, many have noted how difficult it is to think of these people as dying, when their faces bear no evidence of the stress and pain of everyday life. On the contrary, in certain phases of the disease they are reported to seem almost carefree and childlike. This tends to enhance the possibility of denial among family and friends.

Weiss (1976) discusses the notion of "situational distress . . . reactions that are so much the product of exposure to a particular situation that they are displayed by almost everyone in the situation" (p. 213). The uniformity in responses to a diagnosis of Alzheimer's disease implies that the reaction of family and caregivers may reflect a form of situational distress. The importance of this construct for helping professionals lies in the differentiation of therapeutic referral that is made to the individual in distress.

Three levels of situational distress are identified (Weiss, 1976), each demanding a different response from the helping professional. A *crisis* is a situation that occurs suddenly, is intensely upsetting, and is time limited. The diagnosis of AD or acceptance of the diagnosis can represent a crisis. Support, from professional and nonprofessional sources, appears to be the only assistance that can be utilized by an individual in crisis.

When change is required following a crisis, this period of change is identified as a *transition* (Weiss, 1976). The individual in transition is thought to be particularly open to suggestions from helping professionals and can profit from information that will facilitate understanding of the situation, guidance in terms of coping strategies, and referral to organizations designed to help individuals who are facing similar issues. A transition may result in a *deficit situation*, which requires ongoing assistance from helpers and other sources of support. For family and caregivers of AD victims, the transition that results from the diagnosis of Alzheimer's disease generally results in a deficit situation.

Strategies for working with family and caregivers relate directly to the level of situational distress they are experiencing and to the level of the disease process. Table 13.2 identifies a series of strategies associated with the developmental continuum.

Transitions are thought to represent especially opportune times for helping people to learn coping behaviors (Weiss, 1976). Because past coping experiences are thought to affect the way people are able to cope in the future (Schlossberg,

TABLE 13.2 Recommended Strategies Associated with the Global Deterioriation Scale (Reisberg et al., 1972) and the Family/Caregiver Response

Level of disease	Caregiver/family response	Recommended strategy
Borderline	Uncertainty; confusion over unexplained changes; anger at irrational behavior; suspicion of alcoholism or extramarital affair; denial.	Probably not yet diagnosed; if diagnosis has been made, support as a form of crisis intervention.
Early	Anger at situation and victim; loss of income results in fear about future financial situation; denial; search for alternate diagnosis, if diagnosed; search for cure.	Legal and finacial counseling; begin transition phase of assistance— information about the disease process, referral to ADRDA support groups; support if still in crisis response.
Moderate	Increased responsibility for household decision making and maintenance; sense of loss; confusion and despair—do not know where to turn.	Provide knowledge; use transition model to make the process more predictable.
Severe	Inability to meet home care demands; may need assistance—semiskilled aide or day care to continue work outside of home, for social activities, and for respite. Maintenance in home increasingly difficult; anger and despair at lack of control over process.	In view of deficit situation, referral to a temporary community for support.
Late	Necessity for skilled care, special diet, and feeding needs may require placement in a nursing home; anger, despair, and fear at loss of independence and mobility.	Assistance/referral to skilled-care service providers for in-home maintenance or selection of nursing home.

1981, 1984; Weiss, 1976), it is suggested that a model for coping with transitions may be particularly useful for working with family and caregivers of AD victims. It should be helpful in alleviating the primary stress of coping with the effects of the disease and the secondary stress (Weiss, 1976) resulting from the confusion and uncertainty that arises when it is not possible to gain a sense of control in life.

A Process for Working Through Transitions

In a model for analyzing adaptation to transition, Schlossberg (1981, 1984) defines a transition as a process of change that results from an obvious life event such as retirement or death of a spouse, or what she terms a *nonevent*, as when an expected event does not occur. Schlossberg identifies three interrelated sets of factors that influence an individual's ability to adapt to a transition: (1) the transition, (2) the pretransition and posttransition environments, and (3) the individual.

She further conceptualizes the ability of an individual to cope with a transition as a ratio of that person's unique combination of assets and liabilities. Characteristics of transitions that may serve either to enhance or impede coping include the perception of role change (gain or a loss), the affective response to this change, and the source of the change (elective or beyond one's control). Other characteristics include timing, onset (sudden or gradual), and duration. Environmental factors that influence coping ability include support systems ranging from friends and family to institutional resources. Characteristics of the individual that Schlossberg (1981, 1984) suggests may affect adaptation are: race/ethnicity, socioeconomic status, health, age and life stage, sex and sex-role identification, value orientation, psychological competence, and previous experience with transitions.

The diagnosis of AD, when described in these terms, becomes a situation that can be described in entirely negative terms—a loss, accompanied by feelings of sadness, confusion, anger, and grief, which is the result of circumstances beyond anyone's control. The diagnosis seems sudden, although the onset is in fact gradual; and the duration is uncertain, although the outcome is inevitable. The response and the coping ability of the individual or family can be negative or positive, depending on the environmental factors and the involved individuals' unique characteristics.

Schlossberg (1984) combines her transition model with Egan's (1975) model of helping to create a three-stage process for working through a transition. The three stages are (1) *exploring*, (2) *understanding*, and (3) *coping*. A helper in this process can be a friend or family member, a professional (e.g., nurse, physician, or mental health practitioner), a person who has gone through a similar situation, or someone who represents a combination of these roles.

In the first stage, *exploring*, the focus is on gaining knowledge about the nature of the transition and the individual or familial response to it. At this level, the caregiver can express his or her feelings about the impact of AD— anger at the disease and at the victim for having incurred it, fear about the future, guilt for being angry and for not being able to do it all. It is also necessary, at this stage, to identify those thoughts and behaviors that impede effective coping. From the helper's perspective, this involves establishing a relationship characterized by respect and trust. Until this relationship is in place, the important work of self-exploration cannot begin.

At the second stage, *understanding*, caregivers gain knowledge about themselves and the personal resources available to them that can tip the balance of their assets-versus-liabilities ratio in favor of effective coping with the effects of AD. They also need to gain knowledge about Alzheimer's disease, the nature of the continuum of development and its implications for the future of the patient, as well as the financial realities the situation entails. A number of written materials discuss the nature of AD and caring for AD sufferers. Two of the most comprehensive are Mace and Rabins' (1981) *The 36-Hour Day* and Reisberg's (1981) *A Guide to Alzheimer's Disease*.

This is also the time for an assessment of assets, both personal and pragmatic. The goal of the helper is to focus on the larger picture as well as the issues of the moment. This involves an integration of the information obtained in stage 1 with an emphasis on how the caregivers' resources fit into this overall pattern or scheme.

In the third stage, *coping*, helper and caregiver together work out an action plan for dealing with the issues identified in stage 2. At this stage, there are some things the helper is uniquely qualified to offer the caregiver; but because of the wide-ranging needs of the individual, the helper can act as a referral agent as well. There is no substitute for a concrete plan for information and referral sources.

1. It is important to put an emphasis on financial and legal issues early in the disease process. Because of the variations among state laws, caregivers should be referred to local legal-aid resources for accurate information.
2. The information provided in the developmental continuum illustration offers a framework for exploring the current status as well as the projected future for both the AD victim and the family and caregivers. It is an effective vehicle for establishing a methodology for staging the patient following diagnosis. It also provides direction for family and caregivers in seeking strategies for coping and for concrete planning for the future.

3. The establishment of an ongoing support system is crucial for effective coping. Family and caregivers should be referred to the local chapter of the Alzheimer's Disease and Related Disorders Association (ADRDA) as well as appropriate social service organizations in your area. The ADRDA is an advocacy organization that provides a variety of services to families and caregivers, including information, support, and referral resources. This will alleviate some of the issues that may arise if family and caregivers perceive themselves to be in a deficit situation. It can provide the *temporary community* of others in a similar situation, identified by Weiss (1976) as a crucial factor in facilitating effective coping.

A RATIONALE FOR CHANGE

A middle-aged woman whose father died of Alzheimer's disease discusses how she coped with the experience:

> The only thing that kept me going was my feeling that what I was doing was important. When I finally accepted that my father had Alzheimer's and he *was* going to lose his abilities, it was actually freeing. I no longer spent my time and energy trying to preserve what was left of him or trying to make him go back to being how he had been before. Instead I focused on doing the things I needed to do to help him and to anticipate changes that would be coming next. I was also convinced that it was important for me to be with him and help him in the same way that he had been there for me when I was an infant. My brother, who never accepted what it meant that my father had Alzheimer's, spent a lot of time trying to restore my father. He now has a sense of total failure, but I feel I did the best, given the situation, and I feel good about myself because of it.

What this person is saying is that she did not change the course of the disease, but rather the way she thought about it. This is the primary strategy and goal of cognitive restructuring.

Cognitive-behavioral psychology has its roots in the writings of the Stoic philosophers. In the first century A.D., Epictetus wrote in *The Enchiridion*: "Men are disturbed not by things, but by the view which they take of them" (Ellis, 1979, p. 190). Theorists in the field of psychology, including Alfred Adler, Albert Ellis and Donald Meichenbaum (Ellis, 1979) have also focused on the interrelationships among the cognitive, affective, and behavioral domains of human functioning. The way you think about something is thought to influence both your feelings and your behaviors.

The technique of cognitive restructuring focuses on changing the way a person thinks about a situation in order to change feelings and behaviors. This is related to what we call *self-talk*. The way a situation affects us depends upon what we tell ourselves about the situation. If we tell ourselves that a loved one with AD is losing all of his capacities and there is nothing we can do about it and we have no control over the situation, we feel hopeless. If, on the other hand, we say yes, she is losing her capacities but we can have some control over the situation by doing things to help her through it, and that this is an important thing to do, then we are less likely to feel helpless. By restructuring our cognitions or thoughts about the situation, we can change our feelings and our behaviors.

Cognitive restructuring has been employed as a strategy for the management of numerous life transitions. For example, there have been some efforts made to examine the social context of dying, and, in essence, it has been suggested that we create a new norm or standard of behavior to deal with an impending death (Riley & Riley, 1986). This new norm revolves around the issues of autonomy and open confrontation with the meaning of death. Basically there are two choices you can make—to turn your back and pretend nothing is happening, or to try to take control of the situation and make some meaning out of an inevitable process. Making meaning is a type of cognitive restructuring.

An example of this new norm, in practice, exists in the hospice movement, where impending death is acknowledged, accepted as part of the life course, and planned for by the dying person, his or her family, and friends. The goal is what is termed a *good death* (Riley & Riley, 1986), where family and friends are given a chance to tie up loose ends, to express love and affection, to make amends for old hurts, and to say goodbye. It is recognized that ushering someone out of this life is an important and valuable thing to do.

The diagnosis of AD sets the context for a similar situation. Our social norm for confronting illness is to seek a cure, or at least to minimize symptoms, and to deny disability. In the presence of a disease for which there is no intervention—no treatment, no cure, only physical maintenance until death, confounded by the loss of the personality—a new norm that addresses the issues of autonomy and making meaning of the process of decline will serve the needs of both patient and caregiver.

Adult Children of AD Victims

For children of AD victims, the transition associated with the diagnosis of AD triggers a change in the nature of the parent-child relationship. Among middle-aged children (aged 40 to 50) and their aging parents, it has been characterized by Cohen and Gans (1978) as "the other generation gap." It occurs when parents reach the point where they need assistance from their children, thus reversing the established parent-child relationship (Blenkner, 1964, 1965; Cicirelli, 1981; Schwartz, 1977). This change in traditional patterns

of interaction is often defined as a role reversal, and is generally characterized by anger—from the child as a result of the loss of a parent figure, and
from the parent, who is resentful of being placed in the role of the child
(Cicirelli, 1981).

It is also argued, however, that the caregiving role may serve as a final
developmental stage for the adult child, within the parent-child relationship.
Termed *filial maturity* (Blenkner, 1964, 1965), this role enables the adult child
to acknowledge that parents exist as individuals with needs and shortcom-
ings independent of their parental roles. It allows for the development of a
different and more mature relationship wherein the child can turn back toward
the parents—a developmental change from the autonomy-focus of young
adulthood—and voluntarily assume the responsibility for parental care within
the affectional bonds of the filial relationship (Blenkner, 1964, 1965; Cicirelli,
1981).

It is suggested that confronting the issues of aging parents in this manner
will help middle-aged children to confront their own aging process from a
more enlightened and active point of view. This response is not characterized
as a role reversal, but is defined rather as a final stage of development in the
relationship between adult children and their parents. Wright, Pratt, and
Schmall (1985) quote the 39-year-old daughter of an AD victim:

> I would not have given up this period to care for my parents for anything. There
> has been combativeness, wandering—lots of frustrations. But I'm learning for
> the first time to take each day at a time. It has been the richest time of our lives—
> not moneywise, by far—but in emotional and spiritual growth. (p. 34)

CONCLUSION

The diagnosis of Alzheimer's disease represents the official beginning of a
process that has been insidious in onset, is unpredictable in duration, and
immutable in terms of outcome for the victim. The commonality of response
among family and caregivers facing this process characterizes what has been
described by Weiss (1976) as a form of situational distress, in that virtually
everyone exposed to this situation responds in the same manner. The question this raises is, if most people respond in the same way, why is it so difficult to help people cope with the effects of this disease?

What we have proposed is a strategy that will not only facilitate coping,
but will also provide a sense of empowerment and direction for those who
must witness the decline of a person who has Alzheimer's disease. In this
chapter, we have also outlined the roles a helper can take in response to the
different levels in this process of decline.

Through cognitive restructuring, family and caregivers may come to realize that they are being victimized by things other than the disease, things over which they can exercise some control. They can reconsider the value they place on the importance of the caregiver role and stop trying to assess the quality of the AD victims' experience from their own more cognitively complex perspectives. They can also work to influence the social policies that affect Alzheimer's disease victims and their caregivers. Even though they cannot change the course of the disease, they can change the way they react to it and, in time, they may be able to begin to change society's responses to this problem as well. The daughter of an Alzheimer patient reflects on her experiences as a caregiver:

> My father died one year ago today. He had Alzheimer's disease and survived just about 3 years after he was diagnosed. Looking back, from this point in time, I can honestly say that the only regrets I have are that he had AD and that he had to die. . . . We tried not to leave him out of any family event. Instead, we made whatever accommodations were necessary to make it possible to include him in our lives. It wasn't always easy or our first choice of things to do. We didn't try to take him places like the movies or fancy restaurants, but he loved to go to places where he could sit and watch people, and he was always ready to go for a drive. We would try to incorporate his interests into our plans. Like any other family venture, sometimes it worked and sometimes it did not. . . . It was after his diagnosis that we made the Philadelphia Flower Show into an annual family event. My husband and I would drive up from Washington with my mother and father for a preview of spring. The first year, on the drive back home, we asked Daddy what he liked best, and he said breakfast in the room. The next year his answer was the same. He found pleasure in the trips, but in his own context. . . . I think the reason I have so few regrets is that I know his life had joy and meaning virtually until his death, but on his terms, not mine. Being able to let go of my expectations for him and his life course enabled me to share in that joy. . . . Although my father could not survive his encounter with AD, our family did.

RESOURCES

The Alzheimer's Disease and Related Disorders Association, Inc. (ADRDA)
70 East Lake Street
Chicago, IL 60601
1-800-621-0379

The ADRDA will provide information about Alzheimer's disease as well as information regarding support groups in your local area.

REFERENCES

Alzheimer's Disease and Related Disorders Association, Greater Kansas City Area. (1985). *Three profiles—coping with Alzheimer's.* Kansas City, KS: Author.

Blenkner, M. (1964). Developmental considerations and the older client. In J. E. Birren (Ed.), *Relations of development and aging* (pp. 247-266). Springfield, IL: Charles C. Thomas.

Blenkner, M. (1965). Social work and family relationships in later life with some thoughts on filial maturity. In E. Shanas & G. F. Streib (Eds.), *Social structure and the family: Generational relations* (pp. 46-59). Englewood Cliffs, NJ: Prentice-Hall.

Cicirelli, V. G. (1981). *Helping elderly parents: The role of adult children.* Boston: Auburn House.

Cohen, S. Z., & Gans, B. M. (1978). *The other generation gap: The middle-aged and their aging parents.* Chicago: Follett.

Egan, G. (1975). *The skilled helper.* Monterey, CA: Brooks/Cole.

Ellis, A. (1979). Rational-emotive therapy. In R. J. Corsini (Ed.), *Current psychotherapies* (pp. 185-229). Itasca, IL: Peacock.

Goldberg, R. T. (1985). Alzheimer's disease: From benign neglect to community living. *Rehabilitation Literature, 46*(5-6), 122-132.

Hagestad, G. D. (1986). The aging society as a context for family life. *Daedalus, 115,* 119-139.

Heckler, M. M. (1985). The fight against Alzheimer's disease. *American Psychologist, 40*(11), 1240-1244.

Kirkland, G. I. (1985, October). *Meeting the challenge of Alzheimer's disease and related disorders.* Paper presented at the Eastern Regional Workshop, Health and Education Council, Essex Community College, Baltimore, Maryland.

Mace, N. L., & Rabins, P. V. (1981). *The 36-hour day.* Baltimore: Johns Hopkins University Press.

Piaget, J. (1952). *The origins of intelligence in children.* New York: International Universities Press.

Powell, L. S. (1984). A burden of love—Alzheimer's disease caregivers. *Choices, 3,* 5.

Powell, L. S. (1985). Alzheimer's disease: A practical psychological approach. *Women and Health, 10,* 53-63.

Reisberg, B. (1981). *A guide to Alzheimer's disease.* New York: Free Press.

Reisberg, B., Ferris, S. H., deLeon, M. J., & Crook, T. (1982). The Global Deterioration Scale for assessment of primary degenerative dementia. *American Journal of Psychiatry, 139,* 1136-1139.

Reisberg, B., Ferris, S. H., deLeon, M. J., & Crook, T. (1985). Age associated cognitive decline and Alzheimer's disease: Implications for assessment and treatment. In M. Bergner, M. Ermini, & H. B. Stahelin (Eds.), *Thresholds in aging* (pp. 255-292). London: Academic Press.

Riley, M. W., & Riley, J. W., Jr. (1986). Longevity and social structure: The added years. *Daedalus, 115,* 51-75.

Roach, M. (1985, August). Reflection in a fatal mirror. *Discover,* pp. 76-82.

Ross, N. L. (1986, April 13). Some elderly may lose Medicaid under new law. *The Washington Post*, p. F2.

Rovner, S. (1986, May 7). Alzheimer's disease: Games and reality. *The Washington Post, Health*, p. 16.

Schwartz, A. N. (1977). *Survival handbook for children of aging parents.* Chicago: Follett, 1977.

Schlossberg, N. K. (1981). A model for analyzing human adaptation to transition. *The Counseling Psychologist, 9*(2), 2-18.

Schlossberg, N. K. (1984). *Counseling adults in transition.* New York: Springer Publishing Company.

U.S. Congress, House of Representatives, Representative Snowe speaking for H. J. Resolution 555, March 6, 1986, *Congressional Record* (p. E664), No. 25. Washington, DC: Government Printing Office.

Vitaliano, P. P., Russo, J., Breen, A. R., Vitiello, M. V., & Prinz, P. N. (1986). Functional decline in the early stages of Alzheimer's disease. *Journal of Psychology and Aging, 1,* 41-46.

Waerness, K. (1978). The invisible welfare state: Women's work at home. *Acta Sociologica* (Suppl.), 193-207.

Weiss, R. S. (1976). Transition states and other stressful situations: Their nature and programs for their management. In G. Caplan & M. Killilea (Eds.), *Support systems and mutual help: Multidisciplinary explorations* (pp. 213-232). New York: Grune & Stratton.

Wright, S. D., Pratt, C. C., & Schmall, V. L. (1985). Spiritual support for caregivers of dementia patients. *Journal of Religion and Health, 24*(1), 31-38.

Personal Statement: Surviving ALS— A Daughter's Perspective

Judy Teplow

BETTY MILLER
BELOVED WIFE, MOTHER, AND GRANDMOTHER
SEPTEMBER 4, 1986   AGE 70 YEARS

In the early spring, when the ground is soft, I will lay a marker on my mother's grave, a permanent marker to commemorate the life of a very special lady. The inscription will be short, impersonal, and incomplete—and somehow not befitting a woman who courageously struggled against a devastatingly cruel terminal illness.

I cannot inscribe her story in stone, but I can set it on paper as a lasting tribute. I hope it will be a comfort to those who are afflicted with a serious or terminal illness, and a help to the families and health professionals who are involved in their care and treatment.

It was going to be an unbearable, oppressive day, but my mother had no intention of sitting in her small, air-conditioned apartment. She set out early with her walking buddies on their 5-mile jaunt and, as usual, took the lead. She was amused that her companions, who towered over her 5-foot frame, could not keep up with her brisk pace.

Everything seemed to be going well for her and my dad. Retirement for them was not sedentary life, but rather one that was full and gratifying. In a few weeks, they would return to their apartment in Boston for 5 months of relief from Florida's intolerable heat.

But for now, Betty was enjoying her walk and thinking about how rich her life was. As she turned the bend, her thoughts were cut off abruptly by a stiffening in her left leg—perhaps a cramp—but she did not have the pain associated with a cramp. Her gait slowed down considerably, and in a minute she found herself lying on her side. She was stunned by this unexpected interruption. She did not stumble over a rock or a crack in the roadside. What should she attribute this weakness to?

It took 5 months for the doctors to make an accurate diagnosis. An electromyogram (EMG) was performed at the Brigham and Women's Hospital, and it was this test that ultimately determined that my mother had amyotrophic lateral sclerosis (ALS), Lou Gehrig's disease, a progressive, degenerative disease that is terminal. It is probably the most dreaded neurological disease, and is one with no known cause or cure.

Within 1 year of the first visible symptom, Betty would be a virtual paraplegic, confined to a wheelchair, unable to talk or to feed herself. Breathing and swallowing would become progressively more difficult. At no time would the disease affect her mental faculties, and she would always be aware of the creeping paralysis.

My initial reaction to the diagnosis was one of disbelief, devastation, and helplessness. How could such an active and health-conscious person be stricken with such a catastrophic illness? I felt a sadness for my parents, and I had real concerns about my dad's health also. It was conceivable to me that this tragedy could destroy him as well, and I prepared myself for the worst.

The family and doctors were in total agreement as to how much to tell my mother. She had always been petrified of doctors and hospitals, and was by nature very nervous and anxious. We knew that she that she could not cope with such outrageous news.

She was told that she had a chronic neuromuscular disease, and that she would need intensive therapy. We did not offer her hope of a cure, nor did we inform her that she was terminally ill. She asked very few questions, wanted to know as little as possible about her disease, and became adept at tuning out whatever she was not ready to hear.

Like my mother, my aunt, my father, and my brother went to great lengths to avoid the truth. Denial became a protective measure they were to use effectively throughout the course of the illness. As much as I tried to beat through this barrier, I was met with resistance. It was this resistance that was to become a great source of frustration and anger for me. My aunt held out the longest, talking about the research, cures, and the possibility of people living several years. My brother, who never coped with adversity too well, did not become an integral part of the team, and his visits to the nursing home were often sporadic and brief.

I had to know all the medical aspects of the disease, so I asked a lot of questions and read many books on ALS, and on death and dying. Someone had to take charge, to plan, and to carry the family through this crisis.

From the Brigham and Women's Hospital, my mother was transferred to the Braintree Rehabilitation Hospital. It was there that she was put on a daily regimen of physical, speech, and occupational therapies. She was extremely tense and frightened, but the staff was very professional and experienced, and knew how to respond to her emotional as well as physical needs. This was really not a time for rehabilitation as much as a time for enormous adjustment. It also allowed the family to make plans for home health care. I wished that my mother could stay at Braintree indefinitely, for I feared that the support systems at home would not be adequate.

My fears were well founded. She was not home 2 months when all systems began to break down. My mother required constant attention and the Visiting Nurse's Association and private-home health professionals were not able to keep up with her demands. Oftentimes, my father was left without help, and he had to assume the role as primary caregiver. Tensions mounted and tempers began to flare, and what was once a very happy marriage now appeared to be very strained. My dad's health was deteriorating as well as my mother's, and they looked to me for a quick solution.

I knew that my mother required round-the-clock care in a skilled nursing facility, but I did not want to be responsible for initiating the search. I could not find it in my heart to do this to her, especially when she threatened to commit suicide before she would enter a nursing home. My grandmother had taken her own life because she could not cope with a painful illness, so I was worried about my mother's intentions. I began to get pressure from her sister, also, in defiance of any plan to move my mom from her home. We were in a crisis and we needed help quickly.

I was fortunate to find a psychologist who would help me accept and confront problems that were difficult and painful. He helped me see issues more clearly when everything seemed overwhelming and confusing; and it was through him that I began to understand the complexities surrounding chronic and terminal illnesses. His continued support and genuine concern were to sustain me through some very difficult times, the first of which was my mother's move to a nursing home.

The transition from the apartment to the nursing home was traumatic for the family. Ostensibly, the home was attractive and meticulous, with spacious rooms and beautiful furnishings. In sharp contrast to this orderliness was a picture of deterioration—of very old people in their 80s and 90s ravaged by debilitating diseases, marked with permanent deformities, hooked up to life-supporting machines, impaired by mental illness—there was an aura of sadness and loneliness, and a sense that many of these people were deserted by their families.

I wished that I could put blinders on my mother's eyes—to shut out a world that was so unreal, but yet only too real and disheartening. My mother was only 69 years old and looked 10 years younger. How could we do this to her! I knew that there was no alternative, but I was stricken with guilt, a guilt that was to stay with me for a long time. It took a good 3 months before I could walk into the nursing home without feeling sick—without feeling very, very shaken.

I don't think my mother ever adjusted to nursing-home life. I think she resigned herself to her fate. I know she often felt very sad, lonely, and misunderstood, but I do not think she felt abandoned. She knew that the family was there for her, and it was this prevailing sense of security that kept her from slipping into a deep depression.

A schedule was worked out wherein one or two family members would visit daily. This was arranged, mostly out of love, partly out of guilt, and out of an acute awareness that strangers would not minister to her needs the way family would. We also knew that if we were going to survive this ordeal we would have to share the responsibilities, for each of us had a history of medical problems. Often, the burden of responsibility rested on my shoulders, and at times I felt overwhelmed. But I also felt that if my mother could cope with the effects of a very disabling disease, I could deal with any problems that arose.

I do not know how she endured all the suffering, and I do not understand what held her together. She certainly did not triumph over her disease—she did not write a book, or paint by mouth, or engage in anything that was extraordinary. She just tried to get through the day. There were many tears and many moments of anguish, but even in her despair she insisted on getting up, getting dressed, and—above all—having her hair done weekly. Thank God there was a hairdresser on the premises, and thank God she still cared about her appearance. Throughout her illness, she never lost her sense of humor or her ability to smile and laugh. But the laughing was done for the staff, and most of the crying was done with the family.

We tried to maintain a sense of equilibrium, but it was difficult to keep control when all systems were failing. The disease was progressing at an alarming rate, and we knew she would need the strong support of the family and the specialized services of many health care professionals. Some services were effective, but most fell short. Many professionals were not familiar with or could not cope with the demands of ALS. They were uneasy in treating a terminally ill patient, or clearly had an attitude problem toward the sick and the elderly. I must acknowledge, though, that most people did try to help, and I cannot fault them for their human limitations in dealing with a very difficult case.

I also believe that my mother's inability to speak had a lot to do with the quality of care she received. This was a great source of frustration for her as well as for the health professionals who worked with her. The family members were the only ones who had the patience to make use of the communication boards. We acted as liaison between my mother and the staff, so our involvement in her care was crucial.

We also acted as her advocates and protectors. There were aspects of nursing-home care that were unsettling, but because we had a very good working relation with the staff, most of our grievances were worked out. I can only think of one incident that was offensive and repulsive, and it was due to a personality conflict between my mother and an aide. An aide had lost control and, out of anger and impatience, threw a sheet over my mother's head. This was a gross violation of my mother's right to be treated as a living human being until the day she died.

The only other situation that disturbed me occurred outside the home. A week before my mother died, her doctor was called to check on her deteriorating condition. To our dismay we learned that the doctor was on vacation and had left instructions for the covering physician. Her doctor had promised to leave explicit directions regarding heroic measures. This was not an insignificant oversight. I had chosen this doctor because he had been highly recommended by another physician and was on staff at a hospital directly opposite the nursing home. Because of his close proximity, I thought that he would be accessible to my mother and the family, but unfortunately we found him to be very impersonal and distant.

Without the encouragement and concern of a handful of people the experience would have been unbearable. There were three exceptionally caring people who made a great impact on my mother.

Janet, a nurse's aide, became my mother's guardian angel, and she was to watch over her and attend to all her needs while she was in the nursing home. There was such a strong attachment between them that on the day my mom died Janet was unable to work.

Margaret, the Assistant Director of Nursing at the nursing home, had lost her mother to ALS, and she was familiar with the disease and its effects on the family. She was always available to us, and it was not unusual for her to interrupt a busy schedule to explain what comfort measures should be used. She was also instrumental in educating the staff about the nature of the disease. She was my inspiration and a great source of strength.

Bobby was a close friend of the family. He had experienced the loss of a loved one, so he was no stranger to personal tragedy. He attended many workshops with Elizabeth Kübler-Ross and was involved in hospice, and he knew how to relate to the terminally ill. Bobby showered my mother with gifts and flowers and made her feel very special. He was the only one who could talk to her about death and life after death, and ultimately helped her accept her mortality. He was a good friend to me, also, and I was able to talk with him about my greatest fear—the use of life-support systems.

The issue of support systems was always a source of great pain and anguish for me. My anxiety was heightened by my mother's refusal to discuss these matters and the inability of family members to agree on a specific course of action. I personally believed that the use of heroic measures, in my mother's case, would be cruel and inhumane—a prolongation of inexorable suffering pain—and an interference with the natural order of things.

But I had to know where my mother stood on these issues for, ultimately, it was her life and her decision. Three months before her death, she began to make her wishes known. She slowly spelled out the word *die* every day. She made it quite clear to me that she could no longer tolerate living. She finally came to terms with her death, knew it was imminent, and had an urgency to express her grief and fears about dying. Once she accepted her death, she became more tranquil.

I did not want my mother to die in the arms of strangers, nor did I want her to experience death alone. I was fortunate to be with her at the final moment of death. My aunt and I sat by her side and held her hands, and except for a brief interruption by staff this was a family affair. We exchanged a few words of support and comfort, but we were mostly caught up in remembering and recollecting. I wondered if my mother saw her life flashing before her, and if she were passing through the dark tunnel toward Omega—but I could not be sure. . . .

PART V: Study Questions and Suggested Activities

1. How would you go about identifying the respite-care opportunities in your community for caregivers of the home-bound elderly?
2. Why is it important to consider the needs of the primary caregiver when doing a family assessment?
3. If you were asked to design a respite-care model, what would be its major components?
4. Identify three disabilities you feel would require respite care. Explain why.
5. As outlined in Chapter 13, Alzheimer's disease has specific stages in its progress. What do you consider are the particular family crises associated with each stage?
6. Considering the coping mechanism of *cognitive restructuring*, discussed in Chapter 13, devise a strategy a caregiver might use that would transform the disability situation into an opportunity that has personal meaning and value.
7. As a helping professional, what would you find most difficult when attempting to make contact with family members of an Alzheimer patient?
8. What are the unique supports required by families of the Alzheimer patient?
9. After reading the personal statement by Judy Teplow, what do you think could have been done to reduce family stress?
10. Considering the intervention model as explained in Chapter 2 of this book, what parts of this model do you feel are most applicable to Judy's situation?
11. Devise a cognitive restructuring technique that Judy could have used to cope with her own situation concerning her mother.

Index

Acquired immune deficiency syndrome, *see* AIDS
Adams, M., 84–87
Adaptation as family resource, 10
Adolescents
  assertiveness training and behavior modification for, 210–211
  awareness of death by, 95
  cancer in, childhood, 78–81; *see also* Cancer
  chronic illness effects on, 79–80
  development of, 78–79
  fear of disability in others, 201, 204, 208–209
  general separation, need for, 206
  indentification with disabled, 202, 204
  impact of handicapped child on sibling, 154, 201–214
  included in planning for disabled sibling, 211–212
  life review at terminal illness, 98
  need and tasks of, 202–206
  participation in own treatment, 80
  peer relations among, 80
  quest for independence, 202–203
  relaxation and desensitization techniques for, 80
  resource for siblings of disabled, 213–214
  role/identity confusion in, 202, 204
  school-to-work transition for disabled, 154, 216–230
  sexual development of, 79, 202–206
  sexual experience with rheumatoid arthritis, 153, 156–162
  with spina bifida, 153–154, 164–179
  therapeutic life-oriented programs for, 80–81
Advocacy, 176, 308
  for disabled women, 246, 249–250
AIDS, 104–118

definition of, 104–105
diagnosis of, 105–107
transmission of, 105
see also HIV-infected children
Alcorn, D. A., 188
Allied health professionals
  counseling on sex, 188–192, 195–196
  role in sibling relations with disabled, 207–212
  role-playing by, 3–4, 6
  self-assessment by, 24–25
Alternatives, exploration of, at diagnosis time, 27
Alzheimer's disease
  adult children of victims of, 299–300
  caregiver concerns, 289–293, 292–293 (tab.)
  characteristics of, 287–289
  cognitive restructuring and, 298–299
  coping strategies for, 293–298, 295 (tab.)
  cost of institutionalization, 285
  demographic trends and, 289–290
  Global Deterioration Scale, 288–289, 292–293 (tab.), 295 (tab.)
  impact on families and cargivers, 263–264, 285–301
  incidence of, 285
  model of helping and transition model for, 296–298
  parent–child relationship in, 299–300
  referral needs, 297–298
  resources list, 301
  respite care and, 270–273
  role reversal in, 300
  situational distress and, 294
  staging of, 287–289
  support system for, 298
  transition periods and, 294, 296–298
Alzheimer's Disease and Related Disorders Association, 285, 286, 298